Better BONES, Better BODY

Keats Titles of Related Interest

Stopping the Clock
by Dr. Ronald Klatz and Dr. Robert Goldman

Making the Estrogen Decision
by Susan M. Lark, M.D.

18 Natural Ways to Look and Feel Half Your Age
by Norman D. Ford

Digestive Wellness
by Liz Lipski, M.S., C.C.N.

Dr. Earl Mindell's Live Longer & Feel Better with Vitamins & Minerals
by Earl L. Mindell, R.Ph., Ph.D.

Menopause Naturally
by Carolyn Dean, M.D.

The Calcium Plus Workbook
by Evelyn P. Whitlock, M.D.

Putting It All Together: The New Orthomolecular Nutrition
by Abram Hoffer, M.D., Ph.D. and Morton Walker, D.P.M.

For Women Only: Chinese Herbal Formulas
by Hong-yen Hsu, Ph.D. and Douglas H. Easer

Junk Food to Real Food: A Blueprint for Healthier Eating
by Carol A. Nostrand

Better BONES, *Better* BODY

A Comprehensive Self-Help Program for Preventing, Halting and Overcoming Osteoporosis

❖
───────

Susan E. Brown, Ph.D.

Medical Anthropologist ~ Clinical Nutritionist

Director, The Osteoporosis Education Project, Syracuse, New York

KEATS PUBLISHING, INC. ◆ NEW CANAAN, CT

BETTER BONES, BETTER BODY

Copyright © 1996 by Susan E. Brown

All Rights Reserved

No part of this book may be reproduced in any form without the written consent of the publisher.

Library of Congress Cataloging-in-Publication Data

Brown, Susan E., Ph.D.
    Better bones, better body / by Susan E. Brown.
        p.   cm.
    Includes bibliographical references and index.
    ISBN 0-87983-700-4
    1. Osteoporosis—Popular works.   I. Title.
RC931.O73B76   1996
616.7'16—dc20   96-637
                                                     CIP

Printed in the United States of America

Keats Publishing, Inc.
27 Pine Street (Box 876)
New Canaan, Connecticut 06840-0876

01 00 99   6   5   4   3

*This book is dedicated to
my father, Lynn, Mikie, Beth and Elisa*

Acknowledgments

While many people have inspired and encouraged me throughout the years I would like to particularly acknowledge the following individuals:

Elisa Buenaventura for all that she has taught me over the years.

Ruby Rohrlich for her endless encouragement of this project and painstaking editing of my early material.

Lynn Miller for her medical and practical insights.

My sister Judy Brown for her right word in the right place at the right time, many times.

My sister Beth Brown for her physical therapy insights and her consistent urging to take care of myself while caring for my projects.

Russ Jaffe for his insights and exquisite scholarship.

Doris Rapp for her enthusiastic support and encouragement.

Ruth Hubbard for her repeated consideration and review of my material.

Lendon Smith for seeing value in the project and his good cheer.

Mary Jackson for her kindness in reviewing the very first draft of this manuscript way back when.

Jean Haag for her boundless commitment to the teaching of deliberate creation.

Bess Path for all those high-energy and good-spirited nights at the computer.

Nina Chiles for her generous and tireless assistance.

Acknowledgments

My father, W.G. Brown, for his constant support of this and other projects.

Joe Jorgensen, Nancie Gonzalez and Marion Greeley who know not even of this project, yet their early caring and interest in my development provided a foundation for all that followed.

Susan Herner for her friendship and enthusiastic promotion of the manuscript.

Phyllis Herman, my editor, who supported this project from its earliest stages on and played a key role in its publication.

Contents

Foreword by Russell M. Jaffe, M.D., Ph.D xv

Introduction
Only a New Seed Can Yield a New Crop

Only a New Seed Can Yield a New Crop 7
About the Better Bones, Better Body Program 10
References 12

PART ONE
Rethinking the Nature of Osteoporosis

Chapter 1
Magical Bodies, Magical Bones

Our Magical Bodies 17
Health Lies in a Self-Maintained Balance Among All Systems ...21
Lifelong Healthy Bones Are Our Birthright...................................22
Our Magical Bones..23
References 33

Chapter 2
Redefining Osteoporosis

Osteoporosis is More Than Just Thin Bones................................35
Osteoporosis is Not Normal Aging Bone Loss 40
Osteoporosis: An Anthropological Perspective..............................41
Osteoporosis is Not Just a Female Disorder.................................45
Osteoporosis is Not a Disorder of Just the Elderly 48
Osteoporosis is Not Faulty Bone Metabolism, or Something
    that "Goes Wrong" With Our Bones.......................................49

Osteoporosis Does *Not* Stand Alone 50
Primary Osteoporosis Versus Secondary Osteoporosis..................52
References 54

PART TWO
Rethinking the Causes of Osteoporosis

Chapter 3
It's Not Just Calcium and Estrogen: Rethinking the Cause of Osteoporosis

Osteoporosis is *Not* Caused Simply by Low Calcium Intake 61
Osteoporosis is *Not* Caused Only by the Lowering of Estrogen
  Levels at Menopause 64
Going Beyond Calcium and Estrogen 67
Rethinking the Cause of Osteoporosis...68
The Total Body Burden Concept 70
Ancient Insights: Traditional Chinese Medicine and
  Ayurvedic Views on Osteoporosis 72
References 74

Chapter 4
Bone-Robbing Nutrient Inadequacies

Calcium is Important to Bone Health, but It Does Not Stand
  Alone..77
Startling Facts About the Standard American Diet 78
The Standard American Diet Versus our Ancestral Diet 79
The 18 Nutrients Essential for Healthy Bones................................80
References 113

Chapter 5
Bone-Robbing Dietary Excesses

The Standard American Diet (SAD) is Both Imbalanced
  and Inadequate 121

Bone Robbing Nutritional Excesses.................................122
Acid/Alkaline Balance: A Crucial Overlooked Factor.............132
References 135

Chapter 6
Bone-Robbing Physical Inactivity

Many Everyday Lifestyle Patterns Damage Bone.........................140
Physical Inactivity Causes Bone Loss..............................141
References 150

Chapter 7
Other Bone-Robbing Lifestyle Factors

Tobacco Harms Bone...153
Alcohol Robs Bone...155
Undernutrition, Dieting and Anorexia Accelerate Bone Loss....157
Many Medications Cause Osteoporosis...............................159
Toxic Metal Exposure Damages Bone 165
Stress is an Unsuspected Bone Killer 167
Weak Digestion Limits Bone Health.................................168
Our Indoor Existence Limits Bone Health...........................171
References 172

Chapter 8
Bone-Robbing Endocrine Imbalance

The Endocrine-Bone Link...178
The Parathyroid Gland 179
The Thyroid Gland 181
The Adrenal Glands 182
The Ovaries 185
The Kidneys...189
References 191

PART THREE
Regaining Bone Health

Chapter 9
Determining Your Risk of Developing Osteoporotic Fractures

Tell-Tale Signs of Bone Loss...200
How Medicine Measures Osteoporosis Risk....................................206
The New Urine Tests for Bone Resorption 213
References 215

Chapter 10
Better Bones, Better Body Program

It is Never Too Late or Too Early to Build Bone........................219
Clinically Proven Bone Building Programs 225
Getting Your Personal Program Started: The First Two Steps 229
References 232

Chapter 11
Maximizing Nutrient Intake

How Adequate is Your Diet?...235
Eating for Better Bones Guidelines 237
Bone is Best Built When All Bone Building Nutrients
    Are Consumed in Adequate Supply..................................246
Designing Your Own Bone Building Supplement Program 248
Special Notes on Maximizing Nutrient Intake for
    Those with Osteoporosis..256
    Perimenopausal Women 259
    Youth Still in Their Growing Years 262
References 263

Chapter 12
Building Digestive Strength

Digestion and Your Magical Body 266
Ten Steps to Stronger Digestion 269
Increasing Hydrochloric Acid Production 271

The Right Food Might Be Wrong for You: Food Allergies
and Osteoporosis Prevention 272
References 275

Chapter 13
Minimizing Anti-Nutrient Intake

Cutting Excess Protein Intake..276
Reducing Your Caffeine Count 278
Curbing Your Sweet Tooth 280
Trimming Excessive Fat..283
Setting Aside Salt..285
Avoiding Tobacco and Alcohol...287
References 289

Chapter 14
Developing An Alkaline Diet

Your Body's Acid-Alkaline Balance is Very Important 290
Diet Can Contribute to Excess Acidity...291
Monitoring Your Acid/Alkaline Balance 292
Developing an Alkaline Diet 293
References 300

Chapter 15
Exercising Into Bone Health

Sample Exercise Programs 302
Developing Your Own Personal Exercise Program 306
Better Bones, Better Body Guidelines for Strength Training 309
Better Bones, Better Body Guidelines for Aerobic
Enhancement 311
Special Exercise Notes for Those with Osteoporosis, for
Women Near Menopause and for Youth..................................313
References 321

Chapter 16
Promoting Endocrine Health

Caring for Your Thyroid, Parathyroid, Adrenals,
Ovaries, Kidneys, Pancreas and Liver 325

Chapter 17
Rethinking the Role of Estrogen Replacement for Osteoporosis

Estrogen Replacement and Osteoporosis 330
The Better Bones, Better Body Perspective on Hormone
    Replacement Therapy 335
Is Postmenopausal Hormone Replacement Worth It? What the
    Experts Now Say 352
The New Natural Progesterone Treatment for Osteoporosis 354
References 360

Chapter 18
Fosamax and Final Thoughts 366

References 371

Appendices

1 Recommended Dietary and Nutrient Guidelines......................375
2 Services of the Nutrition Education and Consulting
   Service...379
3 Wholesome Food Sources of Selected Nutrients......................382
4 Product Suppliers...395
5 Additional References..401

Index 405
About the Author..413

List of Illustrations

Chapter 1

Illustration 1.1   Mineral Movement In and Out of Bone.......28
Illustration 1.2   Bone Repair and Remodeling Processes.......30

Chapter 2

Illustration 2.1   Normal Bone vs. Osteoporotic Bone..............36
Illustration 2.2   Development of the "Dowager's Hump".....37
Illustration 2.3   Aging Bone Loss: Normal vs. Excessive.......41
Illustration 2.4   Osteoporosis Rates Cross-Culturally..............43
Illustration 2.5   Causes of Secondary Osteoporosis.................52

Chapter 3

Illustration 3.1   Bone-Building Factors vs. Bone-Thinning
                    Factors..69
Illustration 3.2   Factors Favoring Osteoporosis
                    Development 70

Chapter 4

Illustration 4.1   Average Dietary Nutrient Intake of
                    Selected Nutrients for American
                    Women Aged 14 to 65.....................................78
Illustration 4.2   RDA for Calcium, 1989.....................................82
Illustration 4.3   NIH Calcium Intake Recommendations........82

Chapter 9

Illustration 9.1   Osteoporosis Fracture Risk Assessment:
                    Your Personal Checklist............................198
Illustration 9.2   The 17 Independent Risk Factors
                    For Hip Fracture...211

Chapter 10

Illustration 10.1   Research Studies on How to Halt and
                     Reverse Osteoporosis.................................227
Illustration 10.2   Research Studies on How to Eliminate
                     New Fractures in Those with Osteoporosis ..228
Illustration 10.3   The Total Body Burden of Bone
                     Depleting Factors 230

Chapter 11

Illustration 11.1   Better Bones, Better Body Eating Guidelines 239
Illustration 11.2   Nutrient Content of a Broad Spectrum Multi-
                     Vitamin and Mineral Supplement 251

Chapter 13

Illustration 13.1   Protein Content of Selected Foods 278
Illustration 13.2   The Caffeine Count......................................279
Illustration 13.3   Sugar Content Of Selected Foods...............281
Illustration 13.4   Fat Content of Selected Foods....................283
Illustration 13.5   Sodium Content of Selected Foods 286

Chapter 14

Illustration 14.1   Food and Chemical Effects on Acid/Alkaline
                     Body Chemistry Balance.........................297

Chapter 15

Illustration 15.1   Dr. Dalsky's Clinically Proven Bone-
                     Building Program 304
Illustration 15.2   My General Exercise Commitment 308
Illustration 15.3   My Strength Training Exercise Program...311
Illustration 15.4   My Aerobic Enhancement Program..........312
Illustration 15.5   Exercises Not Recommended for Those
                     with Osteoporosis 315
Illustration 15.6   Safe Beginning Exercises for Everyone 316

Chapter 17

Illustration 17.1   Estrogen Use and Breast Cancer Risk.......343
Illustration 17.2   Potential Side Effects of Provera 350

Foreword

My 50-year-old cousin Cathy has a 50 percent chance of an osteoporotic fracture. While many fractures, such as a wrist fracture, are usually self-limiting and merely inconvenient, others may be life-threatening. A hip fracture, for example, not only involves six or more months of physical rehabilitation and life disruption, but it is frequently complicated by excessive blood clots which may travel to the lungs, kidneys, brain, liver or intestines. More than 300,000 hip fractures were reported in 1995 and each case cost at least $35,000.

This crisis situation shows no signs of improving despite the millions of dollars being poured into pharmaceutical research and promotion annually. Perhaps what is needed is a fresh new approach.

Dr. Susan Brown, a brilliant anthropologist and nutritionist, gives us just that in her comprehensive, beautifully written and impeccably researched book. She offers many important concepts and breakthroughs which lead us to rethink this debilitating disease: Why do people in poor countries have healthy bones and people in the richest countries have tremendous bone loss? What is the real nature of osteoporosis and what are the real causes? Given this new understanding, how can we prevent osteoporosis in future generations and how can we best treat those already suffering with it?

Dr. Brown answers these tough questions, drawing on the latest research, challenging old ideas and offering us a step-by-step self-help program for lifelong bone health. Finally, and perhaps most importantly, Dr. Brown offers both insight and hope: insight that bone health development and maintenance is natural and spontaneous for those living a life of healthful balance and hope that individuals can actually prevent needless fractures and even regain enough bone mass to take them out of the high risk zone.

My cousin Cathy (and millions like her) would do well to read and act on the life-saving information and guidelines provided in *Better Bones, Better Body.*

Russell Jaffe, M.D., Ph.D.
Fellow, Health Studies Collegium
Director, Serammune Physicians Lab

Better BONES, Better BODY

Introduction

. . . .

Only a New Seed Can Yield a New Crop

GENERAL STATISTICS

✦ Excessively thin bone, known as osteoporosis, is the most common bone disorder in the United States. An estimated seven to eight million people in the United States have osteoporosis and another 17 million are at high risk for the disease due to low bone density.

✦ 1.5 million osteoporotic fractures occur each year in the United States. This includes over 538,000 vertebral (spinal) fractures and over 300,000 hip fractures and 200,000 wrist fractures.

YOUR LIFETIME RISK OF SUFFERING AN OSTEOPOROTIC FRACTURE

✦ Overall half of all Caucasian American women aged 50 will suffer one or another osteoporotic fracture during her lifetime. Some of these will be as inconsequential as slight spinal fractures that go unnoticed. Others will be potentially life-threatening, such as hip fracture in an elderly person.

✦ By age 65, one-third of all Caucasian American women will experience at least one spinal vertebral fracture.

✦ By age 70, 40 percent of all Caucasian American women will suffer an osteoporotic bone fracture, whether of the spine, wrist, arm, rib or hip.

✦ By age 85, the majority of Caucasian women in the United States will have at least one partial deformity in their spine.

✦ A 50-year-old Caucasian American woman has a one in six chance of experiencing a hip fracture during her lifetime. Of those women surviving into their late 80s and beyond, the figure rises to one in three. The lifetime risk of hip fracture among African American women is much lower than among Caucasian women at six percent. The risk for Asian American, Native American and Latino women is believed to be between these two extremes. Of men surviving into their 90's and beyond, one in six will fracture a hip. All in all, osteoporosis is a common chronic condition with serious consequences for one third of older females and perhaps 15 to 20 percent of all older males in this country.

The Consequences of Osteoporotic Fractures

✦ Spinal fractures result in untold spinal deformation and painful crippling.

✦ Hip fractures, however, are the greatest threat: up to one-half of those who fracture a hip need permanent help with daily living; 20 to 30 percent enter into long-term care; 20 percent die shortly after the hip fracture.

✦ Currently osteoporosis costs the health care system some $18 billion each year. Hip fractures represent 80 percent of the total expense, averaging $35,000 per patient.

Future Prospects

✦ The aged sector of the population is growing. By the year 2000 nearly 15 percent of the United States population will be 65 or older, and by the year 2050 nearly 25 percent of all United States residents will be 65 plus.

✦ More people are fracturing more bones more often. By the turn of the century hip fractures alone will climb to 350,000 per year, costing the nation $30 to $40 billion annually. Some authorities estimate that that increase alone will be enough to bankrupt the Medicare system.

These are the startling, yet standard facts about the current United States bone health crisis. As an anthropologist, however, the most striking fact about this disorder is not even listed above: the disease of osteoporosis is a needless disorder. It is a disease, in fact, that barely exists in much of the world. As we shall see, it is a disease we have created and one we can eliminate. Like coronary heart disease, diabetes mellitus, hypertension, obesity, diseases of the colon, dental and periodontal disease, gallstones and kidney stones, it also is a disease of Western civilization created by our lifestyles. All these disorders are unknown or uncommon among indigenous and traditional peoples living their time-honored lifestyles as fellow anthropologists have documented.[15,16]

Looking cross-culturally we begin to see that osteoporosis, like the other diseases listed above, is a "degenerative disease." Its cause stems from a breakdown, a degeneration, of normal physiological functioning. When functioning normally the body builds and maintains lifelong healthy bones. This is a natural, effortless process in vertebrate animals all over the world. Bone is built spontaneously; it requires no conscious effort. This generative process is natural, simple and automatic. It is only when the body is forced to adapt to less-than-ideal circumstances that it builds weak and fragile bones.

A dozen years ago my grandmother fell in her home and broke a hip at the age of 101. Looking back it is clear to me that she had long suffered the effects of osteoporosis, although none of us even thought about it. She had broken a wrist bone several years before, lost a lot of height and developed a hump on her back from accumulated vertebral fractures. It was at the time of her death, one year after her hip fracture, that my interest in osteoporosis peaked. Over the years this interest actually grew into a compulsion as I doggedly sought to understand why the disease existed and what we could do about it. At that time I was an established anthropologist and a budding nutritionist. Looking into the cross-cultural anthropological data, I soon discovered that osteoporosis is not a disorder we naturally or inevitably develop as we age; instead it is a degenerative disease, as mentioned above. My next question was, "If osteoporosis is largely created by human or cultural factors, why can't we eliminate it just as we created it?" If we have knowledge and technology to rendezvous astronauts in distant space, transplant a human liver and split the atom, why can't we learn how to recover our body's innate ability to build and maintain lifelong healthy bones? And so my compelling search for answers began.

Thousands of research hours later several things became clear to me. Specifically, I now know that osteoporosis is preventable and that it can be halted once begun. I also know that it is to some degree reversible, even though science has not yet determined the extent of this reversal potential. Moreover it is clear that the natural lowering of estrogen levels at menopause is not *the* cause of osteoporosis, and that we have seriously misunderstood the menopause-osteoporosis link. Several dangerous implications, in fact, flow from this faulty assumption. Nor does the answer simply concern low calcium intakes. I also now know that we have failed in our attempts to halt or prevent, much less reverse, osteoporosis because we do not adequately understand the true nature and causes of this disorder. Hard as we may try, we cannot build a strong and effective program to eliminate a disease which we do not truly understand.

❖ ONLY A NEW SEED CAN YIELD A NEW CROP

As the ancient Vedic saying goes, "Only a new seed can yield a new crop." To recover our natural birthright of life-long bone health we need something new. The new knowledge required to conquer osteoporosis and regenerate natural bone health is vast. Specifically we need to more fully explore the following questions:

1. **What is the true nature and extent of osteoporosis?**
   Is osteoporotic bone really normal or just thin bone? Is osteoporosis the result of the normal aging bone loss? Does it occur all over the world? Has our osteoporosis rate always been so high? Is it mainly a woman's disease? Does osteoporosis *per se* cause osteoporotic fractures or is there something else involved?

   Part I of this book explores these issues, rethinking the nature and distribution of osteoporosis.

2. **What are the true causes of osteoporosis? Are calcium and estrogen really to blame?**
   Does low calcium intake really cause osteoporosis? What about other nutrients? What about lifestyle and environmental factors? Does the natural lowering of estrogen levels at menopause really cause osteoporosis? Is there a difference between "estrogen deficiency" and the natural lowering of estrogen levels at menopause? Can estrogen deficiency be corrected naturally, without hormone replacement? Currently 25 percent of American women experience surgical menopause and by age 65 a woman has almost a 50-50 chance of having

lost her reproductive organs. How does all this surgery relate to our current osteoporosis incidence?

Part II of this book challenges our current assumptions about the causes of osteoporosis and rethinks the true causes of this disorder from the wider cross-cultural perspective.

3. What are the proven life-supporting methods to prevent, halt and reverse osteoporosis?

What do the latest scientific studies tell us about preventing osteoporosis? What should be done at the different life stages? What programs are best for children? Do young adults present special needs? What light does science shed on the critical menopausal period? What is best for older folks and those already afflicted with osteoporosis? Can bone loss be halted? Can lost bone be rebuilt?

Part III of this book rethinks the optimum prevention and treatment of osteoporosis, developing a unique, comprehensive program capable of eliminating most osteoporosis. This Better Bones, Better Body Program is designed to normalize and optimize bone mass at all ages.

Being fully life-supporting, the program introduced in Part III does not endorse the widespread use of estrogen replacement hormones. Here you will also find the latest scientific findings on the pros and cons of estrogen therapy. With this data you can make more informed decisions about your personal bone building program.

4. How can we better utilize our magical bodies and optimize our innate "regeneration response"?

Just how complex is our physical body? How does it function? What holds it together and organizes its vast functioning? What directs its activities and maintains order? What is the role of internal balance and how does the body maintain it? What are the causes and effects of imbalance? Is it possible to restore balance? What are the underlying sources of health and disease?

The goals of this book are threefold. The first is to rethink the nature and causes of osteoporosis, moving from the common simplistic explanations to deeper, truer understandings. Among other things I will demonstrate that osteoporosis is not something that "goes wrong" with our body, but rather it is a useful, actually essential, survival mechanism on the part of an infinitely intelligent body. Allied to the first, the second goal is to impart a sense of appreciation for the truly magical nature of our bodies. Each detail of our mysterious body/mind has been crafted and perfected by nature over millions of years. Each detail is incomprehensibly intertwined one with all others. Here the goal is to impart an appreciation that will stimulate you to seek ways to work with your magical body to fulfill your optimum health potential. The third and final goal is to create a comprehensive new self-help program capable of preventing, halting and even beginning to reverse osteoporosis. The program is fully life-supporting. This means that every aspect of our osteoporosis program is good not only for bone, but also good for the entire body. It is a program capable of building vastly better bones, a better body and better overall health.

At first glance these might seem like overly ambitious goals. As you move through this book, however, you will see that these goals are not so difficult to achieve. In fact in many cultures whose lifestyles work with nature, lifelong healthy bones already are, and have always been, the norm. We need merely to set the stage, provide the life-supportive raw materials and environment and let nature do the rest. By working with nature, by capitalizing on the vast intelligence and organizing power of life itself, we can accomplish these goals. Most of us have unwittingly come to confuse our current state of degeneration with normal human functioning. We have come to expect poor health and in particular anticipate declining health as we age, as if it were normal. *The aim of this book is to illuminate the journey from where and what we are to where and what we can be.*

❖ ABOUT THE BETTER BONES, BETTER BODY PROGRAM

This book represents both an invitation for personal initiative and a call for scientific research. Currently about one-third of all women in this country and 15 to 20 percent of men will in their lifetime experience a "meaningful" consequence of osteoporosis.[17,19] The most significant of these, of course, are hip fractures which one in six American women and men will suffer. My research as both an anthropologist and nutritionist has led me to propose the following:

- ✦ If Americans followed most of the Better Bones, Better Body Guidelines from youth, osteoporosis could be eliminated as a major public health concern in the U.S.
- ✦ If most people of any age today started the Better Bones, Better Body Program we could quickly and significantly reverse the ever-growing trend of increasing osteoporotic fractures.
- ✦ If the 18 million Americans considered to be at high risk of osteoporosis due to low bone density

were to engage in this program the majority would never actually become osteoporotic.

✦ If the seven to eight million people in this country with osteoporosis were to incorporate the Better Bones, Better Body Program as an adjunct to their medical therapy program, the number of them who actually come to suffer an osteoporotic fracture could be cut by one half or more.

Also, I would like to emphasize that the Better Bones, Better Body Program is not necessarily exclusive. For the majority of individuals it will be all they need to maintain life-long healthy bones. For others, however, it will serve as an adjunct to their pharmaceutically-based therapy program. For all, hopefully it will provide useful information and inspiration.

It is also important to note that while the Better Bones, Better Body Program is a proposal for us as a culture to go beyond estrogen drug therapy for osteoporosis, estrogen therapy is still important to millions of individual women for various reasons. For those women, incorporation of The Better Bones, Better Body Program will enhance the benefits of estrogen therapy.

Finally, if you are at high risk for suffering an osteoporotic fracture I encourage you to work with a health professional to monitor the success of your bone building program, whatever it may be. Today there are reliable means available for testing changes in both bone density and the rate of bone breakdown. As the old Chinese saying goes, "If we continue in the same direction we will end up right where we are headed." I suspect that in regards to osteoporosis neither you as an individual nor we as a culture want to end up "right where we are headed."

❖ References

1 National Osteoporosis Foundation, *National Objectives for Disease Prevention and Health Promotion for the Year 2000*, (Washington D.C.: National Osteoporosis Foundation, 1988).

2 National Osteoporosis Foundation, Audrey Singer, Personal Communication October 20, 1995.

3 Nevitt, Michael C., "Epidemiology of Osteoporosis," *Rheumatic Disease Clinics of North America* 20.3 (1994): 535-559.

4 Riggs, B.L., "Differential Changes in Bone Mineral Density of the Appendicular and Axial Skeleton with Aging Relationship to Spinal Osteoporosis," *J. Clin. Invest.* 67.February (1981): 328-35.

5 Riggs, B., and L. Melton, "Involutional Osteoporosis," *New England Journal of Medicine* 26 (1986): 1676-1686.

6 Heaney, R., and J. Barger-Lux, *Calcium and Common Sense*, (New York: Doubleday, 1988).

7 Ettinger, B., "Preventing Postmenopausal Osteoporosis with Estrogen Replacement Therapy," *International Journal of Fertility* Supplement (1986): 15-20.

8 Ettinger, B., "Estrogen Replacement Therapy Symposium: Introduction," *Obstetrics and Gynecology* 72.5 (1988): 1S.

9 Lindsay, Robert, "The Burden of Osteoporosis Cost," *American Journal of Medicine* 98 (1995).

10 Snider, Mike, "Lives don't heal after hip fractures," *USA Today* February 19, 1993.

11 Cummings, S., et al., "Epidemiology of Osteoporosis and Osteoporotic Fractures," *Epidemiol Rev* 7 (1985): 178-208.

12 Holbrook, T., et al., *The Frequency of Occurrence, Impact and Cost of Selected Musculoskeletal Conditions in the United States*, (Chicago: American Academy of Orthopedic Surgeons, 1984).

13 Farmer, M., et al., "Race and Sex Differences in Hip Fracture Incidence," *Am J Public Health* 74 (1984): 1374-1380.

14 Heaney, Robert P., "Prevention of Osteoporotic Fracture in Women," *The Osteoporotic Syndrome*, (New York: Wiley-Liss, Inc., 1993) 89-107.

15 Eaton, S., and M. Konner, "Paleolithic Nutrition," 312 (1985): 283-289.

16 Trowell, H., and P. Burkitt, ed., *Western Diseases: Their Emergence and Prevention,* (Boston: Harvard University Press, 1981).

17 Slemenda, Charles, and C. Conrad Jr. Johnson, "Osteoporotic Fractures," *Nutrition and Bone Development,* ed. David Jason Simmons. (New York: Oxford University Press, 1990) 131-147.

18 NIH, "Optimal Calcium Intake," *National Institutes of Health* 12.4 (1994): 1-24.

19 Meuleman, J., "Beliefs about Osteoporosis: A Critical Appraisal," *Arch Intern Med* 147.4 (1987): 762-765.

PART ONE

❖ Rethinking the Nature of Osteoporosis

Chapter **1**
. . . .

Magical Bodies, Magical Bones

❖ OUR MAGICAL BODIES

The moment one gives close attention to anything, even a blade of grass, it becomes a mysterious, awesome, indescribable, magnificent work in itself.—Henry Miller

*I*n our busy daily lives we rarely pause to ponder the mystery of such a simple thing as a blade of grass. Yet if we did we might well wonder. What holds this blade of grass together? How does it know how to produce chlorophyll, starch, protein and fats from air, water, sunlight and soil? What oversees its exquisitely ordered reproduction? What was in the seed from which it came that made possible a dynamic, self-repairing, self-maintaining, living entity?

If we turn our attention to the human body the mystery magnifies many times. Each of us is composed of some 60 trillion plus independently functioning parts—cells which miraculously function together to create the most sophisticated creature on earth. Although so tiny that 100 cells fit on the head of a pin, each cell is comprised of systems within systems. Each of our billions of cells is a whole world unto itself.

No matter which layer of our physiology we choose to look at, whether a single cell or an entire organ, we find that the body is composed of untold systems within systems. For example, something as simple as one square inch of skin contains approximately 250 sweat glands, 25 hairs, 40 oil glands, 7.5 feet of blood vessels and 30 feet of nerves with 7,500 sensory cells at their ends. Each sweat gland, each hair, each oil gland, each blood vessel, each nerve is in turn a world unto itself.

The human body, however, is not just a collection of independently operating systems. All systems, each layer of our physiology, functions together, one in relation to all others. Guided by an invisible, all-pervasive, organizing intelligence, all systems are coordinated by a series of seemingly infinite feedback loops. For example, if the calcium level in our blood gets low, a complex series of feedback loops is activated and again many balance-maintaining systems are involved. A vast array of biochemical reactions occur in response to low blood calcium. Some of the more major compensating actions are carried out by the parathyroid hormone and vitamin D. Parathyroid hormone stimulates the kidney to convert vitamin D to its active form: it directs that calcium be extracted from the bones and sent for use in the blood (first from the calcium pool on the surface of bone and later from other reserves); it also retards mineralization. Activated vitamin D moves to increase intestinal calcium absorption, to encourage kidney reabsorption of calcium and to facilitate mobilization of calcium from the bone. As soon as the amount of calcium in the blood again returns to an acceptable level, these feedback mechanisms are reversed. Other hormones and chemical messengers are then sent to signal a cessation of these processes. They tell the intestines to stop absorbing more calcium, the kidneys to resume excreting calcium in the urine, and the parathyroid to cease taking calcium from the bones.

An even more complicated feedback system is that aimed at providing each bone location with sufficient bone tissue, with appropriate material properties, advantageously placed to withstand the functional load put on that location. One fascinating component of this system is the adaptive response to a loading strain as from exercise or strenuous activity. As it appears, the osteocyte (the basic bone cell) acts as a strain gauge sensor, evaluating the amount of stress and strain on the bone at its location. With this information it can then calculate the amount of new bone needed. These osteocytes then somehow stimulate the production of prostaglandins which in turn lead to increased production of a substance known as G6PD, which in turn affects RNA production ultimately resulting in new bone formation.

The mechanics of how this all happens is unknown. The story, however, becomes even more fascinating when we look at where this new bone is placed. Interestingly enough the maximum amount of new bone formation does not seem to occur at the site of greatest strain. Rather the bone cells make an area-wide evaluation of where new bone should be placed and where redundant tissue should be removed in view of the overall mismatch between the actual and desirable strain distribution for the entire area, not just at the local site of the peak strain.[1] Thus bone is not simply rebuilt and reduced at the point of strain or inactivity, but somehow our all-encompassing internal computer calculates where to strengthen or reduce bone in regard to the needs of the entire body.

You might well be wondering how bone cells make this "area-wide evaluation" of where to build new bone and where to reduce existing bone mass. This determination involves a vast communication network among bone cells. Within each cubic millimeter of bone, that is a cube about the size of a head of a pin, there lie buried some 25,000 such bone cells each nestled in its own tiny lacunae. Although independent, each of these bone cells communicates with other bone cells through a network of tentacle-like structures called cell processes. Out from each bone cell these tentacles extend contacting the tentacles of other bone cells, forming a network connecting all bone cells. Using this vast body-wide communication network bone cells effectively evaluate where to reinforce and where to reduce bone.

How a feedback system is shut off can be even more intriguing than how it is initiated. For example, when looking at the unique mineralization process which allows bone tissue to harden, the most interesting question becomes, "What stops this process, what keeps the body from crystallizing all its calcium and phosphorus into solid tissues?" In this case it appears that the same bone forming cells (the osteoblasts) that initiate the intricate crystallization process are also responsible for controlling the crystallization and bringing a halt to the process at the appropriate time.

Feedback loops such as these are the mechanisms which enable the complicated systems within systems to work together. They are the mechanisms by which these systems talk to one another. Such communication between all of the many systems in our body allows the systems to stay in balance, each with all others.

❖ HEALTH LIES IN A SELF-MAINTAINED BALANCE AMONG ALL SYSTEMS

Why is it important for all the systems of the body to be in balance with one another? Consider New York City with its few million cars. What would happen without traffic signals or driving regulations? Obvious chaos. Imagine how much more chaotic it would be if each of the trillions of independent cells in our body lacked coordination. The body would be quickly rendered a heap of useless protoplasm.

Balance and coordination among every body system are necessary for full and spontaneous functioning. We simply cannot survive without the proper level of sugar in our blood, if blood calcium drops too low or goes too high, if the temperature of our body is not within a small range, and on and on. Balance is necessary for even the lowest level of physical functioning and a very refined level of balance is necessary for optimum physical and mental functioning. Ideal bone health, the concern of this book, depends upon the balanced functioning of many systems. In the truly healthy individual, there is a self-maintained state of balance within and between all systems. *Our degree of health depends on the degree of balance. Perfect balance equals perfect health; conversely, imperfect balance equals imperfect health.*

This equation applies to our bones. Unhealthy bones speak of imbalance, as we shall see in detail. The current epidemic of poor bone health stems directly from our contemporary lifestyle. Unwittingly we have adopted a way of living which imposes great stress and forces great imbalance upon the layers of systems within systems which compromise our bodies. Presented with these stresses and imbalances, the body does its best to compensate, to remain in balance and continue functioning.

Most of today's degenerative diseases, and certainly osteoporosis, actually represent noble, life-saving coping mechanisms the body resorts to in order to maintain a minimal required level of internal balance. For the body to do better, for it to return to normal optimum functioning, it must be provided with a more nourishing, life-supporting environment. We must restore the balance which allows for the spontaneous flow of our all-pervading bodily intelligence.

❖ LIFELONG HEALTHY BONES ARE OUR BIRTHRIGHT

The human body is an unfathomed organism beautiful and complex. Guided by an organizing intelligence, countless systems within systems operate with exacting elegance to create our fully integrated, self-repairing human body. A strong skeletal system providing us with lifelong healthy bones is but one of its smaller accomplishments. It is only natural to enjoy lifelong healthy bones effortlessly, just as every animal in the forest does. The growing epidemic of weak and fragile bones among young and old alike is unnatural and totally preventable.

Even the slightest glance at our magical body leaves one wide-eyed with wonder. In my case, the study of how we build and maintain bone has left me with a deep appreciation for the intelligence and organizing power of nature. I now know that the best way to build bone health is by working with and maximizing nature's intelligence, rather than by trying to override or improve upon it. Hopefully

23

. . . .
Magical Bodies, Magical Bones

this book will convey a sense of that wonder and appreciation while showing you how to work with nature to guarantee your birthright of life-long healthy bones.

❖ OUR MAGICAL BONES

Bone is Vital, Living, Ever-Changing Tissue

While our bodies might seem to be static, solid and rather slow to change, nothing could be further from the truth. Our bodies are constantly changing as we exchange atoms with the universe through such processes as breathing, eating, elimination, sweating and sloughing off skin. In just one year 98 percent of all the atoms in our body are replaced. Every five weeks we make a new skin, a new liver each six weeks. Even our fat cells are filled with fat and emptied out constantly, so that their contents are fully exchanged every three weeks.[2]

The skeleton is no exception. Bone is living tissue which undergoes constant transformation. Bone might appear static, but its basic components are continually renewed. At any given moment in each of us, there are from one to ten million sites where small segments of old bone are being dissolved and new bone laid down in its place. Every atom in our skeleton is replaced within a three month period. At any given time within the average adult there are from one to ten million sites where small bits of bone are being broken down by these specialized cells, later to be replaced with new bone or other cells dedicated to this rebuilding task. Thus while bone appears "dead" and inactive, it is really extremely vital, active tissue. Bone is living tissue, nourished and detoxified by blood vessels, in constant exchange with the whole body.[3,4]

The Life Cycle of Bone

The skeleton develops rapidly through infancy, childhood, puberty and adolescence, reaching its maximum size and density between the owner's 25th and 30th birthdays. This state of maximum bone density is called the "peak bone mass." At this point the bones are their strongest and their densest. From this point on, sooner or later, most people begin to lose bone mass. Studies conducted in the United States suggest that over a lifetime a woman might lose 38 percent of her total peak bone mass, and a man 23 percent of his. This includes a 50 percent loss in the spongy type of bone known as trabacular bone and about a 35 percent loss in the harder type of bone known as cortical bone.[5,6] Some people, however, lose little or no bone mass at all as they age. A study from 1970, for example, reported that 38 percent of the men and 22 percent of the women aged 55 to 64 lost little or no bone over an 11-year period.[7,8]

Bone loss generally begins in the later 30s, and in women can accelerate around menopause. Many Western scientists report a so-called "menopausal effect" in which a woman might lose some two to four percent of her bone mass per year in the first two to five years after menopause.[9-11] This is not a consistent finding, however. Not all researchers report an acceleration of bone loss at menopause.[12-16] This is an important controversy which we will discuss later. Even researchers reporting the "menopausal effect" note that rapid bone loss slows a few years into menopause and by the mid or late 50s the rate of bone loss returns to less than one percent per year, or ceases altogether, depending on type of bone studied. In men, accelerated bone loss is reported to begin in the late 60s.

Bone Fulfills Many Functions for the Body

Bone Gives the Body Form, Rigidity, Protection and Locomotion

Bone is a pretty amazing tissue, a clever creation of nature which gives more than structure to the body. Our bones, all 206 of them, are the hardest of all our tissues. As such, they give form and rigidity to our bodies allowing us to sit, stand straight and walk. Without bones, we wouldn't have a leg to stand on! Bone also serves to protect our vital organs and soft tissue from damage from external sources. A sort of armor, the ribs, for example, protect the heart and lungs from blows and injury just as the skull acts as a bony box protecting the fragile brain.[17] In addition to shaping, stabilizing and protecting the body, our bones serve many other essential functions.

Bones Serve as an Incubator for Red Blood Cells

Each second, our body produces some 2.4 million red blood cells. These red blood cells are produced inside bone, in the nine ounces of bone marrow our body contains. Bone is an active manufacturing plant requiring a constant supply of nutrients to produce this extraordinary number of red blood cells. Nutrients flow in and out of bone ceaselessly in this essential process.

Bones Serve as the Mineral Bank for the Body

Ninety-nine percent of the body's total calcium is stored in the bones, 85 percent of the phosphorus, 60 percent of the magnesium, and 35 percent of the sodium. Why are these minerals in bone?

Their most obvious job is to give strength and rigidity to the bone. In this fashion, these minerals directly serve bone. Less obvious is that these minerals also serve the body at large. Bones store these minerals, keeping them available for use anywhere in the body. The level of blood calcium, for example, must be kept within a very precise range. Many essential functions, from heartbeat and nerve transmission to blood clotting and enzyme activation, depend on precise blood calcium levels. For example, even a small drop in blood calcium causes the nerves and muscles to go into autonomic discharge, producing involuntary muscle spasms. Calcium, in fact, is reported to be the most fundamental regulator of intracellular processes and bone's role as regulator of calcium metabolism supersedes its structural roles. In evolutionary terms the physiological function of calcium precedes the evolution of bone and still holds a higher priority.[18] Thus, when the level of calcium in the blood drops, a myriad of reactions occur aimed at drawing the mineral from the bone and depositing it into the blood.[17]

Other minerals are tucked away in bone and stored there until needed, just like calcium. Phosphorus, another major bone constituent, is essential for DNA and RNA structure, plays a major role in energy production and is needed to maintain proper acid/base balance of body fluids. Magnesium, also stored in bone, is indispensable to the body. It is involved in transmitting impulses among nerve cells and muscle cells and is required as a cofactor by many enzymes involved in producing energy and protein and in using calcium.[19] Minute by minute, minerals flow from the bone into the blood and back again.

How are these vital minerals transferred in and out of bone? As we shall see, it is the role of specialized bone cells, known as osteoclasts, to break down small bits of bone releasing calcium, phosphorus, magnesium and other nutrients for use in the blood. Each day some 360 mg or more of calcium are dissolved from the bone and deposited in the blood. In this fashion each year 20 percent of an adult's bone calcium is replaced. Another group of bone cells, the osteoblasts, carries out the reverse process, absorbing minerals and placing them back into bone while building new segments of bone. These opposing processes must be carried out in precise balance to maintain a stable bone mass. If more minerals are taken out of the bone than are deposited back into the bone, the end result is thin, weak bones.[4]

The Basic Bone Structure

The architecture of bone gives it strength and resistance, yet it is also designed for flexibility. The hip, for example, must be strong enough to withstand up to 600 pounds of force, yet it must also be flexible enough to tolerate twisting and bending without breaking. Bone contains an elastic living matrix made of protein. This living part of bone is called collagen and it comprises about 22 percent of all bone. On its honeycombed protein matrix, crystalline minerals are deposited. The collagen imparts flexibility and the crystalline minerals impart rigidity and strength.[17]

Illustration 1.1

MINERAL MOVEMENT IN AND OUT OF BONE

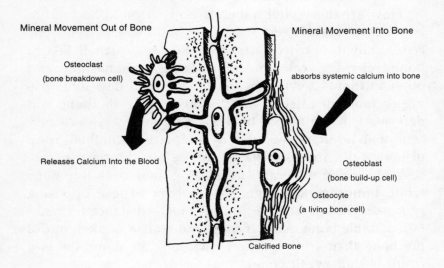

Mineral Movement Out of Bone

Osteoclast
(bone breakdown cell)

Releases Calcium Into the Blood

Mineral Movement Into Bone

absorbs systemic calcium into bone

Osteoblast
(bone build-up cell)

Osteocyte
(a living bone cell)

Calcified Bone

The Unique Architecture of Bone

The unique architecture of bone also provides for two types of bone structures. One type of bone structure is called "cortical" or "compact" bone. This is the dense compact bone seen on the outside. It forms a tough outer protective layer of bone. The other type of bone is found inside the bone and it is called "trabecular bone." Trabecular bone has a much looser lattice weave and appears "spongy." Some 80 to 90 percent of compact cortical bone is calcified and thus it is very dense, solid bone with a low surface-to-volume ratio. On the other hand, only 15 to 25 percent of the spongy trabecular bone is calcified, the rest is marrow. Trabecular bone with its loose web-like weave has a much greater surface area than the more solid cortical bone. As the breakdown of bone always occurs on the surface of bone, the spongy trabecular bone undergoes more loss than cortical bone. Also, given its greater loss of both minerals and of the protein matrix which holds the minerals, fractures occur most commonly in bones with high trabecular content.

About 80 percent of our bone is of the cortical type and 20 percent is trabecular. The spine is nearly all trabecular bone, while the arms and legs are nearly all cortical bone. The lower part of the wrist which often fractures is two-thirds trabecular. The ribs are all high in trabecular bone, as is the jaw bone. The hips overall are composed of roughly half trabecular and half cortical bone. Given this distribution of trabecular and cortical bone we find that most commonly the first osteoporotic fractures to occur are in the wrist, spine and ribs while hip fractures occur later in life.

The Self Repair Capability of Bone

Because of the wear and tear it undergoes, bone needs to heal and repair itself constantly. As such, unique self-repair mechanisms have evolved for the healing and regeneration of bone. These repair processes are conducted by the same "osteoclast" bone-breakdown cells and the "osteoblast" bone-building cells already mentioned. The osteoclasts eat up old, weakened segments of bone, while the osteoblasts, lay down fresh new segments of bone. The process is much like that of the highway repair. A damaged area of the road is picked for repair; the site is excavated removing the old weakened asphalt, and then new material is put down. In like fashion bone heals and renews itself in a process called "bone remodeling." This self-repair capability is extremely important: imbalances in bone remodeling cause osteoporosis. When more old bone is eaten up than new bone is laid down bone loss occurs. In actuality this is exactly how bone loss occurs. Scientists estimate that for every

Illustration 1.2

BONE REPAIR AND REMODELING PROCESSES

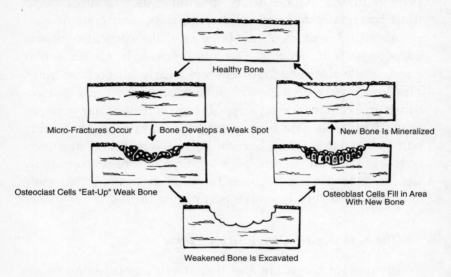

Healthy Bone

Micro-Fractures Occur   Bone Develops a Weak Spot   New Bone Is Mineralized

Osteoclast Cells "Eat-Up" Weak Bone   Osteoblast Cells Fill in Area With New Bone

Weakened Bone Is Excavated

30 parts of bone resorped only 29 new parts are laid down in replacement. Bone loss becomes excessive as the difference between the amount of bone removed and that replaced grows or when the bone turnover rate is high. High bone turnover means that little bits of bone are lost more frequently.[3] There are new urine tests for bone breakdown, which are discussed in Chapter 9. Given the above explanation, you can see why it is important to know if you are breaking down bone more rapidly than normal.

In an evolutionary sense there is a constant balancing act between the strength and the weight of bone. The evolutionary advantage, so to speak, is in having the lightest possible bones capable of doing the job that needs to be done. In fact, the whole architecture of cortical and trabecular bone individually, and their unique combination in each type of bone, was designed through evolution to this end. In this sense it is also interesting to note that bones continue evolving and adapting day by day, always with the same efficient goal of being no more heavy than necessary. If we put more stress on them, if we do a lot of exercise, if we build muscle or have a heavier body to move around, bones will be stronger. They grow stronger in response to demands we place upon them. If on the other hand, we are inactive and don't put very much stress and strain on the body, then bones tend to get lighter and thinner.

Factors Regulating Bone Remodeling

As you might imagine, remodeling is a very complicated process which is not yet fully understood. It involves untold cellular functions directed toward the resorption of old bone and formation of new bone. Both systemic hormones and local factors play important roles in this process. The systemic hormones at work include parathyroid hormone for the parathyroid glands, calcitonin and thyroxin from the thyroid, insulin from the pancreas, growth hormone from the pituitary and vitamin D as synthesized and activated by the kidney, as well as glucocortical adrenal hormones and the sex hormones, estrogen and androgen. The role of each of these many hormones in bone remodeling is multifaceted and complex.

While it was once thought that the systemic hormones were the major regulators of remodeling, it is now clear that various locally produced factors such as growth hormones, vitamin B_2, microglobulins and transferrin are also of great importance.

Our Bones are Designed to Last Us a Lifetime

By nature's design, our bones were meant to last us a lifetime. Spontaneously, without any thought or effort, all animals build and maintain lifelong healthy bones. So it should be with humans.

Throughout human history, as people aged, their bones tended to thin and get somewhat weaker but there remained enough bone mass and bone strength to withstand the stresses and strains of daily activities. Cross-culturally osteoporotic fractures have been rare as we detail in the next chapter. Today, however, the situation is different. Currently, the most modernized countries are experiencing a virtual epidemic of poor bone health. In many areas such as the United States, Sweden, Denmark, England and France, large numbers of aging people and a growing number of the young have bones so thin and brittle that they fracture under the common stress and strains of everyday activity. In these countries bone health is degenerating and the osteoporosis rate is soaring.

❖ References

1 Lanyon, L. E., "Skeletal Responses to Physical Loading," *Physiology and Pharmacology of Bone*, ed. Gregory R. Mundy, and John T. Martin. (Berlin: Springer-Verlag, 1993) 107: 485-505.

2 Chopra, Deepak, *Perfect Health*, first ed. (New York: Harmony Books, 1990) 327.

3 Frost, H., "The Pathomechanics of Osteoporosis," *Clin Orthop* 200 (1985): 198-225.

4 Heaney, R., and J. Barger-Lux, *Calcium and Common Sense*, (New York: Doubleday, 1988).

5 Riggs, B., et al., "In Women Dietary Calcium Intake and Rates of Bone Loss From Midradius and Lumbar Spine Are Not Related," *J Bone Min Res* 1(suppl) (1986): 167.

6 Genant, Harry K., and et al, "Osteoporosis: Assessment by Quantitative Computed Tomography," *Orthopedic Clinics of North America* 16.3 (1985): 557-568.

7 Adams, P., and et al, "Osteoporosis and the effects of aging on bone mass in elderly men and women," *J. Med. New Series* 39 (1970): 601-615.

8 Avioli, L., *The Osteoporotic Syndrome: Detection, Prevention, and Treatment*, (New York: Grune and Stratton, Inc., 1983-A).

9 Lindsay, R., et al., "Bone Loss During Oestriol Therapy in Postmenopausal Women," *Maturitas* 1 (1979): 279-285.

10 Horsman, A., et al., "The Relation Between Bone Loss and Calcium Balance in Women," *Clin Sci* 59 (1980): 137-142.

11 Horsman, A., et al., "Non-linear Bone Loss in Oophorectomized Women," *Br J Radiol* 50 (1977): 504-507.

12 Hansson, Tommy, and B. Roos, "Age changes in the bone mineral of the lumbar spine in normal women," *Calcif Tissue Int.* 38 (1986): 249-251.

13 Harris, S., and B. Dawson-Highes, "Rates of change in bone mineral density of the spine, heel, femoral neck and radius in healthy postmenopausal women," *Bone Miner* 17.1 (1992): 87-95.

14 Riggs, B., et al., "Rates of Bone Loss in the Appendicular and Axial Skeletons of Women: Evidence of Substantial Vertebral Bone Loss Before Menopause," *J Clin Invest* 77 (1985): 1487-1491.

15 Trotter, M., and B. Hixon, "Sequential Changes in Weight, Density and Percentage Weight of Human Skeletons from an Early Fetal Period through Old Age.," *Anat Rec* 179 (1974): 1-8.

16 Leichter, I., et al., "The Effect of Age and Sex on Bone Density, Bone Mineral Content and Cortical Index," *Clin Orthop Rel Res* 156 (1981): 232-239.

17 Shipman, Pat, and et al, *The Human Skeleton*, (Cambridge, Massachusetts: Harvard University Press, 1985).

18 Stini, William A., "Osteoporosis: Etiologies, Prevention, and Treatment," *Yearbook of Physical Anthropology*, (NY: Wiley-Liss, 1990) 151-194.

19 Brown, Judith, *The Science of Human Nutrition*, (New York: Harcourt Brace Jovanovich, Inc., 1990).

Chapter 2
....

Redefining Osteoporosis

OSTEOPOROSIS IS NOT:	RATHER OSTEOPOROSIS IS:
Just Thin Bones	Thin and Substandard Bone
Normal Aging Bone Loss	A Degenerative Disease
Common All Over the World	Common Only in Westernized Countries
A Female Disorder	A "Feminist Issue" in Westernized Countries
A Disorder of Just the Elderly	Becoming More Common Among the Young
Faulty Bone Metabolism, Something that "Goes Wrong" With Our Bones	An Intelligent Bodily Response to the Stress of Long-Term Imbalance
An Isolated Disorder	One Manifestation of Systemic Breakdown

❖ OSTEOPOROSIS IS MORE THAN JUST THIN BONES

"*O*steo" means bone, "porosis" denotes porosity. The word osteoporosis literally means porous bones. In osteoporosis, bone density is low and the bones are thin.

35

Illustration 2.1
NORMAL BONE VS. OSTEOPOROTIC BONE
(*as viewed by electron micrograph*)

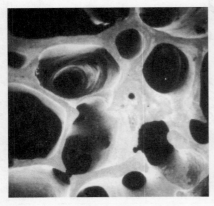 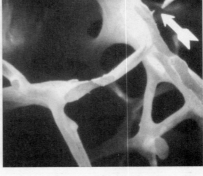

Normal Bone   Osteoporotic Bone

(Scanning electron micrographs courtesy of Dr. David W. Dempster with permission from the Journal of Bone Mineral Research 1:15-21, 1986, Mary Ann Liebert, Inc., Publishers.).

Having less substance the bones become weak and it is assumed they will fracture more easily.[1] Indeed, osteoporotic bone looks thin and weak as viewed under a high power microscope.

Weak spinal vertebrae, for example, can actually collapse entirely resulting in what is known as a "compression" fracture, or collapse on just one side causing a "wedge" fracture. When several vertebrae are crushed, the spinal column becomes deformed. This causes a loss of height, side-to-side curvature and development of a hump on the upper back known as the "Dowager's Hump" and subsequent stooping.

Over the decades it has been assumed that the osteoporotic process of bone thinning was in itself the cause of osteoporotic fractures. The central assumption has been that once bone reaches a certain level of thinness, it becomes subject to fracture more easily. It is now clear, however, that this is *not* the full story. *Bone does not fracture due to thinness alone; that is, osteoporosis by itself does not cause bone fractures.* This is documented simply by the fact that half of the people with thin osteoporotic bones, in fact, never fracture. As noted osteoporosis researcher, Lawrence Melton of the Mayo Clinic noted as early as 1988, "Osteoporosis alone may not be sufficient to produce such (osteoporotic) fracture, since many individuals remain fracture-free even within the sub-

Illustration 2.2

DEVELOPMENT OF THE "DOWAGER'S HUMP"

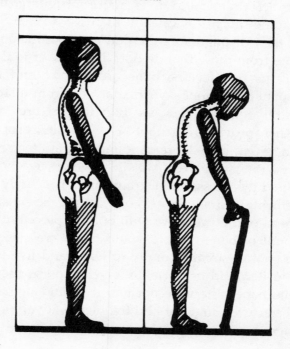

groups of lowest bone density. Most women aged 65 and over and men 75 and over have lost enough bone to place them at significant risk of osteoporotic fracture, yet many never fracture any bones at all. By age 80 virtually all women in the United States are osteoporotic with regard to their hip bone density, yet only a small percentage of them suffer hip fractures each year."[2]

This suggestion that thinness of bone alone is not enough to cause osteoporosis is further substantiated by the intriguing fact that older folks in many other cultures, ranging from France and Germany to China and Japan, have lower bone density that do we, yet they suffer less osteoporotic fractures. The Japanese case is particularly striking. There aging hip density is markedly lower than in the United States, yet their incidence of hip fractures is two and one half times less than ours.[3] Even more intriguing, the Japanese consume much less calcium than we do.

What then distinguishes the thin osteoporotic bones that do fracture from those that do not? The answer to this question concerns two factors, bone architecture and the self-repair capability of bone. When analyzed from a structural-architectural point of view we find that nature in all her wisdom has provided each of us with plenty of surplus bone. We have such a large bone mass safety factor, in fact, that even with osteoporosis we still have enough bone mass to withstand the stresses and strains of daily activity without ever fracturing a single bone. For example, scientists report that an osteoporotic vertebra with only 50 percent of its normal amount of bone (which would be severe osteoporosis) is strong enough architecturally to withstand five times the strain load it would be normally given. And as they report, "Were the bone otherwise normal, it should not fracture." But such fractures do occur and frequently at very low strain levels thus, ... "osteoporosis must involve more than reduced bone mineral density; the bone cannot be normal in quality."[4]

We now know that osteoporotic fractures involve more than osteoporosis. Bones that fracture are not only osteoporotic, but they also lack the ability to repair themselves properly from the microfractures that regularly occur due to normal stress and strain. Thus, bone which fractures isn't only thin, but also of poor quality with diminished self-repair capabilities.[4-8]

Given this new understanding the most accurate osteoporotic fracture equation is as follows:

THE NEW OSTEOPOROSIS FRACTURE EQUATION

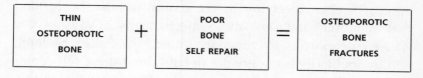

| THIN OSTEOPOROTIC BONE | + | POOR BONE SELF REPAIR | = | OSTEOPOROTIC BONE FRACTURES |

Many factors contribute to the breakdown of our bones' self-repair mechanisms. First, a wide range of nutrients is necessary for bone repair, as we shall see in Chapter 4. Inadequacies of these nutrients inhibit the self-repair processes. Chemicals and pollutants toxic to bone such as chemotherapy, heavy metals or radiation also damage bone repair mechanisms. We know exercise builds bone and doubtless plays a major role in enhancing bone repair. Lack of exercise reduces the self-repair capability of bone.

The benefits of exercise are particularly intriguing. Recent research shows that exercise increases various bone building factors, including a bone building protein and vitamin D metabolites. Other mechanisms by which exercise stimulates bone building and repair processes involve the "body electric" concept, as elaborated so well by Dr. R. Becker in his research.[9] Becker was one of the first to point out that electricity and electromagnetic fields are vital to life, and that the human body itself is largely electrical in nature. His experiments documented that the healing and growth of bone could be stimulated by the application of electrical currents. While there is much left to learn about the role electrical currents play in bone maintenance and healing, we do know that under the stress of exercise, electrical potentials are generated within the bones. A substantial body of evidence indicates that this electrical activity promotes bone growth and repair.[9-11] Conversely, reduced physical activity brings about less electrical activity which manifests itself in lessened growth and repair.

Already, many scientists are beginning to realize that bone self-repair mechanisms are central to bone health and that the breakdown of these mechanisms always occurs where osteoporosis fractures are found.[4, 11-14] Future research will undoubtedly bring greater details about these self-repair processes. For now it seems reasonable to assume that everything we do to maintain or restore the internal balance necessary for strong bones will also enhance the natural, automatic self-repair mechanisms of bone.

❖ OSTEOPOROSIS IS *NOT* NORMAL AGING BONE LOSS

Cross-cultural studies show that throughout the world most individuals lose bone mass as they age.[15] The remaining bone, however, is healthy and capable of constant self-repair. This is normal aging bone loss and this process leaves one with bones sufficiently dense and strong to withstand the stresses and strains of daily activity. In osteoporosis, bone loss goes beyond that of normal aging. It is an

Illustration 2.3

AGING BONE LOSS: NORMAL VS. EXCESSIVE

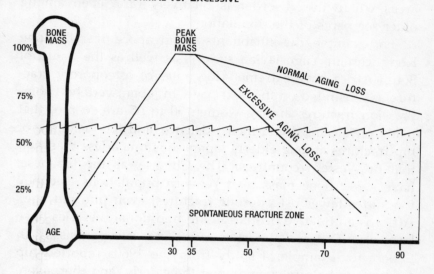

abnormal condition in which bone becomes excessively thin due to a loss of mineral. In addition, we now know that another factor is at play in osteoporosis and that is a reduction in bone's natural self-repair capacity. No matter what the self-repair capacity is, however, osteoporosis is excessive bone loss, not normal aging loss.

❖ OSTEOPOROSIS: AN ANTHROPOLOGICAL PERSPECTIVE

Looking at the anthropological data from around the world, we see that osteoporosis is a degenerative disease that occurs in some areas much more than it does in others, just as does cancer, heart disease and diabetes. It is not a natural artifact of aging. While the United States has one of the highest osteoporosis rates in the world, there are other areas where this disorder is relatively rare, even among older segments of the population.

For example, the inhabitants of Singapore overall, Hong Kong, certain Yugoslavian sectors, as well as the Bantu of South Africa have extremely low rates of osteoporotic fracture as illustrated on the next page. In Japan, vertebral compression fractures among women 50 to 65 are so rare that many physicians doubt their existence, and the incidence of hip fractures among elderly Japanese is much less than half that of Western countries.[3] The Chinese, as the Japanese, have lower bone mass than Western populations, yet they too suffer fewer osteoporotic fractures, even into old age.[3] Africans and native peoples living traditional lifestyles have been classified as "almost immune" to osteoporosis.[16-18] In Sudan, for example, a study from the 1960s reported hip fractures to be rare even among the elderly, and there were no cases of osteoporosis to be seen in a large teaching hospital. In Gambia, hip fractures were very infrequent. Only about one case annually was admitted to Victoria Hospital in Bathurst, even though the total population at risk was about 300,000.[19]

Around the world, osteoporotic hip fracture rates vary 30-fold for women and 16-fold for men. As illustrated on the next page, the highest osteoporosis rates are found in the most prosperous and technologically advanced societies. Conversely, the lowest rates are typically found in poorer, less technologically advanced societies.

Less cross-cultural data exist on the incidence of osteoporotic spinal fractures, partly because these often go unreported. Nonetheless it is held that their incidence parallels that of hip fractures and that countries with high hip fracture rates have high spinal fractures rates.

Illustration 2.4

OSTEOPOROSIS RATES CROSS-CULTURALLY: AVAILABLE DATA
Yearly Hip Fracture Rates Per 100,000 People Age 35 And Older

	Females	Males
USA (Rochester, MN)	319.7	177.0
USA (District of Columbia)		
whites	231.8	82.0
blacks	118.8	109.7
Finland	212.8	136.1
Norway (Oslo)	421.0	230.5
Sweden (Malmo)	237.2	101.4
Holland	187.2	107.9
United Kingdom (Oxford-Dundee)	142.2	69.2
Yugoslavia		
high calcium intake area	43.5	44.5
low calcium intake area	105.3	93.9
Israel (Jerusalem)		
American/European-born	201.8	113.9
Native-born	168.0	107.5
Asian/African-born	141.7	109.2
Hong Kong	87.1	73.0
Singapore (total)	42.1	73.1
Indian	312.9	131.4
Chinese	59.0	106.1
Malay	24.2	35.4
New Zealand		
whites	220.4	98.6
Maori	104.4	84.0
South Africa (Johannesburg)		
whites	256.5	98.8
Bantu	14.0	14.3

(adapted from Riggs and Melton, 1983; 59)

The United States appears to have the highest spinal fracture rate in the world, although a study of Danish women suggests that their vertebral fracture rate now approximates that of women in the United States.[20] Among American women aged 65 and older, 25 to 33 percent have detectable vertebral fractures. By age 80–85 Mayo Clinic researchers Drs. Riggs and Melton report that the majority of Caucasian women have at least one partial deformation in their spine.[21-26]

Although even less data is available on the cross-cultural incidence of osteoporotic wrist and arm fractures, these too appear much more common in the highly technological Westernized countries. For example, the female wrist fracture of Norway and Sweden is some 12 times that of Singapore.[25, 27]

Osteoporosis is on the Rise

It is commonly said that our dramatic increase in osteoporotic fractures is simply due to a longer life expectancy. People in Westernized countries, it is argued, are living longer thus suffering more osteoporotic fractures. This is not accurate. The osteoporosis rate is growing well beyond that which can be explained by population growth alone. As one researcher puts it, "More people are fracturing more bones more often".[28] For example, in Oxford, England the hip fracture rate increased six times between 1938 and 1955 while the population at risk increased only 12 percent. Continuing to grow, the Oxford hip fracture rate was about 75 percent greater in 1983 than it was in the 1954-58 period. In Sweden also there has been a documented increase in fracture incidence in the last decade.[28] The age-adjusted hip fracture rate for the United States Caucasian population also has increased dramatically going from 24.3 fractures per 100,000 in the period 1928-1932 to 114.8 in 1978-1982.[29] All this would suggest that the bones of those living in Westernized countries are growing weaker, and in fact scientists have found this to be true. British researchers recently untombed and analyzed the bone density of 87 females buried between 1792 and 1852. After comparing their findings with bone density measurements of nearly 300 present-day women the researchers found that women living two and three hundred years ago had stronger bones than contemporary women.[30] Going back to the Near Eastern populations of some 12,000 years ago anthropologists report that their bone mass was nearly 20 percent higher than ours today.[31]

❖ OSTEOPOROSIS IS *NOT* JUST A FEMALE DISORDER

In the United States and other Westernized countries, more women have osteoporosis than do men, and osteoporosis is held to be largely a disorder of women. This, however, is not accurate. Looking around the world we see that men are far from immune to excessive bone thinning.

In this country, older men suffer roughly one-sixth the spinal fractures, one-half the hip fractures and many more rib fractures than do elderly women.[21, 32, 33] The osteoporosis pattern in less industrialized countries, however, is strikingly different. In Hong Kong, the hip fracture rate is the same for men and women 55 years old and older, while among the Chinese in Singapore, the rate is even greater for men. Men also are known to suffer more osteoporosis than do women in some parts of Yugoslavia and even among peoples like the Bantu of South Africa who experience very few osteoporotic fractures.[17, 18, 27]

The question of why women in the United States and other westernized countries suffer so much osteoporosis is a fascinating one. As it turns out, social and cultural factors, not genetic factors are responsible for the current osteoporosis epidemic among American women. Let's briefly outline the major factors making osteoporosis a feminist issue in Westernized countries. Many of these factors will be detailed more fully in subsequent chapters.

You can never be too thin.

For decades our culture has let us know that to be thin is attractive and desirable. Embroiled in a "thinness mania" millions of women, young and old, persist in following misguided attempts at attaining and maintaining thinness, often at a terrific cost to their bones. It is virtually impossible to consume the nutrients required for bone maintenance, much less those needed for bone growth, on a low calorie diet. During periods of inadequate nutrient intake, bone is robbed of precious minerals. Undernutrition causes osteoporosis in young and old alike. Additionally, excessive weight loss and extreme reduction of body fat causes a cessation of menstrual periods and associated bone loss.

Females consume fewer nutrients than males.

In the United States young children, girls, adult women and older women are the populations at highest risk of suffering inadequate nutrient intake.[34] A recent government study of mineral consumption, for example, found the diets of teenage girls and adult women low in six minerals (calcium, magnesium, iron, zinc, copper and manganese). The diet of teenage boys, however, was low in only magnesium and copper and adult men were found to have a deficient intake only of copper. The diet of older women was found low in calcium, magnesium, zinc, copper and manganese while their male peers experienced low intakes of only magnesium and copper.[34] A full one-half of all United States women consume less than 1,493 calories a day, a level where it is almost impossible to create meals providing RDA levels of the essential nutrients.[35]

Nice girls don't build muscle mass.

Frequently girls and women are taught that is not proper to exercise heavily enough to build visible and defined muscle mass. Strong muscles are a good indicator of strong bones and it takes strenuous activity to build strong muscles. Also girls and women don't spend as much time outdoors in manual labor or vigorous exercise as do their male counterparts. For example a recent large study found that while half of the male 12th graders exercised regularly, only 17 percent of the girls did so.[36]

Women also undergo much more surgery. One-quarter of all surgical procedures performed in United States hospitals are on female reproductive organs, induced abortions excluded. Many of these cause or contribute to osteoporosis. Let's look at these surgical procedures one by one.

Ovary removal is the fourth or fifth most common surgical procedure performed in the United States. The vast majority of women lose bone rapidly after "castration," as this procedure is referred to in medical texts. In fact, most young women will show beginning signs of osteoporosis four years after ovary removal if hormone replacement is not given.[37] Women who have had their ovaries removed at 30 frequently have been found to have the bones of a 70-year-old by the time they reach 50.[38] Over one half million United States women undergo ovary removal each year.

Hysterectomy, the removal of a woman's uterus, ranks as the second most commonly performed major operative procedure in the United States, second only to Cesarean sections. The United States has the highest hysterectomy rate in the world, and the majority of such operations are performed on women between the ages of 19 and 44.[39] Even though a woman's ovaries remain intact, the removal of her uterus can cause osteoporosis. This is because anywhere between 16 and 57 percent of all women who undergo uterus removal suffer from premature loss of ovarian function with its associated rapid bone loss.[40-43] Given existing trends, 60 percent of all women in this country will have undergone a hysterectomy by age 65 and some 35 to 45 percent of all women will be without a uterus at the age of natural menopause.[7, 42, 44]

Finally, even tubal ligation has been found to cause a lowering of estrogen levels and thus may well be expected to contribute to the development of osteoporosis.[45]

❖ OSTEOPOROSIS IS *NOT* A DISORDER OF JUST THE ELDERLY

Osteoporosis is becoming more common among the young. More and more we are finding that even the young are not free from the specter of osteoporosis. Currently the disease is being rather widely documented among young people. Among the groups most affected are anorexic individuals, training ballet dancers and other athletes who underconsume nutrients trying to remain very slim. Women who suffer from menstrual irregularities, those who have undergone ovary and/or uterus removal and persons on long-term steroid therapy are also affected. Dr. Lazarro, a radiologist at Upstate Medical Center in Syracuse, New York is one of the many clinical practitioners to notice this new trend. He reports they are finding a growing number of young women and even young men with excessively low bone mass.[46]

❖ OSTEOPOROSIS IS *NOT* FAULTY BONE METABOLISM OR SOMETHING THAT "GOES WRONG" WITH OUR BONES

Osteoporosis is really our magical body's intelligent response to long-term imbalances and stressors. While we might tend to think that osteoporosis occurs when something "goes wrong" in the body's automatic pilot responsible for bone maintenance, the truth is quite to the contrary. Osteoporosis is really a long-term negative effect of an essential positive short-term coping mechanism. Without these coping mechanisms the body would have long since fallen into intolerable imbalance and perished.

If we were to divide our body's many systems into givers and takers, bone would be classified as a great giver. To cope with low levels of blood minerals, nutrients are drawn out of the bone. Without adequate calcium, phosphorus, magnesium or sodium, the body cannot survive. The immediate effect of drawing minerals out of the bone is a most positive one. Blood mineral levels are returned to normal and the body is able to continue its functioning. If the minerals are not redeposited into the bone, however, osteoporosis ensues as a long-term negative effect of such repeated, short-term, positive coping processes. The first bones to give up their minerals for use in the blood are those that have a high trabecular content, such as the jaw, wrist and spine. Receding gums are often the first sign of systemic bone loss. The vertebrae and wrist, also high in trabecular bone, fracture earlier in life than does the hip. This is because the hip has more cortical bone, and cortical bone is lost later in life than trabecular bone.

The more we learn about osteoporosis, the more we appreciate its complex and dynamic nature. Far from being a simple disorder of bone thinning among older women, osteoporosis is a very complex disorder increasingly found among a wide range of Westernized populations. It involves not only the thinning of bone, but also a loss in the natural self-repair mechanisms of bone. Cross-cultural data confirms that osteoporosis is a degenerative disease, not a universal artifact of aging or an inevitable outcome of being born female. Osteoporosis is really the end product "disorder" of our body's lifelong attempt to maintain a crucial internal "order." In this light, osteoporosis is seen as a positive, life-supporting, coping mechanism which allows the body to maintain the necessary degree of internal balance under less than ideal, perhaps even life-threatening, circumstances. Even in osteoporosis we see evidence of our magical body's intelligence!

❖ OSTEOPOROSIS DOES *NOT* STAND ALONE

As we have seen above, osteoporosis is not just a dreadful disease that randomly strikes some of us. Also, osteoporosis does not stand alone. It is not an isolated disease process that happens to fully healthy people. Excessive bone thinning and the development of weak bones does not occur without due cause and the due cause of osteoporosis is often associated with other health problems. Lifelong patterns of poor eating, little exercise, smoking, irregular periods, surgeries and medication use, toxic exposure, excessive stress and the like take their toll on the whole body, not just the bones. In fact one study found that women with moderate to severe spinal deformities were more likely to consider themselves limited in their activity by overall poor health rather then by their back problems.[26]

Most recently a ground-breaking four year study of nearly 10,000 older United States women found an increased risk of hip fractures among those who rated their own health as fair to poor and indeed were less fit than others of their age. In practical terms, selected fitness factors were found associated with a greater risk of hip fracture. Interestingly enough these risk factors significantly raised a women's risk of hip fracture regardless of her bone density. These independent fitness risk factors for hip fracture included:

+ Being unable to rise from a chair without using one's arms.
+ Being on one's feet for less than four hours a day.
+ Not walking for exercise as opposed to walking for exercise.
+ Having poor depth perception and/or poor contrast sensitivity.
+ Having a resting heartbeat of 80 or greater beats per minute.[47]

The more closely we look and the more variables we study, the more interesting becomes the osteoporosis story. From the above cited study alone, it is clear that osteoporosis does not stand alone and that bone density is but one risk factor.

❖ PRIMARY OSTEOPOROSIS VS. SECONDARY OSTEOPOROSIS

As we conclude this chapter on redefining osteoporosis it is important to acknowledge the Western medical distinction between "primary" and "secondary" osteoporosis. Primary osteoporosis is held by Western medicine to be osteoporosis of relatively unknown origin that occurs with aging and accelerates at menopause. There is no direct or singular cause for this primary osteoporosis. Secondary osteoporosis, on the other hand, has a direct cause. This type of osteoporosis is secondary to, or caused by, some other event. The table below lists the well recognized direct causes of such secondary osteoporosis. These direct causes of osteoporosis should be ruled out anytime excessive bone loss occurs.

Illustration 2.5
CAUSES OF SECONDARY OSTEOPOROSIS

ENDOCRINE CAUSES

✦ Hyperparathyroidism
✦ Cushing's syndrome
✦ Hypogonadism
✦ Hyperthyroidism
✦ Prolactinoma
✦ Diabetes mellitus
✦ Acromegaly
✦ Pregnancy and lactation

BONE MARROW DISORDERS

✦ Plasma cell dyscrasias
✦ Systemic mastocytosis
✦ Leukemias
✦ Lymphomas
✦ Chronic anemias: sickle cell disease
✦ Lipidoses: Gaucher's disease
✦ Myeloproliferative disorders

CONNECTIVE TISSUE DISORDERS

✦ Osteogenesis imperfecta
✦ Ehlers-Danlos syndrome
✦ Marfan's syndrome
✦ Homocystinuria
✦ Menke's syndrome
✦ Scurvy

DRUG-INDUCED

✦ Corticosteroids
✦ Heparin
✦ Anticonvulsants
✦ Methotrexate, cyclosporin A
✦ GnRH agonist or antagonist therapy
✦ Aluminum-containing antacids

IMMOBILIZATION
RENAL DISEASE

✦ Chronic renal failure
✦ Renal tubular acidosis

NUTRITIONAL AND GASTROINTESTINAL

✦ Malabsorption
✦ Prolonged total parenteral nutrition
✦ Postgastrectomy
✦ Hepatobiliary disease
✦ Chronic hypophosphatemia

MISCELLANEOUS

✦ Familial dysautonomia (Riley-Day disease)
✦ Reflex sympathetic dystrophy

Adapted from Mundy and Martin, 1993

❖ References

1 Slemenda, Charles W., and Conrad C. Johnston, "Epidemiology for Osteoporosis," *Treatment of the Postmenopausal Woman*, ed. Rogerio A. Lobo. (New York: Raven Press, 1994) 161-168.

2 Mazess, R., Personal communication, Continuing Education Course on Osteoporosis: Harvard University (1987).

3 Fujita, T., and M. Fukase, "Comparison of osteoporosis and calcium intake between Japan and the United States," *Proceedings of the Society of Experimental Biology & Medicine* 200.2 (1992): 149-152.

4 Frost, H., "The Pathomechanics of Osteoporosis," *Clin Orthop* 200 (1985): 198-225.

5 Biewener, A.A., "Safety factors in bone strength," *Calcified Tissue International* 53 (1993): S68-74.

6 Heaney, R., "Prevention of Age-Related Osteoporosis in Women," *The Osteoporotic Syndrome: Detection, Prevention, and Treatment*, ed. L. Avioli. (New York: Grune and Stratton, Inc., 1983).

7 Heaney, R., and Barger-Lux, *Calcium and Common Sense*, (New York: Doubleday, 1988).

8 Chappard, D., et al., "Spatial distribution of trabeculae in iliac bone from 145 osteoporotic females," *Maturitas* 10 (1988): 353-360.

9 Becker, R., and G. Selden, *The Body Electric: Electromagnetism and the Foundation of Life*, (New York: William Morrow & Co., 1985).

10 Peck, W., and W. Woods, "The Cells of Bone," *Osteoporosis Etiology, Diagnosis and Management*, ed. B. Riggs, and L. Melton. (New York: Raven Press, 1988) 1-44.

11 Heaney, R., R. Recker, and P. Saville, "Menopausal Changes in Bone Remodeling," *J Lab Clin Med* 92 (1988): 964-970.

12 Parfitt, A.M., "Bone Remodeling and Bone Loss: Understanding The Pathophysiology of Osteoporosis," *Clinical Obstetrics and Gynecology* 30.4 (1987): 789-811.

13 Peck, W., et al., "Research Directions in Osteoporosis," *The American Journal of Medicine* 84 (1988): 275-282.

14 Melton, L., E. Chao, and J. Lane, "Biomechanical Aspects of Fractures," *Osteoporosis Etiology, Diagnosis and Management,* ed. B. Riggs, and L. Melton. (New York: Raven Press, 1988) 111-132.

15 Garn, S., "Nutrition and Bone Loss: Introductory Remarks," *Fed Proc.* Nov/Dec (1967): 1716.

16 Luyken, R., and R. Luyken-Koning, "Studies on the Physiology of Nutrition in Surinam VIII. Metabolism of Calcium," *Trop Geogr Med* 13 (1961): 46-54.

17 Chalmers, J., and K. Ho, "Geographical Variations in Senile Osteoporosis," *Journal of Bone and Joint Surgery* 52B (1970): 667-675.

18 Matkovic, V., et al., "Bone Status and Fracture Rates in Two Regions of Yugoslavia," *The American Journal of Clinical Nutrition* 32 (1979): 540-549.

19 Nordin, B., "International Patterns in Osteoporosis," *Clin Orthopaed* 45 (1966).

20 Jensen, G., et al., "Epidemiology of Postmenopausal Spinal and Long Bone Fractures: A Unifying Approach to Postmenopausal Osteoporosis," *Clinical Orthopaedics and Related Research* 166 (1982): 75-81.

21 Cummings, S., et al., "Epidemiology of Osteoporosis and Osteoporotic Fractures," *Epidemiol Rev* 7 (1985): 178-208.

22 Smith, R., and J. Rizek, "Epidemiological Studies of Osteoporosis in Women of Puerto Rico and Southeastern Michigan With Special Reference to Age, Race, National Origin and to Other Related or Associated Findings," *Clinical Orthopedics and Related Research* 45 (1964): 31.

23 National Institutes of Health, *Osteoporosis: Cause, Treatment, Prevention,* National Institute of Arthritis, Diabetes, and Digestive and Kidney Disease, 1986).

24 Cummings, S., and D. Black, "Should Peri-menopausal Women Be Screened for Osteoporosis?," *Ann Intern Med* 104 (1986): 817-823.

25 Melton, L., "Epidemiology of Fractures," *Osteoporosis Etiology, Diagnosis and Management,* ed. B. Riggs, and L. Melton. (New York: Raven Press, 1988) 133-154.

26 Ettinger, B., et al., "An examination of the association between vertebral deformities, physical disabilities and psychosocial problems," *Maturitas* 10 (1988): 283-296.

27 Melton, L., and B. Riggs, "Epidemiology of Age-related Fractures," *The Osteoporotic Syndrome: Detection, Prevention and Treatment,* ed. L. Avioli. (New York: Grune and Stratton, 1983) 45-72.

28 Johansson, C., et al., "Prevalence of fractures among 10,000 women from the 1900 to 1940 birth cohorts resident in Gothenburg," *Maturitas* 14 (1991): 65-74.

29 Melton, L., W. O'Fallon, and B. Riggs, "Secular Trends in the Incidence of Hip Fractures," *Calcif Tissue Int* 41 (1987): 57-64.

30 Lees, B., et al. 1993. Differences in proximal femur bone density over two centuries. *Lancet* 341:673–675.

31 Eaton, S. Boyd, and Dorothy A. Nelson, "Calcium in evolutionary perspective," *Am J Clin Nutr* 54 (1991): 281S-7S.

32 Seeman, E., et al., "Risk Factors for Spinal Osteoporosis in Men," *Am J Med* 75 (1983): 977-983.

33 Holbrook, T., et al., *The Frequency of Occurrence, Impact and Cost of Selected Musculoskeletal Conditions in the United States*, (Chicago: American Academy of Orthopedic Surgeons, 1984).

34 Pennington, J., et al., "Mineral Content of Food and Total Diets: The Selected Minerals in Foods Survey, 1982 to 1984," *J Am Diet Assoc* 86 (1986): 876-891.

35 Krehl, "Vitamin Supplementation," *The Nutrition Report*. May (1985): 36.

36 Elias, Marilyn, "Fewer teens exercise their workout option," *USA Today* November 8, 1994.

37 Cutler, W., C. Garcia, and D. Edwards, *Menopause: A Guide for Women and the Men Who Love Them*, (New York/London: W. W. Norton & Company, 1983).

38 Richelson, L., et al., "Relative Contributions of Aging and Estrogen Deficiency to Postmenopausal Bone Loss," *N Engl J Med* 311 (1984): 1273-1275.

39 Polister, and Cunico, "Socio-economic Factbook for Surgery," *American College of Surgeons* (1988).

40 Cutler, W., *Hysterectomy: Before & After*, (New York: Harper & Row, 1988).

41 Siddle, N., P. Sarrel, and M. Whitehead, "The Effect of Hysterectomy on the Age at Ovarian Failure: Identification of a Subgroup of Women With Premature Loss of Ovarian Function and Literature Review," *Fertil Steril* 47.1 (1987): 94-100.

42 Garcia, C., and W.B. Cutler, "Preservation of the Ovary: A Reevaluation," *Fertil Steril* 42.4 (1984): 510-514.

43 Ranney, B., and S. Abu-Ghazaleth, "The Future Function and Control of Ovarian Tissue Which is Retained in Vivo During Hysterectomy," *Am J Obstet Gynecol* 128 (1977): 626-634.

44 Shainwald, Sybil, "A Legal Response to Hysterectomy Abuse," *The Network News* May/June (1985): 6.

45 Cattanach, J., "Oestrogen Deficiency After Tubal Ligation," *Lancet* (1985): 847-849.

46 Lazarro, Juan Carlos, "Personal Communication," Upstate Medical Center, Radiology Department - Syracuse, NY, 1994).

47 Cummings, Steven, et al., "Risk Factors For Hip Fracture In White Women," *The New England Journal Of Medicine* 332.12 (1995): 767-774.

PART TWO

❖ Rethinking the Causes of Osteoporosis

3
....

It's Not Just Calcium and Estrogen: Rethinking the Cause of Osteoporosis

❖ OSTEOPOROSIS IS *NOT* CAUSED SIMPLY BY LOW CALCIUM INTAKE

*W*e have all heard and read that osteoporosis is caused by low calcium intake. This, in fact, has been the opinion of Western researchers for decades, and was reaffirmed by the National Institutes of Health (NIH) Consensus Development Conference on Osteoporosis.[1] Because bone is composed largely of calcium, it might appear logical to link calcium intake with bone health. A true correlation between calcium intake and osteoporosis, however, is more difficult to establish than it appears. *Even a glance at the cross-cultural data shows that most areas of the world have lower calcium intakes* *than we do, and lower rates of osteoporosis.* In less developed countries fewer dairy products are consumed and less total calcium ingested yet osteoporosis rates are much lower than in Western countries.[2]

For example, daily calcium intake among the Bantu is estimated to range from 175 to 476 mg,[3,4] yet they rarely experience osteoporosis. In Japan calcium intakes have been traditionally low with an average daily consumption of 300 mg in 1952. Slowly this has increased to reach an average daily intake of 540 mg in 1989. Yet osteoporosis is much less common in Japan than in the United States. The early postmenopausal spinal fractures so common in the United States are almost unheard of in Japan, and overall their spinal fracture rate is one-half that of the United States. Equally surprising, the Japanese hip fracture rate is two-and-a-half times less than that of the United States.[5] All this is true even though the Japanese have one of the longest lifespans of any population. This defies the conclusion that osteoporosis is a normal consequence of aging.[5, 6] Similarly, the Chinese consume only one-half the calcium Americans do, yet they experience very little osteoporosis even though their average life expectancy is 70 years. Gambian women consume about one-half the calcium we do, yet even as they age few osteoporotic fractures are reported.[7]

Other studies report that children in Ceylon and Surinam maintain adequate growth and a positive calcium balance on intakes of about 200 mg calcium per day.[8] Most strikingly, no difference in skeletal development was found in groups of Surinam children consuming higher amounts of calcium than in groups consuming the more typical low calcium diet.[9] A study of Peruvian inmates found considerable variation in the amount of calcium needed to produce a positive calcium balance. Half of the men studied needed less than 200 mg per day, while others needed more. These researchers concluded, "The minimum calcium requirement of adult males is probably so low that deficiency is unlikely in most natural diets".[10, 11] Moving from single small studies to a much larger scale, we find the work of anthropologist Stanley Garn who measured bone loss over a period of 50 years on large numbers of individuals in both North and Central America. His comprehensive, long-term studies also failed to find a link between calcium intake and bone loss.[12, 13] How do we reconcile these cross-cultural findings with the growing body of current United States data suggesting a strong link between calcium intake and osteoporosis?

All researchers agree that adequate calcium is absolutely essential for development and maintenance of bone health. The question, however, is just what comprises an adequate calcium intake. Cross-cultural analysis indicates that there is no one standard ideal calcium intake, neither is high calcium intake necessary. The anthropological data suggests that adequate calcium can vary from culture to culture. For example, a recent study of elderly Japanese women found that among the normal non-osteoporotic women a positive calcium balance was maintained on only 550 mg of calcium daily and the osteoporotic aged needed 648 mg a day. In the United States, on the other hand, 1,241 mg calcium were found necessary to maintain calcium balance in normal perimenopausal women and this need is documented to increase with age. Nearly one-quarter of all American post-menopausal women would still be in negative calcium balance with a calcium intake of 1500 mg a day.[14, 15] The adequate level for any given population, as we shall see, varies based on a number of other coexisting factors. These include: intake of other bone building nutrients; consumption of potentially bone damaging substances like excess protein, salt, fat and sugar; the use of some drugs, alcohol and tobacco; the level of physical activity; exposure to sunlight; environmental toxins and stress; ovary and uterus removal; and many other factors that limit endocrine gland functioning.

As much as Western medicine would like to locate a single, simple cause of osteoporosis, the cross-cultural data does not support the notion that low calcium intake *per se* is the cause of osteoporosis. Calcium is important to bone health, but osteoporosis cannot be reduced to low calcium intake either here or abroad. Why we in this country need such high calcium intakes to build and maintain bone health is an interesting question to be explored in the next chapters.

❖ OSTEOPOROSIS IS *NOT* CAUSED ONLY BY THE LOWERING OF ESTROGEN LEVELS AT MENOPAUSE

In the late 1940s, German researchers noted that post-menopausal women and women who had undergone ovary removal suffered a greater incidence of osteoporosis than menstruating women. Administering estrogen hormones seemed to reduce the problem, thus they concluded that osteoporosis was caused by estrogen deficiency.[16] Over time this theory has come to gain wide acceptance in Western medicine and in 1984 the N.I.H. Consensus Development Conference on Osteoporosis concluded that menopausal estrogen deficiency was one of the two probable causes of osteoporosis; calcium deficiency was the other.[1] At menopause, it is said, women suffer "ovarian failure" and as a result the female body becomes estrogen deficient, which, in turn, leads to excessive bone loss.

The idea that a natural lowering of estrogen at menopause causes osteoporosis is worthy of further analysis. Such a proposal suggests that nature made a mistake in her design of female physiology, and that women should have been provided with lifelong high estrogen levels. On the other hand, a broader anthropological perspective leads us to consider the idea that a woman's estrogen production is gauged by her body's needs. As such, the normal universal decrease in estrogen production after a woman's reproductive years would be of survival benefit and not prove a detriment to her overall health. In fact, from this wider perspective we see that less estrogen is produced because less is needed. After childbearing years, the main function of estrogen, which is to allow and regulate reproduction, is no longer necessary or beneficial. Furthermore, prolonged exposure to high levels of estrogen is actually harmful, as we shall detail in Chapter 17.

Is this natural menopausal reduction in ovarian estrogen the cause of osteoporosis? Again, taking a comparative, cross-cultural perspective we see that the answer quite simply is *no*. In the first place, if the universally experienced lowering of estrogen levels at menopause *per se* did cause osteoporosis, all women around the world would develop osteoporosis. This does not occur. Looking around the world we find that postmenopausal women do not always, or even generally, suffer osteoporosis as found in the Western countries. Cross-culturally, the normal decrease in estrogen production at menopause is not necessarily associated with the development of osteoporosis. Furthermore, in various cultures, postmenopausal women have been found to have lower estrogen levels than women in this country yet they experience much less osteoporosis. This is true for the Japanese as well as the Mayan Indians.[5] Even in the United States, where osteoporosis is common, many older women remain free from the disorder. In addition, the higher male and lower female osteoporosis rates found in some cultures do not support the notion that excessive bone loss is due to declining ovarian estrogen production. Adding another dimension, we find that vegetarian women have lower serum estrogen levels, yet higher bone density than their meat-eating peers.[17, 18]

Recent medical research also supports the argument that osteoporosis cannot simply be attributed to postmenopausal "estrogen deficiency." If osteoporosis is due to estrogen deficiency, then we would expect to find lower estrogen levels in women with osteoporosis than in women without the disorder, but sex hormone levels were found to be similar in postmenopausal women both with and without osteoporosis.[19, 20]

The link between menopause and osteoporosis was also questioned by Mayo Clinic researchers in 1985. Setting aside the old assumption that osteoporosis began at menopause, they asked the question, "Just when, in fact, did excessive bone loss begin?" In response to this new question they uncovered the fact that one half the total vertebral bone loss a woman in this country will experience during her lifetime occurs *before* she undergoes menopause.[19] Other studies have since supported this finding.[21]

Finally it is noteworthy that while some may report a significant decrease in bone mass at menopause, other studies failed to find this association. For example, a North Carolina study of 217 women aged 40 to 55 found no significant difference in spine or hip density between pre- and perimenopausal women and their postmenopausal counterparts.[22] Research at the USDA Human Nutrition Research Center on Aging on 288 women aged 41 to 71 also failed to detect any accelerated rate of bone loss in the hip or wrist among women close to menopause. Neither did they find any significant adjusted change in bone mineral density in the group of women as a whole.[23] Similarly a Swedish study of women aged 35 to 80 reported a continuous aging decrease in bone mineral after age 35 with no clear acceleration of bone loss noted around the time of menopause.[24] Personally I suspect this may be the case for a good number of healthy women around the world living wholesome lifestyles who have not had any of their sex organs removed. Keep in mind that osteoporosis authority Dr. Robert Heaney hypothesizes that only 10 to 15 percent of women's skeletal mass is affected by estrogen.[25]

While estrogen plays an important and complex role in bone health maintenance, osteoporosis cannot simply be attributed to lower estrogen levels. Numerous dietary, lifestyle and endocrine factors contribute to the development of excessive bone loss; osteoporosis is not simply produced by the lack of one single hormone.

❖ GOING BEYOND CALCIUM AND ESTROGEN

Osteoporosis is a very complicated problem which Western medicine has tried to make very simple. It is not caused by low calcium levels *per se,* even though calcium intake may be critical if other nutrients are low and there are other calcium depleting factors at play. Neither does the natural lowering of estrogen levels at menopause by itself cause osteoporosis.

It is important we resist these superficial explanations as to the causes of osteoporosis for several reasons. First, we simply cannot successfully prevent such a complicated disorder without understanding it fully. Secondly, in settling for superficial explanations of the cause of osteoporosis we fail to appreciate both the complexity and perfection of nature's design. Nature did not make a mistake in gradually ceasing to produce ovarian estrogen after the reproductive years, by giving women smaller bones, by limiting calcium absorption with age, or even by allowing for bones to thin.

On the contrary, osteoporosis begins as a very positive survival strategy, a strategy which draws minerals from the bones into the blood so that the body can continue to survive under less than ideal circumstances. Nature provides us with the capacity for accumulating tremendous bone mineral reserves so that we would have life-long healthy bones as well as a constant source of minerals for transfer to the blood in times of need. Unfortunately, our lifestyles do not enable us to return these essential minerals to our bones. Our unhealthy habits deplete our bones of their precious stores of life-supporting minerals. The price we pay for these excesses is osteoporosis.

❖ RETHINKING THE CAUSE OF OSTEOPOROSIS

Just as a myriad of factors work to maintain bone, so many factors also contribute to bone loss. From the broader anthropological perspective, osteoporosis occurs only when the whole series of bone-building forces are overpowered by a series of bone-depleting factors.

Bone-Building vs. Bone-Thinning Factors

The bone-building forces include adequate quantities of all essential nutrients, healthy and well balanced endocrine gland functioning, appropriate levels of exercise and activity and a well-balanced body chemistry. The bone robbers are many. As of today dozens of factors are known to contribute to excessive bone thinning. Some of these bone-burdening factors are illustrated on page 230. Keep in mind, however,

Illustration 3.1

BONE-BUILDING FACTORS VS. BONE-THINNING FACTORS

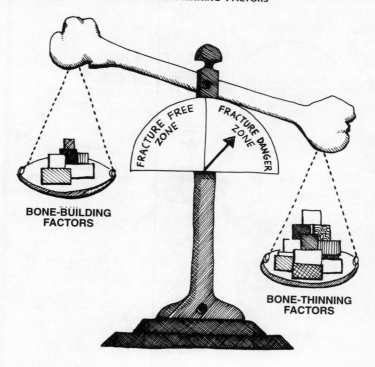

that this list grows almost daily as we expand our understanding about bone and its dynamic relationships with the rest of the body and the surrounding environment.

The importance of any given bone breakdown factor varies from culture to culture, as well as from individual to individual. Each culture and each individual has its own profile of bone-depleting factors. No matter what the individual bone-depleting factors are, however, osteoporosis only occurs when the total bone breakdown forces overpower the total bone-building forces.

Illustration 3.2

FACTORS FAVORING OSTEOPOROSIS DEVELOPMENT

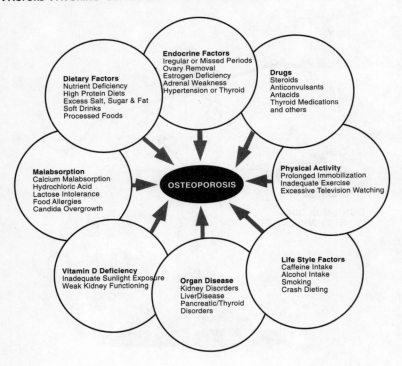

❖ THE TOTAL BODY BURDEN CONCEPT

The first key concept for our new understanding of osteo-porosis is that of a balance between bone-building and bone depleting forces. The second key concept is that of the cumu-lative nature of bone-depleting factors. Looking at the illus-tration on page 230 you can see that each bone-depleting factor is another straw on the camel's back. Adding one drain on bone integrity to the next, we pile straw upon straw. Eventually our bones become weak, fragile and susceptible to fracture, breaking the camel's back and quite literally our own back as well.

The "Total Body Burden" concept illustrates the true complex nature of this disorder. Reviewing it we realize why it is simplistic to suggest that osteoporosis is due simply to low calcium intakes or lower estrogen levels. It also sheds light on the question of why one two-pack-a-day smoker gets osteoporosis and another does not, or why some women undergoing youthful ovary removal suffer early fractures while others remain fracture-free. For one individual a high caffeine intake on top of all her/his other bone-depleting factors might represent the last straw dropping their bone mass into the fracture danger zone. Another person may be able to maintain adequate bone density and integrity in the face of high caffeine use or even after ovary removal. Each individual's total body burden of bone-depleting factors is the ultimate issue of concern.

The "Total Body Burden" concept also illustrates why any step you take to improve your bone health is useful. You might choose to start by reducing your sugar or meat intake, adding just a one mile walk daily or by beginning an individualized supplement program. Each step you take will decrease your total load and give the body a little more opportunity to restore its all important internal balance. Chapter 10 presents a step-by-step program for building and rebuilding bone health.

❖ ANCIENT INSIGHTS: TRADITIONAL CHINESE MEDICINE AND AYURVEDIC VIEWS ON OSTEOPOROSIS

While the total load concept and the idea of collective imbalance leading to disease are somewhat new ideas to Western medicine, they have long been the central premises of Eastern medicine. For example, in both Traditional Chinese Medicine (TCM) and the ancient medical science of India known as Ayurveda, perfect health is said to lie in perfect balance and long-standing imbalances are the cause of all disease, including poor bone health. Their theories are both fascinating and profound and this traditional approach has yielded lifelong strong bones for those who follow both TCM and Ayurveda. In Part 3 we will incorporate some of their approaches and therapies into the Better Bones Program.

In both TCM and Ayurveda the central focus is on non-material concerns like the flow of vital energy and internal balance, rather than on material concerns such as this or that nutrient or hormone. Osteoporosis in both systems is seen as the result of long-term imbalances and energy depletion.

In Traditional Chinese Medicine the kidney and its energy are responsible for the utilization of minerals and the associated health of bone. The kidney is also the organ system where one's vital energy is stored and depletion of this energy leads to aging and general debilitation, as well as to weakened bones. As such TCM stresses lifestyle habits and herbal therapies to tonify and nourish the kidneys, especially as one ages. Around 45 or 50 years of age it is common for the Chinese to begin herbal therapy aimed at enriching and rejuvenating their kidney energy. Interestingly enough, within this medical system menopause is seen not as "ovarian failure" but rather as a very positive mechanism aimed at preserving a woman's vital kidney energy. As Honora Lee Wolfe explains, "From the Chinese medical point of view, menopause is an intelligent homeostasis mechanism. Menopause brings an end of the unnecessary loss of blood each month via the menses. Holding on to this blood is a way of slowing the aging process."[26, 27]

Ayurveda also holds that the flow of energy and information and the maintenance of internal balance are central to good health. In Ayurveda a major focus is placed on the three basic elements or operating principles which manifest in the human body and in the entire universe for that matter. The three operating principles in Ayurveda are an amalgamation of the five basic elements or humors recognized as ether (space), air, fire, water and earth. In Ayurveda the three basic elements which govern all biological, psychological and physiological functions are known as Vata, Pitta and Kapha. Each person, it is held, is born with a specific balance of these three elements. Maintenance of this balance provides for good health; imbalance creates distress and, if prolonged, disease arises.

Vata is the element of space and air and it controls movement; it is cold and dry. Pitta is the element of fire and water and it controls metabolism; it is hot. Kapha is the element of water and earth; it controls structure and suggests solidity and stability. In Ayurveda one first determines his or her constitution type and through diet, lifestyle, herbal therapy and detoxification techniques attempts to maintain a state of internal balance. With age, however, the Vata element naturally tends to increase, leading among other things to increased coldness, dryness and frailty. Osteoporosis from this perspective is associated with excesses and imbalances in the Vata element. With age a Vata imbalance can lead to the development of dry, frail and weak bones. The prevention of osteoporosis then involves balancing or "pacifying" the Vata element. Among the many Vata-pacifying actions are regularity of lifestyle, such as going to bed regularly at 10 and rising at 6; eating meals at regular times; daily meditation and relaxation. Adequate rest, nourishing hot food, avoidance of cold temperatures, full-body hot sesame oil massages to reduce dryness, and the avoidance of stimulants such as coffee and excess sugar are also recommended. Carrot juice and ghee (clarified butter) in particular are considered beneficial to bones as are various herbal preparations.[28, 29]

Those interested in more information on either Ayurveda or Traditional Chinese Medicine can refer to Appendix 5. These medical systems offer simple self-help techniques as well as sophisticated, individualized therapeutic programs to enhance bone health at any age.

❖ References

1 NIH, "Consensus Development Conference on Osteoporosis," (Washington, D.C.: National Institute on Aging, 1984).

2 Melton, L., and B. Riggs, "Epidemiology of Age-Related Fractures," *The Osteoporotic Syndrome: Detection, Prevention and Treatment* ed. L. Avioli. (New York: Grune and Stratton, 1983) 45-72.

3 Walker, A., "The Human Requirement of Calcium: Should Low Intakes Be Supplemented?" 25 (1972): 518-530.

4 Davidson, S., *Human Nutrition and Dietetics*, 7th ed. (New York: Churchill Livingstone, 1979) 90-98.

5 Fujita, T., and M. Fukase, "Comparison of osteoporosis and calcium intake between Japan and the United States," *Proceedings of the Society for Experimental Biology & Medicine* 200.2 (1992): 149-152.

6 Hirota, Takako, et al., "Effect of diet and lifestyle on bone mass in Asian young women," *Am J Clin Nutr* 55 (1992): 1168-73.

7 Junshi, Chen, T. Colin Campbell, et al, *Diet, Lifestyle and Mortality in China: A Study of the Characteristics of 65 Chinese Counties,* (Oxford: Oxford University Press, 1990).

8 Ballentine, R., *Diet and Nutrition,* (Honesdale, Pennsylvania: Himalayan International Institute, 1978).

9 Luyken, R., and F. Luyken-Koning, "Studies on the Physiology of Nutrition in Surinam VIII. Metabolism of Calcium,"*Trop Geogr Med* 13 (1961): 46-54.

10 Hegsted, D., I. Moscoso, and C. Collazos, "A Study of the Minimum Calcium Requirements of Adult Men," 46 (1952): 181-201.

11 Hegsted, D., "Mineral Intake and Bone Loss," *Fed Proceedings* Nov/Dec (1967): 1747-1763.

12 Garn, S., "Nutrition and Bone Loss: Introductory Remarks," *Fed Proc.* Nov/Dec (1967): 1716.

13 Garn, S., *The Earlier Gain and Later Loss of Cortical Bone in Nutritional Perspective,* (Springfield: Charles O. Thomas, 1970).

14 Heaney, R., R. Recker, and P. Saville, "Calcium Balance and Calcium Requirements in Middle-aged Women," *Am J Clin Nutr* 30 (1977): 1603-1611.

15 Heaney, R., and R. Recker, "Distribution of Calcium Absorption in Middle-aged Women," *Am J Clin Nutr* 43 (1986): 299-305.

16 Albright, F., and E. Reinfenstein Jr., *The Parathyroid Glands and Metabolic Bone Disease,* (Baltimore: Williams & Wilkins, 1948).

17 Albanese, Anthony A., "Diet and Bone Fractures," *The Nutrition Report* November 1986: 84-85.

18 Anderson B, J., and F. Tylavsky, *Diet and Osteopenia in Elderly Caucasian Women,* , ed. C. Christiansen, and C. Arnaud. Proceedings of the Copenhagen International Symposium on Osteoporosis, 1984: 299-304.

19 Riggs, B., and L. Melton, "Involutional Osteoporosis," *New England Journal of Medicine* 26 (1986): 1676-1686.

20 Taelman, P., et al., "Persistence of increased bone resorption and possible role of dehydroepiandrosterone as a bone metabolism determinant in osteoporotic women in late post-menopause," *Maturitas* 11 (1989): 65-73.

21 Buchanan, J.R., et al., "Early vertebral trabecular bone loss in normal premenopausal women," *J Bone Miner Res* 3.5 (1988): 583-587.

22 Carter, M.D., et al., "Bone mineral content at three sites in normal perimenopausal women," *Clin Orthop* 266 (1991): 295-300.

23 Harris, S., and B. Dawson-Highes, "Rates of change in bone mineral density of the spine, heel, femoral neck and radius in healthy postmenopausal women," *Bone Miner* 17.1 (1992): 87-95.

24 Hansson, Tommy, and B. Roos, "Age changes in the bone mineral of the lumbar spine in normal women," *Calcif Tissue Int.* 38 (1986): 249-251.

25 Heaney, R.P., "Estrogen-calcium interactions in the postmenopause: a quantitative description," *Bone Miner* 11 (1990): 67-84.

26 Wolfe, Honora Lee, "Traditional Chinese Medicine," *A Friend Indeed* No.6 (1993): 1.

27 Buenaventura, Elisa, L.Ac., Fairfield, IA, Personal communication, (1995).

28 Cravatta, Mary Jo, D.C., San Raphael, CA. Personal Communication, (1995).

29 Chopra, Deepak, *Perfect Health*, first ed. (New York: Harmony Books, 1990).

Chapter 4

Bone-Robbing Nutrient Inadequacies

❖ CALCIUM IS IMPORTANT TO BONE HEALTH, BUT IT DOES NOT STAND ALONE

*I*t is common knowledge that calcium is essential for bone health, and we have all heard about the importance of consuming adequate calcium. What we are generally not told, however, is that at least 17 other nutrients are also essential for bone health. If our diets are low in any of these nutrients our bones suffer.

THE 18 NUTRIENTS ESSENTIAL FOR BONE HEALTH

Minerals: Calcium, Phosphorus, Magnesium, Zinc, Manganese, Copper, Boron, Silica, Fluoride
Vitamins: D, C, A, B_6, B_{12}, K, Folic Acid
Essential Fatty Acids
Protein

❖ Startling Facts About the Standard American Diet (SAD)

Despite our wealth and prominence as a nation, our nutrient intake is largely inadequate. Most of us do not consume adequate quantities of many essential nutrients. For example, a recent United States Department of Agriculture (USDA) survey studied the three day food intake of 21,500 people. Not a single person consumed 100 percent of the Recommended Daily Allowance (RDA) for the 10 nutrients included in that survey.[1] The RDAs are best understood as the minimal recommended values needed to prevent deficiency diseases in healthy people. For a further discussion of the RDAs as opposed to optimum health-promoting intakes, see Appendix 1.

In particular we frequently underconsume many, if not most of the 18 key bone building nutrients. Illustrated on the next page is the average nutrient intake of several important bone building nutrients of women in the United States aged 14 to 65. Note that many women have a markedly deficient intake of several key nutrients.

Many males in America also underconsume several key nutrients, and looking at our total population as a whole we see an undeniable tendency toward nutrient inadequacy.

Illustration 4.1

**AVERAGE DIETARY INTAKE OF SELECTED
NUTRIENTS FOR AMERICAN WOMEN AGES 14-65[2-9]**

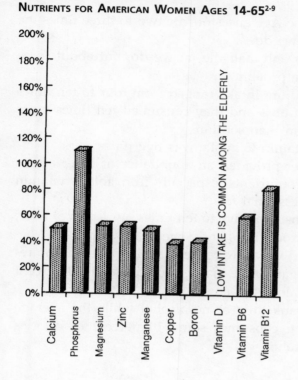

❖ THE STANDARD DIET VS. OUR ANCESTRAL DIET

So accustomed are we to today's standard way of eating that we rarely pause to consider what things were like in the past. What was our nutrient intake like for the first million or so years of human existence?

As anthropologists look back to the Stone Age and reconstruct the diet of modern human ancestors they find patterns of nutrient intake strikingly different from ours.

Our Ancestral Diet Compared to the Standard American Diet[10, 11]

+ Our Stone Age ancestors ate two to three times the calcium we do.
+ They ate only half the fat we do, but about three times the protein.
+ Their sodium intake ranged from four to ten times less than ours and they consumed ten times more potassium than sodium.
+ Their vitamin C intake was five times ours.
+ Their diet provided an abundance of other essential micronutrients, especially iron, folate, vitamin B_{12} and essential fats.
+ They consumed five to ten times our levels of fiber, mostly from fruits and vegetables.
+ They had very few concentrated sweets and no refined sugar, while many of us consume 20 percent of our calories as sugar.
+ They drank little or no alcohol while the average American consumes some 10 percent of calories from alcohol.

❖ THE 18 NUTRIENTS ESSENTIAL FOR HEALTHY BONES

There are at least 18 key bone-building nutrients essential for optimum bone health. Let's look at them one by one. What role do they play in bone health? How much of each nutrient should we be getting? What are the best food sources of these bone builders?

Remember, if you do not consume adequate amounts of

81

. . . .
B o n e - R o b b i n g   N u t r i e n t   I n a d e q u a c i e s

every one of these nutrients, you are not playing the bone building game with a full deck.

Calcium

Role in Bone Health:

The body contains more calcium than any other mineral. Approximately two percent of an adult's body weight is calcium and the vast majority of the body's calcium is found in the bones and teeth. Bone is made of a mineral compound embedded in a living protein matrix. This mineral compound is a crystalline structure, called hydroxyapatite, formed of calcium and phosphorus. Calcium, and the hydroxyapatite crystal it forms with phosphorus, is essential to bone development and maintenance, giving it strength and rigidity. The loss of calcium from bone or demineralization leads to the development of thin, porous bones.

Numerous, but not all, studies on those consuming the standard American diet report low calcium intake to be associated with lower bone density and an increased risk of fracture at all ages. Higher calcium intakes within our population are correlated with greater bone mineral content and less fracture. Overall, experiments providing calcium supplements show a consistent, if modest, reduction in bone loss in postmenopausal women. Numerous studies also document the ability of calcium supplementation to significantly reduce spine and hip fractures among the osteoporotic aged.[12-15] More about these studies in Chapter 10.

Recommended Intake:

The RDA for calcium is summarized below.[16]

Illustration 4.2
RDA FOR CALCIUM, 1989

POPULATION	CALCIUM RDA
Children aged 1-10	800 mg
Adolescents aged 11-24	1200 mg
Adults aged 25 and up	800 mg
Pregnant and lactating women	1200 mg

However, recent guidelines from the National Institutes of Health (NIH) go further. They suggest:

Illustration 4.3
NIH Calcium Intake Recommendations

POPULATION	NIH RECOMMENDATION
Birth to 6 months	400 mg
6 months to 12 months	600 mg
Children aged 1-5 years	800 mg
Children aged 6-10 years	800 to 1200 mg
Adolescents and young adults	1200 to 1500 mg
Pregnant or lactating women	1200 mg
Premenopausal women ages 25-50	1000 mg
Postmenopausal women not on estrogen drugs	1500 mg
Postmenopausal women on estrogen drugs	1000 mg
All women and men over 65 years of age	1500 mg

NIH Consensus Statement - Optimal Calcium Intake, 1994

In the United States some 80 percent of our calcium comes from dairy sources. In many other parts of the world most dietary calcium comes from vegetable sources. Appendix 3 provides a complete list of wholesome food sources of calcium.

Average Intake:

✦ All Americans, except infants and young men, consume much less than what is recommended by our RDA. The Second National Health and Nutrition Examination found 42 percent of our total population, particularly girls and females older than 11 years of age, consume less than 70 percent of the RDA for calcium.

✦ During the years of peak bone mass formation calcium intake is low. The General Mills Dietary Intake Study found 95 percent of the 11- to 18-year-old girls and 79 percent of the 11- to 18-year-old boys consumed less than the RDA for calcium. Also, more than 66 percent of American women aged 18 to 34 fail to consume even the RDA for calcium.

✦ Postmenopausal women average 511 mg of calcium per day, barely one-third of the 1500 mg recommended by the National Institutes of Health

✦ One out of four women consumes less than 300 mg of calcium on a typical day. Thirty percent of all school children consume less than two-thirds the RDA.

References: [2, 12, 17]

Phosphorus

Role in Bone Health:

Phosphorus is the second most abundant mineral in the body; fully one-fourth of all the mineral material in the body is phosphorus. Phosphorus plays a role in almost all chemical reactions within the body and thus is important to every cell. It is essential for a myriad of biochemical processes including cell growth and repair; energy production; heart contraction; nerve and muscle activity; calcium, glucose, fat and starch metabolism; and pH buffering. Of special interest to us is the fact that phosphorus combines with calcium to form a mineral salt which gives strength and structure to the bones and teeth. Eighty percent of our total body phosphorus is found in the bones and teeth.

While phosphorus is essential for bone health, in excess it is detrimental. Within both bone and blood, phosphorus works in delicate balance with calcium. Too little or too much phosphorus in relation to calcium can be a problem for bone.

Recommended Intake:

The current RDA for phosphorus has been matched to that of calcium. Large amounts of phosphorus are found in meat and meat products, soft drinks, processed foods such as baked goods and cheeses to which phosphorus compounds have been added.

Average Intake:

The average American actually consumes much more phosphorus than calcium. While the recommended calcium to phosphorus ratio is 1 to 1, in the United States consumption ranges from one part calcium to two, three or even four parts or more phosphorus due to diets high in meat, soft drinks and processed foods. This high phosphorus-to-calcium ratio can be detrimental to bone.[18, 19]

Magnesium

Role in Bone Health:

Magnesium participates in an astonishing variety of bio-chemical reactions and thus it should not come as a surprise that it is essential for healthy bones and teeth. Adequate magnesium is required for absorption and metabolism of calcium. Magnesium stimulates the thyroid's production of calcitonin, a bone preserving hormone. It also regulates parathyroid hormone, a bone breakdown force. Magnesium is also necessary for the conversion of vitamin D into its active form and a deficiency of magnesium can produce a syndrome known as "vitamin D resistance."[20] Alkaline phosphate, an enzyme required for forming new calcium crystals, also requires magnesium for its activation.[21] Overall, magnesium assures the strength and firmness of the bone and makes the teeth harder, and low magnesium levels have been correlated with abnormal bone crystal formation. Even mild magnesium deficiency has been reported to be a leading risk factor for osteoporosis.[21-24]

Sixty percent of our total body magnesium is found in the bones. As with calcium, the bones provide a reservoir of magnesium guaranteeing adequate supplies of this important mineral for transfer into the blood in times of need. When we do not consume enough magnesium, the magnesium stored in our bones is drawn out for use in the blood. Long-term loss of magnesium from the bone causes disturbances in bone building and bone repair and low magnesium intake is associated with poor bone health. Recent studies, for example, found magnesium intake and magnesium red blood levels to be significantly lower among women with osteoporosis than among similar women without osteoporosis. Equally, trabecular bone magnesium content was found to be lower than normal in women with osteoporosis. In one study 16 of the 19 women with osteoporosis studied were found to have low whole body content and low bone concentration of magnesium. All 16 of these women with low magnesium had abnormal crystal formation.[22, 23, 25, 26]

Dietary intake of magnesium has been found to be a significant predicator of bone mineral content for both pre- and postmenopausal women. In 595 Caucasian women aged 23-75 forearm mineral bone density was positively correlated with dietary magnesium intake. Increased magnesium consumption led to stronger bones.[27]

Furthering this concept, magnesium supplementation has been shown effective in rebuilding bone mass. A study at Tel Aviv University's Sackler School of Medicine, for example, found that almost two-thirds of the 31 women who took 250 to 750 mgs of magnesium daily for two years showed a bone density increase of one to eight percent while similar women not supplementing with magnesium lost between one and three percent bone during this same period.[28] Also, U.S. researcher Guy Abraham, M.D. of Torrance, California has found magnesium to greatly enhance bone density of postmenopausal women, especially when used in conjunction with a full range of bone-building nutrients. His research is discussed further in Chapter 10.

Often overlooked is the fact that magnesium and calcium function together so that a deficiency of one markedly affects the metabolism of the other. Increasing calcium supplemen-

. . . . *87*

Bone-Robbing Nutrient Inadequacies

tation without increasing magnesium supplementation can actually increase magnesium losses. Furthermore, the use of calcium supplementation in the face of a magnesium deficiency can lead to a depositing of calcium in the soft tissue such as the joints promoting arthritis, or in kidney, contributing to kidney stones. Asthma is also worsened by imbalanced calcium and magnesium intake.[25] [29, 30]

Recommended Intake:

The 1989 revised RDA for magnesium has been lowered to 280 mg per day for adult females (from 300 mg) and kept at 350 mg for adult males.[16] Recent large scale balance studies, however, indicate that we might actually need about 450 mg of magnesium per day. Magnesium is a very important nutrient, being an essential co-factor in 80 percent of all cellular enzymes. Why authorities would lower the magnesium RDA for women in the face of declining intakes and increased nutrient need is unclear. I believe this decision was unwise.

Calcium and magnesium are closely linked and when supplemented, magnesium should be taken along with calcium to reach at least the daily recommended intake for magnesium as well as for calcium. Those suffering from kidney impairment, however, should use calcium and magnesium supplementation only under medical supervision.

While magnesium is high in many whole grains and vegetables, much of it is lost in food processing. Appendix 3 lists wholesome food sources of magnesium.

Average Intake:

✦ Numerous studies show our intake of magnesium to be clearly inadequate, largely due to our high consumption of processed, fast and sugared foods.

Not only do these foods contain little magnesium, but they cause magnesium wasting, and their consumption increases the need for magnesium.[2, 22, 31]

✦ Except for children, females and males of all ages do not receive adequate magnesium, the average intake being 60 to 76 percent the RDA. 40 percent of the general population and 50 percent of all adolescents consume less than two-thirds of the RDA. As a subgroup women consume much less magnesium that the population at large.[31-34]

Fluoride

Role in Bone Health:

Fluoride is another mineral important for healthy bones and teeth. Through the action of fluoride, bone and teeth become harder, larger, more uniform and display greater resistance to decay and demineralization. The intake of excessive fluoride, however, be it from fluoridated water or medication, can have adverse effects, including the weakening of bone. Some studies suggest that high fluoride intake actually increases the risk of osteoporotic fractures.[35, 36, 38] Some scientists suggest that artificial fluoridation even in low amounts increases the risk of hip fractures.[36]

As currently used, fluoride as a treatment for osteoporosis has largely lost favor. A recent Mayo Clinic study concluded that fluoride should not be used to treat osteoporosis as the new bone growth stimulated by fluoride treatment is structurally unsound and fluoride treatment actually leads to a threefold increase in the number of hip fractures.[38]

Recommended Intake:

Fluoride was recently added to the RDA tables. The RDA for adults was set at 1.5 to 4.0 mg. Fluoride is found in small amounts in many foods. Fish, oysters, tea, milk and eggs are usually fair sources of fluoride as are lettuce, cabbage, radishes, lentils, whole wheat, oats and other foods. Some public water supplies contain fluoride. There is, however, a great controversy surrounding the use of fluoridated water and recently such fluoride use has been linked to increased hip fractures and bone cancer.[36, 39]

Average Intake:

Fluoride intake in the United States is estimated at 2.6 mg for those with a fluoridated water supply and 0.9 mg for those with a nonfluoridated water supply.[40]

Silica

Role in Bone Health:

Silica is the earth's most abundant mineral. While the full range of its functions within the human body are poorly understood, we do know that this mineral is high in the strong tissues of the body such as the arteries, tendons, skins, nail ligaments, teeth, hair, connective tissue and collagen. Bone collagen is reported to increase with silica supplementation and the mineral appears to strengthen the connective tissue matrix by cross linking collagen strands. Dietary silicon appears to increase the rate of mineralization particularly when calcium intake is low. Additionally, a concentration of silica is found in the areas of active bone mineralization and silica combines with calcium in the bone-building cell. Overall silica plays an important role in initiating the calcification process, thus helping maintain strong, flexible bones.[26, 41-43]

Recommended Intake:

There is no established RDA for silica, although some researchers suggest that the daily need for silica ranges from 20 to 30 mg. Silica is found in mother's milk; in the fiber fraction of brown rice, barley, oats and leafy greens such as lettuce, dandelions and spinach; in bell peppers, parsnips, cucumbers, leeks and onions. Other whole grains, fruits, nuts, seeds and beans are also good sources. The shiny outside bran layer of grain and the skins of fruits, vegetables, nuts, seeds and grasses are especially high in silica. Herb teas made from horsetail grass, oat, wheat or rice straw are also good sources of organic silica.

Average Intake:

Although we do not have statistics on exact silica consumption, the high uses of processed foods brings with it lower silica content. As nutrition educator Betty Kamen reports, when food is processed fiber is usually the first to go, and along with the fiber goes the silica. Remember, today over 80 percent of the food we consume is processed compared with a mere 10 percent at the turn of the century.[44]

Zinc

Role in Bone Health:

The two or three grams of zinc found in the body function as a co-factor in over 200 enzymatic reactions.[45] In bone metabolism, zinc is needed to produce the matrix of collagen protein threads upon which is deposited the bone-forming calcium-phosphorus compound. Zinc is also required for proper calcium absorption. A deficiency of zinc prevents full absorption of calcium. Equally zinc enhances the biochemical activity of vitamin D. Low zinc levels have been closely linked with osteoporosis. Blood zinc was found to be 30 percent lower in osteoporotic women as compared to non-osteoporotic women. Bone zinc levels were also 28 percent lower.[46] Low serum zinc levels were also found in individuals with advanced jawbone loss. Zinc is essential for bone healing and increased amounts are found at the sites of bone repair.[47]

Recommended Intake:

In 1989 the daily adult female RDA for zinc was lowered from 15 mg to 12 mg with slight increases during pregnancy and lactation. The adult RDA for males was kept at 15 mg. As with magnesium, authorities have seen fit to lower zinc requirements in the face of declining intakes and growing deficiencies. Appendix 3 lists the best food sources of zinc.

Average Intake:

✦ Some authorities estimate that as little as eight percent of United States diets provide the adult RDA (15 mg) for zinc.

✦ Recent studies from the Massachusetts Institute of Technology estimate that the average zinc consumption in this country ranges from 46 to 63 percent the RDA. Another dietary survey found 68 percent of all adults to consume less than two-thirds the RDA for zinc.[48] The Second National Health and Nutrition Examination Survey reported Caucasian and black women to have zinc intakes of only 9.8 mg and 7.8 mg respectively. Black men were also well below the RDA at 12.3 mg. Only Caucasian men meet their RDA.[49]

✦ Within the general population, women and teenage girls have even lower zinc intakes.[2]

Manganese

Role in Bone Health:

Manganese has been shown to play a special role in the maintenance of bone health only recently. Its importance was uncovered by researchers trying to understand why the professional basketball player Bill Walton suffered from joint pain, frequent broken bones and an inability to heal fractures. His bones were becoming osteoporotic even though he was a young athlete! Searching for an answer scientists found Walton's diet to be deficient in many trace minerals including zinc, copper and manganese. Much to their surprise there was no detectable level of manganese in his blood. Dietary supplementation with manganese, zinc, copper and calcium corrected his mysterious bone problem.[50]

Research subsequent to this incident has documented that manganese plays an essential role in bone cartilage and bone collagen formation and is required for bone mineralization.[50, 51] Osteoporotic changes in bone can be brought about by manganese deficiency, which appears to increase bone breakdown while decreasing new bone mineralization. On the other hand, greater serum manganese concentrations are associated with decreased bone breakdown.[52] In one recent study osteoporotic women were found to have one-quarter the manganese levels of the non-osteoporotic woman.[53]

Recommended Intake:

Although no RDA has been established for manganese, the officially recommended "safe and adequate" level of manganese consumption ranges from 2.0 to 5 mg for adults. Recent studies, however, suggest that our manganese intake ideally should be higher than this because so many of our dietary patterns limit manganese absorption. For example, large intakes of calcium, phosphorus, iron and zinc depress manganese absorption.[54-56]

Leading researchers now propose that a better "safe and adequate" recommended adult manganese intake would be of 3.5 to 7.0 mg.[57]

Manganese food sources include liver, kidney, red meats, fish, poultry, spinach, lettuce, dried peas and beans, nuts and whole grains. Manganese intake is greatly reduced when whole grain is replaced by refined flour.[53, 58] Appendix 3 lists your best wholesome food sources of manganese.

Average Intake:

Females of all ages consume inadequate amounts of manganese and the average male intake is rather marginal.[2, 57]

Copper

Role in Bone Health:

Like manganese, copper is an essential trace mineral which has only recently been found to play an important role in bone health maintenance. Once again it was Bill Walton's easily fractured bones that led scientists to look at copper's link to bone health. Although the role copper plays in bone health is not fully understood, we do know that copper aids in the formation of collagen for bone and connective tissue. As with manganese, inadequate copper levels have been associated with the development of osteoporosis.[51, 53, 59]

Like many other minerals, copper excretion is increased on a diet high in sugar, sweetners and refined flour.[56] Also some researchers suggest that the milk sugar, lactose, might interfere with copper metabolism making high dairy intake less than ideal for copper utilization.[59]

Recommended Intake:

The recommended intake for copper is 1.5 to 3 mg for everyone over 11 years of age. Foods that contain significant amounts of copper include liver, oysters, lamb, pork, legumes, walnuts, filberts, pecans and peanuts.

Average Intake: [2, 32, 60]

✦ Copper is among the minerals most often deficient in the American diet.
✦ The typical American diet contains only about 50 percent of the RDA for copper.
✦ One recent study concluded that 75 percent of U.S.

diets failed to contain the recommended dietary allowance of copper.

✦ A large-scale survey found all segments of the United States population to have low dietary copper intakes ranging from 50 to 83 percent of the RDA.

Boron

Role In Bone Health:

Only recently, and quite by accident, did scientists discover that boron plays a role in bone health. The body requires boron for proper metabolism and utilization of various bone-building factors including calcium, magnesium, vitamin D, estrogen and perhaps testosterone.[61]

Studies conducted by Dr. Forest Nielsen of the U.S. Department of Agriculture Research Service in Grand Forks, North Dakota reported that when postmenopausal women were supplemented with boron their metabolism of calcium and magnesium improved. After taking 3 mg of boron for seven weeks, the post-menopausal women studied lost 44 percent less calcium from their bodies, 33 percent less magnesium and slightly less phosphorus as compared to the women who did not receive the boron supplement. In addition, blood levels of the bone-building hormones estrogen and testosterone nearly doubled after eight days of boron supplementation. In fact, the use of boron brought the estrogen levels of postmenopausal women up to the level of the two women in the study using estrogen replacement. The mineral conserving and estrogen enhancing effects of boron supplementation were reported to be most striking for women with low magnesium intakes. Needless to say, the results of this study stimulated a great deal of media attention and boron supplements quickly began appearing on the shelves of health food stores.

As of the late fall of 1995 Dr. Nielsen reports that studies subsequent to his first research of 1987 have not duplicated his original findings that boron reduced calcium and magnesium excretion in the urine. Nonetheless, his ongoing research on boron has reconfirmed his belief that boron is a trace mineral of importance to bone health and osteoporosis prevention. Even though the exact mechanism of its action is unknown, Dr. Nielsen considers boron to play an important role in the utilization and metabolism of calcium and vitamin D.

Basically the jury is still out on to what extent and just how boron affects mineral utilization. Boron's effect on estrogen, however, seems somewhat more consistent since subsequent studies have found boron supplements to raise 17-B estradiol levels of women on estrogen replacement therapy. Dr. Nielsen's original finding that boron raised estrogen also in postmenopausal women not on estrogen replacement therapy, however, has not been reproduced to date. Asked if boron supplements might raise estrogen levels excessively in women on estrogen drugs Dr. Nielsen replied that he did not feel this to be the case. Those on hormone therapy, however, might be able to use less estrogen medication if they consume adequate boron.[62] To me this represents an exciting possibility well worth research attention.

Intrigued by the possibility that boron might mimic or maximize endogenous estrogen, Dr. Nielsen and colleagues experimented with giving boron to menopausal women checking to see if hot flashes and other common symptoms of estrogen deficiency might improve with boron supplementation. In this study some 25 percent of the women experienced a reduction of symptoms from 3 mg of boron; in another 50 percent symptoms got worse; and in the remaining 25 percent no changes were noted. Again the boron story takes a complicated turn. There is obviously an important boron-estrogen link yet to be uncovered.

Once considered to have nutrition value only as a food preservative, today boron is a trace mineral on the rise. It is clear we will be hearing more about boron and its role in bone and endocrine health within the near future.[61]

Recommended Intake:

To date there has been no minimal RDA set for boron. It is clear that our ancestors consumed much more of this nutrient than we do. Even today those consuming plenty of fruits, vegetables and nuts may consume up to 10 mg per day. A high boron intake might account for a lower osteoporosis rate among vegetarians. Recent U.S. research indicates that 2 to 3 mg of boron might well be a more optimum intake than our current 0.50 to 1 mg intake.[61]

Excessive boron supplementation can be toxic and animal studies suggest that high boron supplementation adversely affects calcium metabolism, so one should not consume more than 3 mg of supplemental boron unless under proper supervision.[62] Boron from food needs no restrictions and it has been suggested that no adverse effects from boron are found in certain parts of the world where as much as 41 mg are consumed daily.[63]

Boron is found in many fruits, vegetables and nuts. A diet rich in natural whole foods such as soy, prunes, raisins, peanuts, almonds, hazelnuts, dates, apples, pears, grapes, leafy greens, rose hips, sea vegetables and honey would contain relatively high amounts of boron. Appendix 3 lists your best wholesome food sources of boron.

Average Intake:

Intake greatly varies according to consumption of fruits and vegetables. Some researchers suggest that the United States diet today might contain 0.50 to 1.5 mg of boron.[61, 62]

Vitamin D

Role In Bone Health:

Vitamin D is a great regulator of calcium and phosphorus metabolism. It mobilizes calcium and phosphorus for release from bone in the presence of parathyroid hormone; promotes intestinal absorption of calcium and phosphate; increases kidney absorption of calcium and phosphorus and carries them into the blood. Without vitamin D the body cannot properly absorb calcium and the bones and teeth become soft and poorly mineralized. Vitamin D deficiency also results in secondary hyperparathyroidism which in turn can lead to osteoporosis

Adequate vitamin D nutrition is of importance lifelong. The disease of vitamin D deficiency in children is known as rickets and in adults as osteomalacia. This condition is generally distinguished from osteoporosis in that osteoporotic bone is normally mineralized but thin while in osteomalacia bone is poorly mineralized. Low vitamin D status, as low calcium status, leads to overactivity of the parathyroid gland. An overactive parathyroid in turn promotes bone loss. This factor is especially important in the elderly.

Numerous studies now document that up to 80 percent of all hip fracture patients may exhibit vitamin D deficiency.[64-67] The vitamin D-osteoporosis link is strong enough to lead one prominent researcher to conclude that in general, the more adequate the state of vitamin D nutrition, the less bone loss among the elderly.[68] Research now indicates that women past menopause can actually halt bone loss and even increase their bone density over the course of the year by consuming adequate calcium and getting extra vitamin D— the "sunshine vitamin"—during the dark days of winter. With just 400 I.U. of vitamin D in addition to 800 mg of calcium postmenopausal women gained hip bone mass at an age when according to Western medicine, they should have been losing it.[68] Equally impressive is the successful French use of vitamin D and calcium to stop bone loss, to reduce fractures and even rebuild some bone amongst elderly osteoporotic persons.[69, 70]

Recommended Intake:

The recommended dietary allowance for vitamin D in adults is 200 I.U. as compared to 400 I.U. during growth. Many authorities, however, suggest that vitamin D requirements should actually rise with age and that people over 65 may need from 600 to 1000 I.U. of vitamin D per day to compensate for decreases in vitamin D absorption.[71-73] For example, Dr. Dawson-Hughes of the USDA Research Center on Aging has found that in Northern latitudes 800 IU of vitamin D (four times the RDA) is needed to reduce hip fracture among postmenopausal women.[73]

The body, however, is not solely dependent on vitamin D from food sources. Technically, the substance we call vitamin D is more of a hormone than a vitamin. As a hormone, most of our vitamin D supply is produced within our own bodies upon exposure to sunlight. Brief, casual exposure of the face, arms and hands to sunlight is thought to be equivalent to the ingestion of 200 IU of vitamin D. Longer sunlight exposure to more of the body would yield higher vitamin D levels and one researcher suggests that 30 minutes of exposure to sunlight per day over one-third of the body would provide a more ideal vitamin D level.[74-76] This internal production of vitamin D, however, also appears to decrease with age and thus it is even more important that older people consume higher amounts of vitamin D through food or supplementation. Liver, eggs and butter contain some vitamin D, as does fortified vitamin D milk.

Vitamin D is actually a very complex substance with many varied forms and uncounted biological functions. Regarding its pivotal role in mineral metabolism it should be noted that as a hormone vitamin D exists in both more active and less active states. It is converted to more active states within the body as needed. The most active metabolite of vitamin D, known as 1, 25-dihydroxyvitamin D, or calcitriol, is produced by the kidney from less active precursors. It is this kidney-activated substance which mediates the many biological effects of vitamin D including calcium absorption. For example, in the absence of activated 1,25-dihydroxyvitamin D, less than 10 percent of dietary calcium may be absorbed.[77] The degree of intestinal calcium absorption, in fact, is directly related to blood levels of this active form of vitamin D.[78, 79] Interestingly, the role of final vitamin D activation by the kidney gives these small glands a big role in bone health maintenance.

Average Intake:

✦ Most older persons in this country do not consume the RDA for this nutrient. Many researchers point to an unrecognized epidemic of vitamin D deficiency among older Americans, suggesting that of those

200,000+ persons who suffer hip fractures each year, a great many are vitamin D deficient.[66, 78, 79]

✦ A study of healthy free-living elderly in New Mexico found that 60 percent had low blood levels of vitamin D.[80] While vitamin D is essential to the maintenance of healthy bones, excessive vitamin D from food or nutritional supplements can be detrimental to bone health.

On the other hand, high levels of vitamin D can be toxic to the body as a whole. In adults levels of 2,000 I.U. per day have occasionally caused toxicity. While vitamin D deficiency is common and vitamin D toxicity rare, the use of more than 800 I.U. vitamin D for adults per day and 400 I.U. for children is not recommended without professional guidance. We do not need to worry about getting too much vitamin D from our body's own internal production. When our levels are adequate, our body simply stops producing vitamin D.

Vitamin C

Role in Bone Health:

Vitamin C is involved in a great variety of complex and interrelated metabolic processes. Among a host of other things, vitamin C is required for the formation of collagen and thus is essential for healthy bones. As described in Chapter 1, bone mineral is laid down over a protein matrix called collagen. Collagen is abundant in the connective tissue of cartilage and bone. Connective tissue, in fact, comprises about 30 percent of our bone, serving as a support structure for mineral deposits and giving bone its resilience. In addition to its role in collagen formation, vitamin C also appears to stimulate the cells that build bone, enhance calcium absorption and enhance vitamin D's effect on bone metabolism. In addition vitamin C is essential for synthesis and optimal functioning of adrenal steroid hormones which also play a role in bone health.[81, 82]

Recommended Intake:

The RDA for vitamin C is a very minimal 60 mg with a slight increase during pregnancy and lactation. Many well-qualified scientists, including the late Nobel laureate, Dr. Linus Pauling, feel that this recommended level is extremely low. A more ideal intake would be at least 250 mg to 2000 mg (2 grams) per day.[83]

Average Intake: [82–85]

+ Even though the RDA for vitamin C is extremely low, great numbers of Americans do not even consume this minimal amount.
+ A U.S. Department of Agriculture food consumption survey reported that 26 percent of the population consumed less than 70 percent of the RDA for vitamin C.
+ Certain groups such a the elderly, the ill, the institutionalized and smokers have been found to be at even greater risk for vitamin C deficiency.
+ Biochemical evidence of vitamin C deficiency was found in 20 percent of elderly women, even though they were consuming more than the RDA of 60 mg of vitamin C per day.

Vitamin A

Role in Bone Health:

Animal experiments document that vitamin A is essential for normal bone development. Vitamin A helps in the development of osteoblasts, the bone-building cells which lay down new bone. A deficiency of vitamin A also limits calcium metabolism which results in poor bone growth.[85]

Recommended Intake:

The adult RDA for vitamin A varies from 4,000 to 5,000 I.U. with slight increases during pregnancy and lactation. The active form of vitamin A is found in animal tissues; thus, some animal products contain vitamin A. Liver is an exceptionally good source of vitamin A containing 45,000 I.U. per serving. Most of the vitamin A in our diet, however, comes from plants in the form of beta-carotene. Beta carotene is a precursor of vitamin A and is converted in the liver to vitamin A. Vegetable sources of beta-carotene, and thus vitamin A, include yellow and dark green vegetables such as carrots, winter squash, sweet potatoes, pumpkin, collards, dandelion greens, kale, spinach, Swiss chard and broccoli. Orange fruits such as apricots, mangos, cantaloupe and peaches are also good sources. Both vitamins A and D are stored in the liver and thus can become toxic if consumed in excessive amounts. This is especially true in pregnancy when vitamin A supplementation should not exceed 8,000 I.U. per day. Because it is water soluble, high beta-carotene intake does not result in excessively high vitamin A levels.

Average Intake:

✦ The last nationwide food consumption survey reported that 31 percent of the United States population consumed less than two-thirds of the RDA for vitamin A.

✦ Adolescents, teenagers and the elderly display even poorer vitamin A status.[7]

Vitamin B$_6$

Role in Bone Health:

B$_6$ is another nutrient which plays an important, yet indirect, role in bone metabolism. Vitamin B$_6$ is necessary for hydrochloric acid production (HCL), and HCL in turn is required for calcium absorption. B$_6$ is also essential for adrenal functioning. In turn, some 30 different hormones are produced by the adrenal glands, some of which aid in maintaining proper mineral balance within the body. B$_6$ is a necessary co-factor in the enzymatic cross-linking of collagen strands which increase the strength of connective tissue. It also helps to break down homocysteine which tends to increase in postmenopausal women. Homocysteine is a metabolite of the protein methionine which interferes with collagen cross-linking leading to a defective bone matrix and osteoporosis. It also contributes to the development of heart disease. All in all, over 50 enzyme systems are directly dependent on vitamin B$_6$ and many others function suboptimally without sufficient amounts of this nutrient.[89]

Animal studies show that the amount and quality of new bone formed is lower in animals deficient in B$_6$ than in those with adequate B_6 levels. A vitamin B_6 deficient diet has been found to produce osteoporosis in rats and a recent British study with humans found B_6 deficiency more common among those who suffer hip fractures.[90]

Recommended Intake:

The adult RDA for B_6 is 2 mg with a slight increase during pregnancy and lactation. Good food sources of vitamin B_6 include various protein foods, such as organ and other meats, poultry, fish, egg yolks, soy and other beans. Peanuts and walnuts are also good sources of B_6. Whole grains, bananas, avocados, cabbage, cauliflower and potatoes also contain significant B_6. Keep in mind, however, that B_6 is destroyed by light and heat and thus much of it is lost in food processing, storage and preparation. In addition, animal protein creates an increased demand for B_6 as do other common B_6 antagonists such as yellow dye #5, oral contraceptives and certain other drugs and alcohol.[87, 92]

Average Intake:

✦ Recent studies indicate widespread inadequate vitamin B_6 consumption among all sectors of the population.[88]

✦ All of 21 "normal American students" studied over a two week period were found to be functionally deficient in B_6[92]

Vitamin K

Role In Bone Health:

While vitamin K is best known for its role in blood clotting, this nutrient also plays an important part in the maintenance of healthy bones. Noted nutrition authority Dr. Alan Gaby suggests that vitamin K is as important to bone as calcium.[63] Let's follow Dr. Gaby's lead and take a closer look at this nutrient.

Vitamin K is required for the synthesis of osteocalcin, the bone protein matrix upon which calcium crystallizes. Osteocalcin provides the structure and order to bone tissue; without it bone would be fragile and easily broken. Vitamin K also aids in the binding of calcium to the bone matrix.[93-95] Circulating vitamin K_1 has been found to be lower in patients suffering from osteoporotic fractures as compared to age-matched individuals who have not suffered such fractures.[96] Furthermore, in a Japanese study vitamin K given to three osteoporotic postmenopausal women reduced their calcium loss by 18 to 50 percent.[95] This work was recently confirmed in the Netherlands. Here 25 percent of the healthy postmenopausal women studied had elevated excretion of calcium in their urine, probably because they were losing bone at an accelerated rate. Administration of vitamin K reduced this unwanted calcium loss by one-third, suggesting that bone loss had been slowed or stopped.[63, 97] Also it was found that in these women the capacity of the bone protein (osteocalcin) to attract calcium was reduced. After administration of 1 mg of vitamin K daily for two weeks this bone protein function normalized.

Just as vitamin K is central to bone formation so it appears to play an important role in fracture healing. In studies with rabbits vitamin K supplementation was found to accelerate healing of experimental fractures.[95] In humans vitamin K levels fall during recovery from a fracture and it appears that this nutrient is actually drawn from the rest of the body to the site of fracture.[63, 96]

Recommended Intake:

A provisional adult RDA has been set for vitamin K at 70 to 140 mcg for adults. Vitamin K is found in many known health-promoting foods, including dark green leafy vegetables such as spinach, kale, parsley, turnip and other greens. Appendix 3 lists your best wholesome food sources of vitamin K.

We should remember that vitamin K is also produced in the body by certain health-promoting intestinal bacteria. In the next section we look in more detail at the importance of maintaining a healthy bacterial environment within our intestines for the absorption and production of many nutrients essential to bone health.

Like vitamins A and D, vitamin K is fat-soluble and not easily excreted from the body. Those who need to increase their vitamin K intake would do well to expand their diets to include daily use of alfalfa, dark green leafy vegetables and other foods high in this nutrient. If you choose to use supplements, Dr. Gaby suggests 150 to 500 mcg daily taken with meals. Those on blood thinning drugs such as coumadin or warfarin should not use vitamin K as it interferes with the effect of these drugs.[63]

Average Intake:

While some researchers suggest that a "normal mixed diet" will contain from 300 to 500 mcg vitamin K daily, another study has reported intakes as low as 48 mcg in young men.[98, 99]

Vitamin K adequacy is threatened by the freezing of foods, mineral oil laxatives, rancid fats, radiation, impaired fat absorption, oral antibiotic use, sulfa drugs and certain liver diseases. For example, in one study 31 percent of patients with gastrointestinal disorders that required the long-term use of antibiotics developed vitamin K deficiency.[100]

Vitamin B_{12}

Role In Bone Health:

Vitamin B_{12} has recently been added to the list of nutrients essential for proper bone metabolism. The bone building cells require an adequate supply of vitamin B_{12} and a deficiency of thus nutrient diminishes their ability to function properly.[101]

Recommended Intake:

The adult RDA for vitamin B_{12} was lowered from 3 to 2 mcg in 1989. As with B_6, however, we find that many researchers suggest that an optimum B_{12} intake would be significantly higher than even the former RDA of 3 mcg.

Animal protein is an excellent source of B_{12}. Organ meats, clams and oysters are especially high in vitamin B_{12}. Other sources include milk, crabs, salmon, sardines and egg yolk, with smaller amounts being found in mussel meats, dairy products, lobster, scallops, flounder, other fish and fermented cheese. This vitamin is not found in plants but is produced by the bacteria in our digestive tract. This again brings us back to the importance of having a healthy gut with balanced intestinal flora.

Average Intake: [7, 101]

✦ Large national surveys report that only two-thirds of the population consume 100 percent of the recommended dietary allowance for B_{12}
✦ Roughly one-fifth consume between 70 and 99 percent the RDA, while 15 percent show intakes of less than 70 percent of the RDA.

Folic Acid

Role in Bone Health:

Folic acid is one of the B vitamins. The most noted role folic acid plays in bone health is in the detoxification of a substance called homocysteine. Homocysteine is a compound produced as a byproduct of the metabolism of the amino acid methionine. It is normally recycled as another substance or eliminated, but excessive blood levels can accumulate due to genetic or nutritional factors. Excess homocysteine promotes both osteoporosis and atherosclerosis. The proper processing of homocysteine requires folic acid. Researchers suggest that around the time of menopause women experience a reduced capacity to properly process homocysteine. It is not known whether this is a universal trait or one that is found in just the developed countries. Supplementation with folic acid has been found to correct this error in homocysteine processing.

Recommended Intake:

The RDA for folic acid is 400 mcg. Researchers suggest that as a preventive measure one might use 800 mcg of folic acid along with vitamins B_{12} and B_6. Those with

diabetes, heart disease and/or vascular problems, or un-
explained weight gain would do well to discuss the appro-
priateness of a homocysteine clearance test with their
physician.

Average Intake:

> ✦ Deficiency of folic acid is extremely common in
> many parts of the world. The average United
> States intake is about one-half the RDA.[6]
> ✦ Women taking oral contraceptives and women
> on estrogen replacement as well as alcohol abus-
> ers and long-term users of anticonvulsants are
> at special risk for drug-induced folic acid
> deficiency.

Folic acid is high in green leafy vegetables, asparagus, black-
eyed peas, peas, broccoli, sweet potatoes and fruits like cantaloupe and oranges as well as grains like oatmeal, wheat
germ and wild rice.

Essential Fatty Acids

Role In Bone Health:

Nutrition authorities regularly remind us that we should
cut the fat in our diet. Indeed Americans consume far too
much fat and this can have a detrimental impact on bone
by decreasing calcium absorption. On average, we consume
nearly 42 percent of our calories in fat. We are seldom told,
however, that our body actually requires certain fats just as
it requires certain vitamins and minerals, fiber and water.

These fats are called "essential fatty acids." They are "essential" because they are not produced by the body and must be consumed in the diet. These fatty acids are necessary for nerve functioning, hormone production, for the maintenance and functioning of the brain and for everyday energy production. Fatty acids also play multiple roles in bone structure, function and development. Fats are required for proper calcium metabolism as detailed in Chapter 5 and they are essential components of all membranes, including those of cartilage and bone.

Recommended Intake:

Overall, we should reduce the total fat intake of our diet from 40 percent of all calories to perhaps 20 to 25 percent. At the same time we need to increase our intake of the essential fatty acids, the "good" fats.

What are the essential fatty acids and where do we find them? The two essential fatty acids are linoleic acid (omega 6) and alpha-linolenic acid (omega 3). An ideal intake of omega 6 essential fats is around 9 to 30 grams per day, while six grams or more is an ideal intake of omega 3s. The best sources of the essential fatty acids are fish oils, flaxseed, pumpkin, walnut and soy oils. One tablespoon of flaxseed oil, for example, contains eight grams of omega 3 linolenic acid and two grams of the omega 6 linoleic acid. A tablespoon of soy oil offers 6.5 grams of omega 6 oil but less than one-fifth that much of the omega 3 oil. The next best oils are safflower, sesame, sunflower and corn. All vegetable oils should be expeller- or cold-pressed (as found in health food stores) and kept refrigerated. The nuts or seeds from which these oils come are also good sources of essential fatty acids.[102, 103]

Average Intake:

Consumption of high quality cis form essential fatty acids is low due to food processing; the exact figure, however, is unknown.

Protein

Role In Bone Health:

The situation with protein is somewhat similar to that with fat. While some protein is essential, too much is detrimental. Protein is needed for the intestinal absorption of calcium and protein is a major building block for bone. By weight, roughly one-third of our bone is living organic protein matrix. Protein malnutrition debilitates bone and can be a significant problem among elderly people in Western countries. For example, in Japan where protein intake among aging women can be extremely low, protein intake is positively correlated with bone mineral density.[104] Excessive protein, however, can lead to bone loss through increasing the acid load which must be buffered through drawing calcium and other alkalizing minerals from the bone.

While adequate protein is essential to bone health, the vast majority of people in the United States consume far too much protein in the form of animal products. Excess protein actually washes calcium out of the body. The protein content of selected foods is listed in Illustration 13.1 in Chapter 13.

Recommended Intake:

The RDA is 44 grams of protein for women and 56 grams for men. It is easy to exceed the RDA with one four-ounce serving of meat yielding 35 grams of protein and each serving of dairy adding 8 to 11 grams of protein.

Average Intake:

Twice the RDA or nearly 100 grams of protein intake is common.

❖ References

1 Crocetti AF, Guthrie HA. Eating behavior and associated nutrient quality of diets. Anarem Systems Research Corporation, New York, NY, 1982.

2 Pennington, J., et al., "Mineral Content of Food and Total Diets: The Selected Minerals in Foods Survey, 1982 to 1984," *J Am Diet Assoc* 86 (1986): 876-891.

3 Underwood, E., *Trace Elements in Human and Animal Nutrition*, 4th ed. (New York: Academic Press, 1977).

4 Kies, C., *Nutritional Bioavailability of Manganese,*, ed. C. Kies (Washington: American Chemical Society, 1987).

5 Spencer, Herta, et al., "The effect of phosphorus on endogenous fecal calcium excretion in man," *The American Journal of Clinical Nutrition* 43 (1986): 844-51.

6 Daniel, W.A., E.G. Gaines, and Bennett, "Dietary intakes and plasma concentrations of folate in healthy adolescents," *Am J Clin Nutr* 28 (1975).

7 Pao, E., and S. Mickle, "Problem Nutrients in the United States," *Food Technology* .Sept. (1981): 58-64.

8 Guyton, A.C., *Textbook of Medical Physiology*, (Philadelphia: Saunders, 1988).

9 Frieden, E., *Biochemistry of Ultratrace Elements*, (New York: Plenum Press, 1984).

10 Eaton, S., and M. Konner, "Paleolithic Nutrition," *New England Journal of Medicine* 312 (1985): 283-289.

11 Eaton, S. Boyd, Marjorie Shostak, and Melvin Konner, *The Paleolithic Prescription: A Program Of Diet & Exercise and a Design for Living*, (New York: Harper & Row, 1988).

12 Heaney, R., and J. Barger-Lux, *Calcium and Common Sense*, (New York: Doubleday, 1988).

13 Heaney, Robert P., "The Prevention of Osteoporotic Fracture in Women," *The Osteoporotic Syndrome*, (New York: Wiley-Liss, Inc., 1993) 89-107.

14 Nevitt, Michael C.,"Epidemiology Of Osteoporosis," *Rheumatic Disease Clinics of North America* 20.3 (1994): 535-559.

15 Riggs, D. Lawrence, et al., "Effect Of the Fluoride/Calcium Regimen On Vertebral Fracture Occurrence In Postmenopausal Osteoporosis," *The New England Journal Of Medicine* 306.8 (1982): 446-450.

16 National Academy of Science, *Recommended Daily Allowances*, (Washington, D.C.: National Academy of Sciences, 1989).

17 O'Neil, R.D., "Research and application of current topics in sports nutrition," *Continuing Education* 86.8 (1986).

18 Worthington, and B. Roberts, "Contemporary Developments in Nutrition," (St. Louis, Mo.: Mosby Co., 1981) 240-53.

19 Linkswiler, H, et al., "Protein-induced hypercalciuria," *FASEB* 40.8 (1981): 2429-2432.

20 Medalle, R, and et al, "Vitamin D resistance in magnesium deficiency," *Am J Clin Nutr* 29 (1976): 854-858.

21 Iseri, L.T., and J.H. French, "Magnesium: nature's physiologic calcium blocker," *Am Heart J* 108 (1984): 188-193.

22 Seelig, M., *Magnesium Deficiency in the Pathogenesis of Disease*, (New York: Plenum Press, 1980).

23 Cohen, L., and R. Kitzes, "Infrared Spectroscopy and Magnesium Content Of Bone Mineral In Osteoporotic Women," *Israel Journal of Medical Sciences* 17 (1981): 1123-1125.

24 Sojka, J.E., "Magnesium Supplementation and Osteoporosis," *Nutrition Reviews* 53.3 (1995): 71-74.

25 Hegsted, D., "Mineral Intake and Bone Loss," *Fed Proceedings* Nov/Dec (1967): 1747-1763.

26 Gaby, Alan R. M.D., and Jonathan V. Wright, M. D., "Nutrients and Bone Health," *Health World* 1988: 29-31.

27 Angus, R. M., et al., "Dietary intake and bone mineral density," *Bone Mineral* 4.3 (1988): 265-78.

28 Vikhansky, Luba, "Magnesium may slow bone loss," *Medical Tribune* July 22, 1993.

29 Landon, R., and I. Young, "Role of magnesium in regulation of lung function," *Am Diet A* (1993): 674-677.

30 Shils, M., "Magnesium," *Modern Nutrition in Health and Disease*, ed. R. Goodhart, and M. Shils. (Philadelphia: Lea and Febiger, 1973).

31 Morgan, K., "Magnesium and Calcium," *J American College Nutrition* 4.2 (1985): 195-206.

32 Pennington, JAT, and BE Young, "Total diet study nutritional elements," *J Am Diet Assoc* 91 (1991): 170-183.

33 Meacham, Susan, L Taper, and Stella Volpe, "Effect of boron supplementation on blood and urinary calcium, magnesium and phosphorus, and urinary boron in athletic and sedentary women," *J Clin Nutr* 61 (1995): 341-5.

34 Lakshmanan, F., "Magnesium Intakes, Balances and Blood Levels of Adults Consuming Self-selected Diets," *The Amer Jrnl of Clinical Nutrition* 40. Dec (1984): 1380-1389.

35 Sowers, M., R. Wallace, and J. Lemke, "The Relationship of Bone Mass and Fracture History to Fluoride and Calcium Intake: A Study of Three Communities," *Am J Clin Nutr* 44.6 (1986): 889-898.

36 Danielson, C., et al., "Hip fractures and fluoridation in Utah's elderly population," *JAMA* 268 (1992): 746-8.

37 Hedlund, L., and J. Gallagher, "Estrogen Therapy for Postmenopausal Osteoporosis: Current Status," *Geriatric Medicine Today* 7.2 (1988): 55-63.

38 Riggs, B.L., et al., "Effect of Fluoride Treatment on Fracture Rate in Postmenopausal Women with Osteoporosis," *N Engl J Med* 322 (1990): 802-9.

39 Hileman, Bette, "Fluoridation of Water," *Chemical Engineering News* 66.August 1988 (1988).

40 Richmond, V.L., "Thirty years of fluoridation: A review," *American Journal of Clinical Nutrition* 41 (1985): 129-138.

41 Davies, S., and A. Stewart, *Nutritional Medicine: The Drug-free Guide to Better Family Health,* (London/Sydney: Pan Books, 1987).

42 Carlisle, E.M., "A Relationship Between Silicon and Calcium in Bone Formation," *Fed Proc* 29 (1970): 265.

43 Carlisle, E., "Silicon with the Osteoblast, the Bond-forming Cell," *Fed Proc* 34 (1975): 927.

44 Kamen, Betty, Ph.D., Si Kamen, and M.D. Benzoza, *Osteoporosis: What It Is, How to Prevent It, How to Stop It.,* (New York: Pinnacle Books, Inc., 1984) 222.

45 Hendricks, K., "Zinc and Inflammatory Bowel Disease," *The Nutrition Report* 66 March (1990).

46 Atik, Sahap, "Zinc and Senile Osteoporosis," *Jr of American Geriatric Society* 31 (1983): 790-791.

47 Teller, E., P. Kimmel, and D. Watkins, "Zinc (Z) Nutritional Status Modulates the 1,25(OH)2D(125) Response to Low Calcium (LC) Diet (D)," *Kidney Int* 31 (1987): 358.

48 Holden, J.M., et al., "Zinc and copper in self-selected diets.," *J. Am. Dietet. Assoc.* 75.23 (1979).

49 Mares-Perlman, Julie A., et al., "Zinc Intake and Sources in the US Adult Population: 1976-1980," *Journal of the American College of Nutrition* 14.4 (1995): 349-357.

50 Strause, L., and P. Saltman, "Role of Manganese in Bone Metabolism," (Washington, D.C.: American Chemical Society, 1987), 46.

51 Strause, L., et al., "Effects of Long-term Dietary Manganese and Copper Deficiency on Rat Skeleton," *American Institute of Nutrition.* Sept 23 (1986).

52 Slemenda, Charles, et al., "Predictors of Bone Mass in Perimenopausal Women," *Ann Intern Med* 112.2 (1990): 96-101.

53 Raloff, J., "Reasons for Boning Up on Manganese," *Science News* 130 Sept (1986): 199.

54 Ricketts, C., C. Kies, and P. Garcia, "Manganese and Magnesium Utilization of Humans as Affected by Level and Kind of Dietary Fat," *Fed Proc* 44 (1985): 1850.

55 Freeland-Graves, J., "Manganese: An Essential Nutrient for Humans," *Nutrition Today*. Nov/Dec (1988): 13-19.

56 Hallfrisch, J., et al., "Mineral Balances of Men and Women Consuming High Fiber Diets with Complex or Simple Carbohydrate," *J Nut* 117 (1987): 48-55.

57 Freeland-Graves, J.H., C. W. Bales, and F. Behmardi, "Manganese Requirements of Humans," (Washington, D.C.: American Chemical Society, 1987), 90.

58 Schwartz, R., B. Apgar, and E. Wien, "Apparent Absorption and Retention of Ca, Cu, Mg, Mn, Zn from a Diet Containing Bran," *Am J Clin Nutr* 43 (1986): 444-445.

59 Strain, J.J., "A reassessment of diet and osteoporosis—possible role for copper," *Med-Hypotheses* 27.4 (1988): 333-338.

60 Klevay, L., "Evidence of Dietary Copper and Zinc Deficiencies," *JAMA* 241 (1979): 1917-1918.

61 Nielsen, F., C. Hunt, and L. Mullen, "Effect of Dietary Boron on Mineral, Estrogen, and Testosterone Metabolism in Postmenopausal Women," *FASEB J* 1 (1987): 394-397.

62 Nielsen, Forrest, personal communication, (1995).

63 Gaby, Alan R. Ph.D., *Preventing and Reversing Osteoporosis*, (Rocklin: Prime Publishing, 1994) 304.

64 Harju, E., et al., "High Incidence of Low Serum Vitamin D Concentration in Patients with Hip Fracture," *Archives Of Orthopedics And Trauma Surgery* 103.6 (1985): 408-416.

65 Lips, P., et al., "Histomorphometric profile and vitamin D status in patients with femoral neck fracture," *Metab Bone Dis Relat Res* 4 (1982): 85-93.

66 Komar, I., et al., "Seniors at Risk for Vitamin D Deficiencies and Fractures," *J Am Ger So* 41 (1993): 1057-1064.

67 Neer, R., personal communication, Continuing Education Course on Osteoporosis: Harvard University, (1987).

68 Dawson-Hughes, et al., "A controlled trial of the effect of calcium supplementation on bone density in postmenopausal women," *New England Journal of Medicine* 323 (1990): 878-83.

69 Chapuy, Marie C., et al., "Vitamin D3 and Calcium to Prevent Hip Fractures in Elderly Women.," *New England Journal of Medicine* 328.23 (1992): 1637-1642.

70 Meunier, P.J., and M.C. Chapuy, "Calcium and Vitamin D Supplementation For Preventing Hip Fractures in the Elderly," *Challenges of Modern Medicine* 7 (1995): 22-227.

71 Kaplan, F., "Osteoporosis: An Update," *Hospital Medicine.* Feb (1986): 173-197.

72 Heaney, R., "Nutritional Factors in Bone Health," *Osteoporosis Etiology, Diagnosis and Management,* ed. B. Riggs, and L. Melton. (New York: Raven Press, 1988) 359-372.

73 Dawson-Hughes, et al., "Rates of Bone Loss In Postmenopausal Women Randomly Assigned to One of Two Dosages of Vitamin D," *Am J Clin Nutr* 61 (1995): 1140-1145.

74 Haddad, John G., "Vitamin D-Solar Rays, the Milky Way, or Both?," *The New England Journal of Medicine* 326.18 (1992): 1213-1216.

75 Lips, P., F. van Ginkel, and M. Jongen, "Determinants of Vitamin D Status in Patients with Hip Fracture and in Elderly Control Subjects," *Am J Clin Nutr* 46 (1987): 1005-1010.

76 Devgun, et al., "Vitamin D Nutrition in Relation to the Season and Occupation," *The American Journal of Clinical Nutrition* 34 (1981): 1501-1504.

77 NIH, "Consensus Statement," (Washington, D.C.: National Institute on Aging, 1994).

78 Gallagher, J., et al., "Intestinal Calcium Absorption and Serum Vitamin D Metabolites in Normal Subjects and Osteoporotic Patients," *Journal of Clinical Investigation* 64 Sept (1979): 729-736.

79 Eufemio, Michael, "Advances in the Therapy of Osteoporosis-Part VIII," *Geriatric Medicine Today* 9.11 (1990): 37-49.

80 Ohmdahl, J.L., et al., *Am J Clin Nutr* 36 (1985): 1225.

81 Freudenheim, J.L., N.E. Johnson, et al., "Relationships between Usual Nutrient Intake and Bone Mineral Content of Women 35-65 Years of Age: Longitudinal and Cross-sectional Analysis.," *Am. Jr. Clinical Nutrition* 44.863 (1986).

82 Goralczyk, R., et al., "Regulation of steroid hormone metabolism requires L-ascorbic acid," *Ann NY Acad* (1992): 349-351.

83 Pauling, L., *How to Live Long and Feel Better,* (New York: Freeman, 1986).

84 Cheraskin, C.E., et al., *The Vitamin C Connection,* 1st ed. (New York: Harper & Row, 1983).

85 Newton, H., et al., "The Cause and Correction of Low Blood Vitamin C Concentrations in the Elderly," *The American Journal of Clinical Nutrition* 42.Oct (1985): 656-659.

86 Vitale, J., *Vitamins*, (Kalamazoo, MI: Upjohn Company, 1976).

87 Brown, Judith, *The Science of Human Nutrition*, (New York: Harcourt Brace Jovanovich, Inc, 1990).

88 Serfontein, WJ, and et al, "Vitamin B_6 revisited," *SA Medical Journal* 66 (1984): 437-40.

89 Dodds, R., A. Catterall, and L. Bitensky, "Osteolytic Retardation of Early Stages of Fracture Healing by Vitamin B6 Deficiency," *Clin Sci* 68 (1985): 21P.

90 Reynolds, T., and et al, "Hip fracture patients may be vitamin B_6 deficient: Controlled study of serum pyridoxal-5-phosphate," *Act Orth Sc* 63 (1992): 635-638.

91 Murray, Michael T., *Menopause: How You Can Benefit from Diet, Vitamins, Minerals, Herbs, Exercise and Other Natural Methods*, (Rocklin, CA: Prima Publishing, 1994).

92 Azuma, J., et al., "Apparent deficiency of vitamin B_6 in typical individuals who commonly serve as normal controls," *Res Commun. Chem. Pathol. Pharmacal.* 14 (1976): 343-348.

93 Feldman, E., *Essentials of Clinical Nutrition*, (Philadelphia: F.A. Davis Company, 1988).

94 Wright, J., "Testing for Vitamin K_1: Osteoporosis "Risk Factor"," *International Clinical Nutrition Review* 9.1 (1989): 14-15.

95 Tomita, A., "Postmenopausal Osteoporosis Ca-47 Study with Vitamin K_2," *Clin Endocrinol (Jpn)* 19 (1971): 731.

96 Hart, J., et al., "Electrochemical Detection of Depressed Circulating Levels of Vitamin K_1 in Osteoporosis," *Journal of Clinical Endocrinology and Metabolism* 60.6 (1985): 1268-1269.

97 Knapen, M.H.J., "The effect of Vitamin K supplementation on circulating osteocalcin and urinary calcium excretion," *Ann Inter Med* 111 (1989): 1001-1005.

98 Dubick, M. A., "Dietary supplements and health aids: A critical evaluation," *Journal of Nutrition Education* 15 (1983): 123-127.

99 Somer, Elizabeth, "Vitamin K: The Sleeping Beauty," *The Nutrition Report* (1993): 58.

100 Krasinski, S.D., et al., "The prevalence of vitamin K deficiency in chronic gastrointestinal disorders," *American Journal of Clinical Nutrition* 41 (1985): 639-643.

101 Carmel, R., et al., "Cobalamin and Osteoblast-specific Proteins," 319.2 (1988): 70-75.

102 Burton, B., and W. Foster, *Human Nutrition,* (McGraw-Hill Book Company, 1988).

103 Erasmus, Udo, *Fats and Oils: The Complete Guide to Fats and Oils in Health and Nutrition,* (Vancouver: Alive Books, 1986).

104 Lacey, J.M., et al., "Correlates of cortical bone mass among pre-menopausal and postmenopausal Japanese women," *Journal of Bone & Mineral Research* 6.7 (1991): 651-659.

Chapter 5

Bone-Robbing
Dietary Excesses

❖ The Standard American Diet is Both Imbalanced and Inadequate

*W*hen it comes to diet and bone health the rule is simple: Maximize intake of nutrient-dense, bone-building whole foods and minimize intake of the substances which limit bone health. In other words, go for the nutrients and avoid the anti-nutrients.

This mandate, of course, was much easier for our ancestors to follow than it is for us. Living off the land offered plenty of nutrient-rich whole foods and a real dearth of anti-nutrients. Even our grandparents could not have located, much less purchased and consumed, a fraction of the unwholesome foodstuffs which crowd our supermarket shelves today. Of the 25,000 products in a typical supermarket only a small number are nutritious, whole foods. Many are not only highly processed, but largely synthetic.

The standard American diet is not only inadequate but it is also imbalanced. The nutrients we do obtain do not come from a well-rounded buffet. On any given day, nearly

50 percent of us eat no fruit and 25 percent eat no vegetables. Fewer than 10 percent of us actually consume five servings of fruit and/or vegetables, an intake that is at the low end of that recommended by the 1990 U.S. Government Dietary Guidelines.[1] As a group we consume over 20 percent of our calories as sugar and sweeteners and around 40 percent as fat. Additionally, many consume at least another 10 percent of their calories as alcohol. What this means is that our bodies are depending on the remaining 30 to 40 percent of our caloric intake to supply us with all the essential nutrients we need.

There is another surprising twist. While our intake of some nutrients is woefully low, others we consume are in excess. Both deficiencies and excesses present significant problems for bone health maintenance. In this chapter we ask, "What are these bone robbers we over-consume and how do they promote bone loss?"

❖ BONE-ROBBING NUTRITIONAL EXCESSES

Excessive Animal Protein Causes Bone Loss

Bone contains a great deal of protein in the form of collagen, and adequate protein consumption is essential for bone health. Too much dietary protein and particularly animal protein, however, is detrimental to bone and contributes to osteoporosis. The need for protein elegantly illustrates the old saying that "more is not always better." In fact, countries with lower protein consumption as a rule have lower osteoporosis rates than Western countries where animal protein is abundant. As a whole, we in the United States consume almost twice the amount of protein that is recommended by our government and nearly four times that recommended by the World Health Organization.

How does a high protein intake cause bone loss? In the process of metabolizing protein, phosphoric and sulfuric acids are produced which must first be buffered with calcium, an alkalizing mineral, before they can be excreted in the urine. There is no other mechanism for our kidneys to remove these acid products than to excrete them with calcium. Calcium is actually drawn out of the bones to reduce or buffer these by-products of protein metabolism. If protein intake is high and calcium intake is low or even moderate, a significant net loss of calcium can result. For example a recent article in the *American Journal of Clinical Nutrition* and other research indicates that the elimination of animal protein from one's diet can cut urinary calcium losses by one-half.[2-5]

Ideally protein intake should be balanced with calcium intake. However we consume too much protein and too little calcium. For example, those consuming 45 grams of protein (one half of what we generally consume) and 500 mg of calcium (the amount we generally consume) have been found to be in positive calcium balance. This means their protein intake did not cause a loss of calcium from the body. When protein intakes increase to a more typical 95 grams, calcium is lost from the body, even on a very high calcium diet.[6-9] As summarized by noted osteoporosis authority, Dr. Robert Heaney, "At low sodium and protein intakes the calcium requirements for an adult may be as little as 450 mg per day, whereas, if her intakes of both nutrients is high, she may require as much as 2,000 mg of calcium per day to maintain balance."[10]

Considerable research suggests that vegetarians who do not eat meat and generally consume a lower protein diet have greater bone density than their meat-eating counter-parts. An early comparison of bone density among British lacto-ovo vegetarians (those who eat dairy products and eggs) and meat-eaters aged 53 to 79 found the vegetarians to have greater bone density at all ages.[11] A similar study in the United States found omnivorous women aged 50 and beyond to have more osteoporosis than vegetarians.[12] Later research found that between the ages of 60 and 89 vegetarian women lost only 18 percent of their bone mass while meat-eating omnivorous women lost 35 percent of their bone mass.[12] Most recently Dr. Simin Vaghefi, a nutritionist at the University of North Florida, found lacto-ovo vegetarians aged 45 to 60 had greater bone mass than their meat-eating counterparts. Among the vegetarians she found that those who were more physically active had the highest bone densities of all. It is also interesting to note that the few vegans in her study (those vegetarians who do not eat dairy products or eggs) had lower bone density than the lacto-ovo vegetarians. While their sample of vegans was too small to draw a definite conclusion, it is clear to me that it would take a very carefully planned vegan diet to obtain all the essential bone-building nutrients. Finally, the vegetarians in this study were found to have an alkaline urine, indicating that their bodies were not drawing on precious bone-building minerals to buffer the effects of an acid meat-based diet.[13]

Conversely, Arctic Eskimos who consume a great deal of meat and relatively low calcium are reported to have a bone loss rate 15 to 20 percent higher than Caucasians. It should be noted however, that not all studies report higher bone density among vegetarians.[18, 19] For example, a 1992 study from the University of Florida found neither cortical nor trabecular bone density affected by a lacto-ovo vegetation diet.[20] Nonetheless, as an anthropologist I find the cross-cultural correlation between low meat consumption and low fracture rates quite convincing.

Excessive Phosphorus Damages Bone

Phosphorus is the second most abundant mineral in the body. Most of the two pounds contained in our body lies within our bones and is tied up with calcium. Phosphorus linked to calcium forms a crystal which gives strength and rigidity to the bones and teeth. As such phosphorus is another nutrient that is absolutely essential for bone health. Like protein, however, excessive intake contributes to bone loss and osteoporotic fractures. Here, too, balance is the central issue. The critical ratio in this case is between phosphorus and calcium.

The official U.S. recommendation is that we consume one part phosphorus to one part calcium. Our diet, however, deviates greatly from this 1:1 ratio, phosphorus intake being much higher than calcium. The American diet currently contains from two to three or even four parts phosphorus to one part calcium.[21] The problem with such high and imbalanced phosphorus intake is that it causes over-activation of the parathyroid gland which pulls calcium from the bones to increase blood calcium levels to match phosphorus levels.[22-25] Another discouraging fact is that excess phosphates also bind bone-building magnesium and prevent its absorption.

Many factors contribute to our imbalanced phosphorus-calcium intake. The first is our high consumption of meat which contains a great deal of phosphorus and protein, but is low in calcium. The second is our widespread use of processed foods, such as soft drinks, baked goods and other packaged foods to which chemical phosphates have been added.

Consider the impact of just colas and carbonated beverages to which phosphoric acid has been added in the processing. For many, a full one-quarter of our phosphorus comes from the nearly 800 servings of soft drinks the average American consumes each year.[26] Recently, the consumption of colas and other sodas containing phosphoric acid has been linked to a higher incidence of bone fractures in young girls.[27]

High Salt Intake Endangers Bone

Sodium, as found in salt, is a mineral of great importance to overall health. Yet, as with protein and phosphorus, we consume far too much of it. Today Americans consume much more salt than is desirable. Even though the United States Senate Dietary Guidelines in 1977 recommended limiting salt intake to 2,000 mg per day, our consumption still averages over 8,000 mg per day.[28] Don't be deceived into thinking your salt intake is low just because you do not use a salt shaker. The salt in our diet comes mostly from processed foods.

Salt is second only to sugar as the most popular food additive. A three piece fast food fried chicken dinner alone contains 2,285 mg of sodium; one-half of a can of soup could have 1,500 mg of sodium; one cup of canned tomato juice has 500 mg; canned carrots have five times the sodium of raw carrots and canned peas have up to 100 times the salt of fresh peas.

Our high salt intake is especially troublesome because it is combined with low potassium and calcium intakes. Here again the key concept is balance, this time between sodium, potassium and calcium. From an anthropological perspective we find that for millions of years of human evolution, dietary sodium was scarce but its counterpart potassium was abundant. The late Paleolithic diet of 40,000 years ago, for example, averaged under 700 mg of sodium daily and 16 times that amount of potassium.[29] In response to low sodium availability, the human body evolved sodium conserving and recycling mechanisms. For modern humans, however, the tables have turned. Today dietary sodium is abundant while potassium is rather scarce.

High salt intake causes the body to lose calcium in the urine, thus contributing to osteoporosis. In Holland, researchers doubled the sodium intake of Dutch students from roughly 3,000 to 6,000 mg a day and found that the kidneys increased calcium excretion by 20 percent. This is significant because most Americans regularly consume over 8,000 mg of sodium per day. This loss of calcium in the urine from high salt intake occurs in the young as well as among older members of the population.[30-32] Thus, anyone on a high sodium diet can reduce bone resorption simply by decreasing their sodium intake. A recent Australian study, in fact, found hip bone loss could be halted in women 10 years or more past menopause by either increasing calcium intake to 1768 mg per day or lowering urine sodium excretion to 2110 mg a day.[33] Limiting ourselves to the 2,000 mg of sodium per day recommended by the 1977 Dietary Guidelines, we will be guaranteed a daily urinary sodium excretion of less than 2110 mg.

The Sugar-Bone Loss Link

Our consumption of sugar and sweeteners represents a dietary pattern unprecedented in all human history. Some researchers suggest that over the last 100 years our sugar intake has increased over 1,000 times! Today Americans typically consume some 20 percent of their calories in sugar and other sweeteners. Our annual per capita consumption of sugar, corn syrups and other sweeteners averages roughly 150 pounds and includes 21 pounds of candy per person.[34] As a whole, over one half of our carbohydrate intake comes from sugar. Evidence now indicates that high sugar intake contributes to a wide range of degenerative diseases, including diabetes, arthritis, tooth decay, heart disease and osteoporosis.[35, 36]

Sugar is basically a worthless food offering just calories with no nutritional value. In the processing of sugar cane little remains of the original cane except the sweetness and the calories. In order to utilize the calories in sugar the body must take from its own storage several nutrients including the B vitamins. Moreover a high sugar intake increases the urinary excretion of essential nutrients like calcium, magnesium, chromium, copper, zinc and sodium.[37]

When sugar is combined with caffeine, as in coffee or soft drinks, even more calcium is excreted.[39] This sugar-caffeine duo is especially detrimental to bone and comprises a significant risk factor for osteoporosis especially because the average American now consumes more soft drinks than water.[38] A third complication is that sugar also limits calcium absorption.[39] In other words, the very presence of sugar saps the body of valuable and often scarce nutrients.

Finally, sugar consumption stimulates the stomach's production of hydrochloric acid. This adds to the overall acid condition of the body, which in turn is also implicated in bone loss. All in all, it is not surprising that much better tooth and bone health is seen in countries where little sugar is available.

High Dietary Fat Robs Bone

Dietary fat can be good or bad for your bones, depending on the amount and type ingested. Before it is possible to absorb minerals like calcium, the mineral must be dissolved in the hydrochloric acid of the stomach. The mineral then combines with fats to form another substance, a sort of soap, which in turn dissolves. In this form, calcium and other minerals are absorbed into the blood. Thus, sufficient high quality fats are necessary for mineral absorption. At the other extreme, however, consuming excessive fat is clearly detrimental to mineral absorption.[40] High fat intake causes poor calcium and magnesium absorption and a loss of other minerals from the body and recent research links higher fat intake with increased incidence of osteoporotic fractures.[41]

Cross-cultural analysis supports these findings as countries with lower fat intakes have lower osteoporosis rates. Estimates of average fat intake in the United States, Denmark and the United Kingdom range from 142 to 186 grams of fat per day and osteoporosis is reaching epidemic proportions. On the other hand, the fat consumption in Thailand is only 20 grams of fat per day, in the Philippines some 30 grams, Japan averages 40 grams and Taiwan 45 grams daily.[42] In these "low fat" countries osteoporosis is much less common.

In the United States some 38 to 42 percent of our calories come from fat. Fat intake among children ranges from 38 to 53 percent of all calories. We now, in fact, consume one-third more of our calories in fat than did our predecessors in the early 1900s.[43] Excessive dietary fat causes a loss of calcium from the body and is a well-known contributor to obesity, heart disease, cancer, diabetes and other degenerative diseases.

The type of fat we consume is as important as the quantity. "Cis form" essential fatty acids from vegetables are essential for humans and should be consumed while drastically limiting fat from animal sources. The common grocery store vegetable oils, however, do not supply enough of the high quality cis form essential fatty acids we need. The commercial processing of such oils with high heat and harsh chemicals alters the structure of these oils converting them into "trans fatty acids." These trans fats are not only useless but harmful to the body. We need to consume fresh cold pressed or expeller pressed vegetable oils and we need to refrigerate them for freshness. Hydrogenation, the process by which we turn liquid fats into solids, as in the making of margarine and vegetable shortening, also destroys the natural beneficial fatty acids, creating instead trans fatty acids.[44]

Caffeine Depletes Bone

It is clear that caffeine intake, even in relatively small amounts, can cause a significant loss of minerals from the bone. Caffeine causes a direct loss of calcium, magnesium, sodium and chlorine in the urine. It has also been found to lower blood calcium and increase parathyroid hormone, both of which signal the body to draw calcium from the bones.[45-49]

Research at Washington State University has shown that 300 mg of caffeine (the amount in two mugs of brewed coffee) can cause an excretion of 15 mg of calcium while also producing a loss of magnesium, sodium and chlorine.[45, 46] Although 15 mg of calcium may appear insignificant, this small loss alone is more than most of us can spare. To put this into perspective, osteoporosis researcher Dr. Robert Heaney of Creighton University calculates that a urinary calcium loss of 40 mg per day adds up to a 10 to 15 percent bone loss per decade. And a 40 mg calcium loss per day is not uncommon. His research found normal premenopausal women to be in a negative calcium balance of 20 mg per day. With the drop in estrogen at menopause an additional 24 mg of calcium was further lost in the urine, making for a total postmenopausal negative calcium balance of some 40 odd mg.[50-52] Given this general tendency for American women to be in negative calcium balance, we can see the potential importance of even 15 mg extra caffeine-induced calcium loss. Finally, additional caffeine-induced magnesium loss, even if small, could pose a serious problem given our already inadequate magnesium intake

The bone-depleting effects of caffeine are especially noted in individuals on a low calcium diet.[50] And finally, caffeine-induced calcium losses become even more significant when these losses are added to the other calcium losses caused by high intakes of protein, sugar, phosphorus, fat and sodium.

As we might expect, coffee consumption has been linked to increased fracture incidence. Women consuming more caffeine have been found to experience more fractures than those consuming less caffeine. When compared with women who almost never drink coffee, those consuming four cups per day triple the risk of hip fracture.[54] Regularly drinking just a few cups of coffee or several servings of soft drinks and teas containing caffeine could have a notable impact on bone health. And then there is the caffeine from chocolate, medications and sodas. The caffeine in soft drinks such as Coca Cola, Tab, Dr. Pepper or Pepsi can almost be as much as that found in a cup of instant coffee. On the average, Americans consume some 43 gallons of coffee and tea together each year and drink more sodas than water.[43] The "Caffeine Count" illustration in Chapter 13 details the caffeine content of common drinks and medications.

❖ ACID/ALKALINE BALANCE: A CRUCIAL OVERLOOKED FACTOR

When taken in excess, each of the substances discussed above imbalances our biochemistry in a direction that promotes osteoporosis just as an inadequacy of nutrients does. Fortunately there is a simple way to tell if your biochemical balance is being overstrained, leaving you at greater risk of excessive bone loss.

The way to monitor the overall biochemical impact of anti-nutrients, and that of your daily diet and lifestyle as a whole is by looking at your alkaline/acid balance. Alkaline/acid balance is expressed in terms of pH. Potential hydrogen, or pH, refers to the acid or alkaline nature of chemicals. In this case it refers to the acid or alkaline nature of the bodily fluids, be they blood, urine, saliva, extracellular or intracellular fluids. Essentially, we evolved in an alkaline ocean environment and our body's internal environment remains alkaline, with a pH just above 7.0. Our metabolic, enzymatic, immunologic and repair mechanisms all function their best in an alkaline environment.

While an internal alkaline balance is optimal, our biochemical functioning, the processes of living and the metabolism of food produce a great deal of acid. For example, when we exercise or move we produce lactic acid and carbon dioxide. Lactic acid is, of course, acid and the carbon dioxide in turn becomes carbonic acid in water. Phosphoric acid and sulfuric acid are likewise produced from the metabolism of the phosphorus and sulfur contained in many foods such as meats. To regain the life-supporting alkaline state, acids from all sources must be buffered or neutralized through combination with alkaline minerals. Acid-forming elements in our food include phosphorus, sulfur, chlorine and iodine. Foods in which these elements predominate leave an acid residue when metabolized. The alkaline minerals are calcium, potassium, sodium, magnesium and iron. This is the point at which bone health enters the story.

Bone contributes to the maintenance of our all-important alkaline/acid balance by buffering a portion of the acid generated from the metabolism of food. Bone contains a large reservoir of potentially mobilizable alkaline salts of calcium, sodium, magnesium and potassium. When our internal pH turns acid, these minerals are mobilized from bone to neutralize excess acidity. Prolonged and repeated utilization of alkaline minerals for acid neutralization can deplete bone and contribute to osteoporosis. Thus those with a more acid chemistry waste mineral reserves in mandatory pH balancing.[55-58]

While the link between an acid pH and osteoporosis has been known for some time, the topic has been the subject of serious investigation only recently. As mentioned earlier, Dr. Vaghefi found that vegetarians (who had the highest bone density) had an alkaline urine while the meat-eaters (with a lower bone density) had an acid urine. Her research confirmed the long-standing observation that the standard American diet high in meat and low in alkalizing fruits and vegetables left an acid residue in the body. This acid residue, in turn, is associated with bone loss and low bone density.

An important step in the direction of alkaline/acid rebalancing was recently taken by Dr. Sebastian and colleagues at the University of California in San Francisco. In a groundbreaking study reported in the *New England Journal of Medicine*[56] they looked precisely at postmenopausal bone loss and its relation to alkaline/acid balance. Their first observation was that postmenopausal women in the United States generally exhibit a low level acid state, rather than the ideal low level alkaline state, due to acids produced in metabolizing our typical high protein diet. Then they speculated that a lifetime mobilization of alkaline minerals from bone to neutralize this acid condition would contribute to a decrease in bone mass. This bone loss, they suggested, could be reduced and bone formation enhanced by neutralization of these acids and subsequent sparing of the body's alkaline minerals.

Their research findings supported these speculations. Women consuming the standard American diet containing some 80 grams of protein were given alkali in the form of potassium bicarbonate. This alkali agent neutralized internal acid production leading to a decrease in calcium and phosphorus excretion thereby stimulating new bone formation and a reduction in the rate of bone resorption.[56] Thus, facilitating a return to the "normal" alkaline state spared bonebuilding minerals and enhanced bone health. Details on how you can monitor your pH and simple ways to reestablish a bone-supporting alkaline state are given in Chapter 14.

❖ References

1 Patterson, B.H., "Fruit and vegetables in the American diet: Data from the NHanes II SURVEY," *Am. J. Public Health* 80.1443-1449 (1990).

2 Remer, Thomas, and Friedrich Manz, "Estimation of the renal net acid excretion by adults consuming diets containing variable amounts of protein," *Am J Clin Nutr* 59 (1994): 1356–61.

3 Heaney, R., "Prevention of Age-Related Osteoporosis in Women," *The Osteoporotic Syndrome: Detection, Prevention, and Treatment*, ed. L. Avioli. (New York: Grune and Stratton, Inc., 1983).

4 Sherman, H., "Calcium Requirement of Maintenance in Man," *J Biol Chem* 44 (1970): 21.

5 Nordin, B., "Osteoporosis With Particular Reference to Menopause," *The Osteoporotic Syndrome*, ed. L. Avioli. (New York: Grune and Stratton, 1983).

6 Anand, C., and H. Linkswiler, "Effect of Protein Intake on Calcium Balance of Young Men Given 500 mg Calcium Daily," *J Nutr* 104 (1974): 695–700.

7 Linkswiler, H., M. Zemel, and M. Hegsted, "Protein-Induced Hypercalciuria," *Fed Proc* 40.9 (1981): 2429–2433.

8 Hegsted, M., et al., "Urinary Calcium and Calcium Balance in Young Men as Affected By Level of Protein and Phosphorous Intake," *J Nutr* 3 (1981): 553–562.

9 Hegsted, M., and H. Linkswiler, "Long Term Effects of Level of Protein Intake on Calcium Metabolism in Young Adult Women," *J Nutr* 3 (1981): 244–251.

10 Heaney, Robert, "Heaney on Why So Much Calcium Is Needed," *New York Times* June 15 1994:

11 Ellis, F., "Incidence of Osteoporosis in Vegetarians and Omnivores," *American Journal of Clinical Research* 25 (1972): 555.

12 Sanchez, I.V., et al., "Bone Mineral Mass in Elderly Vegetarian Females," *Am J Roentgenology* 131 (1978): 542.

13 Vaghefi, Simin, personal communication (October, 1995).

14 Anderson, J., F. Tylavsky, and P. Jacobsen, "Aging and Clinical Problems in Calcium Regulation Hormones," ed. E. Ogata, and H. Orimo. (Amsterdam: Excerpta Medica Publishers, 1984).

15 Anderson, J., F. Tylavsky, and P. Jacobson, "Diet, Athletic Performance and Bone Mineral Measurements of Post-Menopausal Vegetarian and Omniverous Women," *International Congress Series 635-Exerpta Medica* 8B (1984-A): 306–309.

16 Marsh, A., T. Sanchez, and D. Mickelson, "Cortical Bone Density of Adult Lacto-Vegetarian and Omnivorous Women," *Jr of Am Dietetic Assoc* 76 (1980): 148–151.

17 Marsh, A.G., et al., "Bone Mineral Mass in Adult Lacto-Ovo-Vegetarian and Omnivorous Males," *AM J Clin Nutr* 37 (1983): 453.

18 Hunt, I.F., et al., "Bone mineral content in postmenopausal women: comparison of omnivores and vegetarians," *Am J Clin Nutr* 50:517–23.37 (1989): 924–9.

19 Lloyd, T., et al., "Urinary Hormonal concentrations and spinal bone densities of premenopausal vegetarian and nonvegetarian women," *American Journal of Clinical Nutrition* 54.6 (1991): 1005–10.

20 Tesar, R., et al., "Axial and peripheral bone density and nutrient intakes of postmenopausal vegetarian and omnivorous women," *American Journal of Clinical Nutrition* 56.4 (1991): 699–704.

21 Worthington, and B. Roberts, "Contemporary Developments in Nutrition," (St. Louis, Mo.: Mosby Co., 1981) 240–53.

22 Bland, J., "Dietary Calcium, Phosphorus and Their Relationship to Bone Formation and Parathyroid Activity," *Jr of the John Castyr College of Naturopathic Medicine* 1 (1979): 3–7.

23 Draper, H., and R. Bell, "Nutrition and Osteoporosis," *Advances in Nutritional Research*, ed. H. Draper. (New York: Plenum Press, 1979) 2:97.

24 Krook, L., et al., "Human Peridontal Disease Response to Calcium Treatment," *Cornell Vet* 62 (1972): 32–53.

25 Pennington, J., et al., "Mineral Content of Food and Total Diets: The Selected Minerals in Foods Survey, 1982 to 1984," *J Am Diet Assoc* 86 (1986): 876–891.

26 Bland, J., *Metabolic Up (Audiotape)*, (Gig Harbor, Washington: Healthcomm, Inc., 1987) (July).

27 Wyshak, Grace, Ph.D., , et al., "Bone Fractures and Diet," *Journal of Adolescent Health* 15 (1994): 210–215.

28 Shank, F.R., et al., "Perspectives of the Food and Drug Administration on Dietary Sodium," *Journal of the American Dietetic Association* 80 (1982): 29–35.

29 Eaton, S., and M. Konner, "Paleolithic Nutrition," *New England Journal of Medicine* 312 (1985): 283–289.

30 Matkovic, et al., "Urinary Calcium, Sodium and Bone Mass of Young Females," *American Journal of Clinical Nutrition* 62 (1995): 417–425.

31 Zaarkadas, M., "Sodium chloride supplementation and urinary calcium excretion in postmenopausal women," *J Clin Nutr* 50.5 (1989): 1088–94.

32 Goulding, A., "Osteoporosis: Why consuming less sodium chloride helps to conserve bone," *NZ Med J* 103 (1990): 120–2.

33 Devine, Amanda, et al., "A Longitudinal Study of the Effect of Sodium and Calcium Intake on Regional Bone Density in Postmenopausal Women," *American Journal of Clinical Nutrition* 62 (1995): 740–5.

34 Visigaitis, Gary, "How much candy we eat every year," *USA Today* June 16 1993.

35 Cleave, T., and G. Campbell, *Diabetes, Coronary Thrombosis and the Saccharine Disease*, (Bristol: John Wright and Sons, 1969).

36 Appleton, Nancy, "How Sweet It Is or Isn't," *Townsend Letter for Doctors* June (1992): 497–499.

37 Anderson, R., A. Kozlovsky, and P. Moser, "Effects of Diets High in Simple Sugars on Urinary Chromium Excretion of Humans," *Fed Proc* 44 (1985): 251.

38 Anon., "Soft Drink Consumption Surpasses Water," *Food Engineering* 58.8 (1986): 21.

39 Holl, M.G., and L.H. Allen, "Sucrose ingestion insulin response, and mineral metabolism in humans," *J Nutr* 117.7 (1987): 1229–33.

40 Weiser, N.M., et al., "High dietary fat decreases calcium absorption as fatty acids form calcium soaps," *Absorption and Malabsorption of Mineral Nutrients*, eds. I.H. Solomons, and I.H. Rosenberg. (New York: Alan R. Liss, 1984).

41 Seelig, M, *Magnesium Deficiency in the Pathogenesis of Disease*, (New York: Plenum Press, 1980).

42 Erasmus, Udo, *Fats and Oils. The Complete Guide to Fats and Oils in Health and Nutrition*, (Vancouver: Alive Books, 1986).

43 Brewster, L., and M. Jacobson, "The Changing American Diet," Washington, D.C. *Center for Science in the Public Interest* (1983).

44 Gittleman, *Super Nutrition for Menopause*, (New York: Pocket Books, 1993).

45 Massey, L., and P. Hollingbery, "Acute Effects of Dietary Caffeine and Sucrose on Urinary Mineral Excretion of Healthy Adolescents," *Nutrit Research* 8 (1988): 1005–1012.

46 Massey, L., and T. Berg, "The Effect of Dietary Caffeine on Urinary Excretion of Calcium, Magnesium, Phosphorus, Sodium, Potassium, Chloride and Zinc in Healthy Males," *Nutr Res* 5 (1985): 1281–1284.

47 Bergman, E, et al., "Effects of dietary caffeine on calcium metabolism and bone turnover in adult women," *Fed Proc* 46 (1987): 1149.

48 Harris, Susan S., and Bess Dawson-Hughes, "Caffeine and Bone Loss in Healthy Postmenopausal Women," *American Journal of Clinical Nutrition* 60 (1994): 573–8.

49 Yano, K., et al., "The Relationship Between Diet and Bone Mineral Content of Multiple Skeletal Sites in Elderly Japanese-American Men and Women Living in Hawaii," *Am J Clin Nutr* 42 (1985): 877–888.

50 Heaney, R., "Nutritional Factors in Postmenopausal Osteoporosis," *Roche Seminars on Aging* 5 (1981): 1–11.

51 Heaney, R., "Calcium Metabolic Changes at Menopause, Their Possible Relationship to Post-Menopausal Osteoporosis," *Osteoporosis II*, ed. U. Barzel. (Miami Beach, Fla.: Grune & Stratton, 1978) 101–109.

52 Heaney, R., R. Recker, and P. Saville, "Calcium Balance and Calcium Requirements in Middle-aged Women," *Am J Clin Nutr* 30 (1977): 1603–1611.

53 Barrett-Connor, Elizabeth M.D., et al., "Coffee-associated Osteoporosis Offset by Daily Milk Consumption," *JAMA* 271.4 (1994): 280–283.

54 Hernandez-Avila, Mauricio, et al., "Caffeine, moderate alcohol intake, and risk of fractures of the hip and forearm in middle-aged women," *Am J Clin Nutr* 54 (1991): 157–63.

55 Jaffe, Russell, and Patrick Donovan, "The importance of an alkaline diet," Serammune Physicians Lab, 1993.

56 Sebastian, Anthony, et al., "Improved Mineral Balance and Skeletal Metabolism in Postmenopausal Women Treated with Potassium Bicarbonate," *New England Journal of Medicine* 330.25 (1994): 1776–1781.

57 Barzel, U., "Acid Loading and Osteoporosis," *Journal of the American Geriatric Society* 30 (1982): 613.

58 Draper, H.H., and C.A. Scythes, "Calcium, phosphorus, and osteoporosis," *Fed Proc* 40.9 (1981): 2434–38.

Bone-Robbing Physical Inactivity

❖ Many Everyday Lifestyle Patterns Damage Bone

*A*s citizens of a contemporary American society we are living a vast experiment. Never before have humans been so physically inactive, eaten so much processed food, spent so much time indoors under artificial lighting, taken so many drugs and medications, undergone so many surgical procedures or exposed themselves to such a vast array of chemical, electromagnetic and informational pollution.

While the full impact of this great human experiment remains unknown, some trends are obvious. To me the most striking of these is the unprecedented ever rising predominance of degenerative disease. Cancer, which did not even rank among the top 10 causes of death at the turn of this century, now kills nearly one in four of us. Heart disease, also not among the top 10 United States causes of death even 100 years ago, now causes over one-third of all deaths. Diabetes, a disease unknown in much of the world, affects over 12 million Americans and its incidence is constantly rising. High blood pressure, which was not even reported until the introduction of commercial salt, now threatens one in four of all Americans and two of three over 65 years of age.[1]

Bone health has also degenerated to the point that after age 50 one of two Caucasian American women will suffer a needless osteoporotic fracture.[2] Many men and growing numbers of the young also have bones too weak to withstand the stresses and strains of ordinary daily activity.

The question I often ask myself is how has all this degeneration and disease come about. What are the processes at work in our culture that so damage our health? How, in particular, did we lose our natural birthright to lifelong healthy bones?

❖ Physical Inactivity Causes Bone Loss

In previous chapters we reviewed the impact dietary excesses and deficiencies, lifestyle factors, smoking, drugs, toxic metals, alcohol and even stress could have on bone health. In this chapter we look at physical inactivity, another of our self-inflicted bone-depleting lifestyle factors. I believe that our sedentary lifestyle ranks right beside inadequate nutrition as a major cause of our current osteoporosis epidemic.

Better Bones, Better Body, Better Exercise

Low levels of physical fitness are associated not only with poor bone health but also with overall poor health. Lack of regular exercise has been scientifically linked to a broad spectrum of chronic conditions including heart disease; hypertension; stroke; cancer of the colon, lung and breast; diabetes; low back pain; obesity; depression and anxiety in addition to osteoporosis.[2] Most studies show, for example, that the risk of having a heart attack or stroke in an unfit individual is some eightfold greater than in a physically fit person.[3] In a large-scale study of male Harvard alumni, those who participated in sports activities of moderate intensity had a risk of dying from any cause that was 23 to 29 percent lower than that of the subjects who never participated in sports. In discussing these findings, the principal author of this study, Dr. Paffenbarger, suggests that each hour of physical activity brings you one, two or even three extra hours of life.[4] Many other studies confirm this finding. For example, a large 16-year study of Norwegian men found the most physically fit men had half the risk of dying from any cause as compared to the least physically fit men. This lower death rate among the fitter men was attributable chiefly to a lower risk of dying of cardiovascular causes.[5]

While many of the fitness studies have been done on men, the benefits of exercise equally pertains to women. By simply walking two to three miles a day at any pace, women experience a 6-percent increase in beneficial HDL, which represents an 18-percent drop in heart disease risk.[6] Women who exercise vigorously at least once a week reduced their risk of adult diabetes by one-third.[6] Also the habit of lifelong exercise has been documented to reduce a woman's chance of stroke by one-half.[7] In another study of Harvard alumni, this time on females, it was found that women who were athletes in college had less risk of developing cancers of the reproductive system including cancer of the uterus, ovary, cervix or vagina as they aged. These former athletes also experienced only half the risk of breast cancer than did their non-athletic counterparts. Looking at breast cancer alone, University of Southern California researchers found that women who spent 3.8 or more hours per week in physical exercise experienced a 58 percent reduction in breast cancer incidence compared to inactive women.[8] Finally, a study from Scripps College in California showed that older people who get plenty of exercise mentally outperform their more sedentary counterparts, even when their overall health levels were the same.

Exercise Builds Bone

Whatever controversies surround our understanding of osteoporosis, there is wide agreement that physical activity, exercise and fitness are foremost factors promoting the creation and maintenance of strong bones. Physical activity builds bone at all ages and bone mass maintenance is a natural response to strain loading placed upon it.[9] Bone density is greater in persons with occupations requiring physical exertion than those involved in sedentary work.[10-12] Athletes have greater bone density than non-athletes. For example a recent analysis of spinal bone density comparing young men who participated in regular, vigorous exercise as opposed to those who did not found a 14 percent greater trabecular bone mineral density in the exercise groups.[13] Even among athletes, the bone density varies according to the amount of strain loading stimulus, as we shall detail. Equally among non-athletic older women, those who are more physically active have higher bone density and suffer fewer fractures.[14,15] If you are looking for a minimum exercise cut-off point, one study reported that women doing vigorous exercise two or more times a week, or total physical activity of four hours a week, had greater bone density than women with lower activity levels.

Keep in mind also that physical activity appears to have a systemic as well as local effect. The stressed bone gains density, yet to some degree the entire skeleton also benefits.[16, 17] Overall, exercise researcher Dr. Gail Dalsky from the University of Connecticut Health Center reports that for the normally active person, an exercise training program can yield as much as 5 to 10 percent increase in bone mass. Even larger gains in bone mass can be experienced by those who have less bone density before beginning the exercise program.[18] Dr. William Evans at the Human Nutrition Research Center on Aging at Tufts University is an even more outspoken advocate of exercise. If women exercise throughout their lives, he comments, they will never have the low bone density that ultimately results in osteoporosis.[19]

Exercise builds and maintains bone at all ages. It is absolutely essential for optimum bone development in the young, and without it aging bone regeneration is limited. Nutrition alone cannot bring about maximum peak bone mass or maintain optimum bone mass as we age. Exercise is not optional.[20]

Inactivity Drains Bone

Just as exercise builds bone, a lack of exercise harms bone. Rapid atrophy of both bone and muscle occurs during prolonged bed rest, paralytic syndromes, immobilization from splints or casts or any period of reduced activity. Adults hospitalized and restricted to bed rest for low back pain lose almost one percent of their lumbar spine mass per week.[21] An even greater rate of bone loss occurs among adolescent girls confined to bed rest after undergoing an operation for scoliosis and in patients with spinal cord injury. Fortunately for those forced into bed rest, the body in all its wisdom provides for an unknown mechanism to limit this excessive bone loss. In such cases, once about 30 percent of one's trabecular bone is lost a new steady state is reached and no further bone mass is lost, even though one remains inactive. Interestingly, standing for two or more hours per day can reverse the loss of bone mass induced by bed rest, while even regular exercise performed in bed, for as much as four hours daily, does not stop bone loss.[22]

Another often-noted observation is that weightlessness, as experienced by astronauts, also leads to rapid bone loss. More relevant to the vast majority of us, however, is the well documented fact that even less extreme forms of inactivity, such as that imposed by a sedentary lifestyle, can also cause bone loss and contribute to osteoporosis.

The Bone-Muscle Link

One of the most useful, yet little mentioned findings is the correlation between muscle mass and bone mass. If we build muscle, we build bone. Conversely, if we lose muscle, we lose bone. Overall skeletal strength correlates directly with total muscle mass, and individual bone strength generally correlates with the strength of the muscles attached to it. Archaeologists, in fact, use bone strength and form to estimate muscle strength of prehistoric peoples.

Recent research comparing middle-aged Seventh Day

Adventist women with non-Adventists clearly demonstrates this relationship between lean body mass, that is muscle, and bone indices.[23] In these studies, lean body mass was found to be the best single predicator of skeletal strength. Probing further into the relationship between muscle mass and bone mass a more recent Mayo Clinic study found a significant positive correlation between bone mineral density and back extensor muscle strength in postmenopausal Caucasian women.[22] Women with stronger back muscles have stronger vertebrae and stronger hip bones as other studies also document.[24] Overall, bone mass correlates well with muscle mass and general fitness level. Less fit people have both less muscle mass and less bone mass just as they have less aerobic capacity. Weight training is a very effective way to build muscle mass.

How Exercise Builds Bone

While the full details of how physical activity actually encourages and even dictates bone development are not yet totally clear, some of the mechanisms are obvious. First, exercise increases the flow of nutrients, energy and information to all segments of the bone from the osteocyte bone cells buried deep inside to cells on the surface of each bone. Second, physical activity transmits pressure and tension to bone by the actions of muscles. Both of these forces appear mediated through electrical signals induced by physical activity. It appears to be these physical activity-induced electrical currents which signal the bone cells to repair and regenerate.[9, 25]

All Exercise Is Not Equal

While any physical activity is better than none, certain types of activity build bone better than others. The more weight-bearing exercises yield greater bone benefits than the lesser weight-bearing exercises. Thus among athletes, weight lifters have the highest bone density, followed by throwers, runners, soccer players and lastly, swimmers.[26] Nonweight-bearing activities like swimming do build some bone mass, but not as much as weight-bearing exercises do.[27]

Less strenuous activities like simple walking can help maintain bone mass, but generally more vigorous activity is needed to actually build bone. All things being equal, the more strenuous the activity, the more bone built. For example, exercising vigorously twice a week builds bone mass a bit, doing the same three times a week builds bone even more. Among women at menopause and beyond high intensity strength-training exercises done only twice a week over one year yielded detectable increases in spinal and hip density. The matched control group of women who did not exercise lost an average of 2.5 percent from the hip and 1.8 percent from the spine.[30] Stepping up the workout schedule yields even greater bone density gains as we shall see in Chapter 15.

Finally it is worth noting that while endurance exercise is most beneficial for the cardiovascular system, bone may respond differently. Scientists now suggest that short periods of dynamic strain have the most stimulating effect on bone. Thus they propose that short periods of diverse weight-bearing exercises should be more effective than long periods of running, bicycling or swimming.[9] Supporting this concept is recent British research reporting that two-legged jumps, jumping up and down 50 times a day can increase bone density and reduce the risk of hip fractures in premenopausal women.[31] It will be interesting to see how experiments with short bursts of dynamic strain loading unfold.

How Many of Us Get the Exercise We Need?

How many of us get enough physical activity? Whether we are talking about preventing heart disease or building bone health, most Americans do not get adequate exercise. According to the National Center for Health Statistics, 58.1 percent of all Americans reported irregular or no leisure time activity in 1991. In addition, data from the U.S. Preventive Services Task Force suggest that only 20 percent of the adult population exercise at a level recommended for cardiovascular benefit while 40 percent claim some exercise and another 40 percent are completely sedentary.

Vigorous exercise is also declining among high school students according to a 1994 government report. Only 37 percent of the 11,631 high school students studied got regular exercise (defined as 20 minutes of vigorous exercise three times a week). Just six years ago the figure was 62 percent. Only 25 percent of the girls surveyed were physically active and by 12th grade this figure dropped to 17 percent. Half of all boys exercised, and unlike the girls, their activity rate did not drop with age.[32] Fitness among children is declining yearly as measured by increasing obesity and decreasing cardiovascular endurance. Since the 1960s obesity has increased 54 percent in children ages 6 to 11 and 39 percent among those 12 to 17. There was also a 98-percent increase in super-obesity among children of all ages.[33] Today some

34 percent of all children are overweight as compared to 24 percent in 1984.[34] Overall 33 percent of all Americans are overweight, a rise from 25 percent in 1980.

Too Much of A Good Thing: Can Exercise Cause Osteoporosis?

You might have heard that excessive exercise can lead to excessive bone loss, but this is not really so. While it is well established that top level female athletes can experience excessive bone loss and a high rate of fractures, the strenuous exercise *per se* is not to blame. Rather it is the strenuous exercise practiced in the face of inadequate nutrition, and the resultant hormonal imbalance manifested as a cessation of menstrual periods that causes the bone loss.

Athletic amenorrhea, not exercise, is the problem. For example, among young athletes spinal bone density was highest in those women who had regular periods, a little lower in those with a history of some irregular periods and much lower in those who never had regular cycles.[35] Overall young women who experience amenorrhea (no periods) average 25 percent less trabecular bone than women with regular periods and 10 percent less cortical bone.[36] Exposed to the stresses of rigorous exercise, bone this thin can fracture needlessly. In 1991 the medical literature documented the first non-traumatic hip fracture in an amenorrheic female. Without traumatic provocation, a 32-year-old woman simply broke her hip in the 13th mile of a marathon run.[37] While physical activity is a foremost stimulator of bone, exercise alone cannot build bone or maintain bone without adequate nutrients.

❖ References

1 Trowell, H., and P. Burkitt, ed., *Western Diseases: Their Emergence and Prevention*, (Boston: Harvard University Press, 1981).

2 National Osteoporosis Foundation, Audrey Singer, "personal communication (October 20, 1995).

3 Powell, Kenneth E, et al., "Physical activity and chronic diseases," *Am J Clin Nutr* 49 (1989): 999–1006.

4 Paffenbarger, Ralph S., et al., "The Association Of Changes In Physical-Activity Level And Other Lifestyle Characteristics With Mortality Among Men," *The New England Journal Of Medicine* 328.8 (1993): 538–545.

5 Sandvik, Leiv, et al., "Physical Fitness As A Predictor Of Mortality Among Healthy, Middle-Aged Norwegian Men," *New England Journal of Medicine* 328.8 (1993): 533–7.

6 Snider, Mike, "A stroll is still good for the heart," *USA Today* December 18, 1991.

7 Laino, Charlene, "Exercise From 25 on Guards Against Stroke," *Family Practice News* August 26, 1993: 20.

8 Bernstein, Leslie, et al., "Physical Exercise and Reduced Risk of Breast Cancer in Young Women," *Journal of the National Cancer Institute* 86.18 (1994): 1403–1407.

9 Lanyon, L. E., "Skeletal Responses to Physical Loading," *Physiology and Pharmacology of Bone*, ed. Gregory R. Mundy, and John T. Martin. (Berlin: Springer-Verlag, 1993) 107: 485–505.

10 Smith, E., W. Reddan, and P. Smith, "Physical Activity and Calcium Modalities for Bone Mineral Increase in Aged Women," *Med Sci Sports Exerc* 13.1 (1981): 60–64.

11 Smith, E., and C. Gilligan, "Effects of Inactivity and Exercise on Bone," *The Physician and Sports Medicine* 15.11 (1987): 91–100.

12 Everett L., et al., "Deterring Bone Loss by Exercise Intervention in Premenopausal and Postmenopausal Women," *Calcif Tissue Int* 44.312–321 (1989).

13 Block, J.E., et al., "Greater Vertebral Bone Mineral Mass in Exercising Young Men," *West Jr Med* 145 (1986): 39.

14 Paganini-Hill, et al., "Exercise and other factors in the prevention of hip fracture: the Leisure World study," *Epidemiology* 1.2 (1991): 16–25.

15 Carter, M.D., et al., "Bone mineral content at three sites in normal perimenopausal women," *Clin Orthop* 266 (1991): 295–300.

16 Rikli, R.E., and B.G. McManis, "Effects of exercise on bone mineral content in postmenopausal women," *Res Q Exerc Sport* 61.3 (1990): 243–9.

17 Brewer, V., B. Meyer, and M. Keele, "Role of Exercise in Prevention of Involutional Bone Loss," *Med Sci Sports Exerc* 15.6 (1983): 445–449.

18 Dalsky, G.P., "The role of exercise in the prevention of osteoporosis," *Compr-Thor* Sep:15 (1989): 30–7.

19 Evans, William, personal communication, (1995).

20 Halioua, Lydia, and John JB Anderson, "Lifetime calcium intake and physical activity habits: independent and combined effects on the radial bone of healthy premenopausal Caucasian women," *Am J Clin Nutr* 49 (1989): 534–41.

21 Krolner, B., and B. Toft, "Vertebral Bone Loss: An Unneeded Side Effect of Therapeutic Bed Rest," *Clin Science* 64 (1983): 537–540.

22 Sinaki, M., "Exercise and Physical Therapy," *Osteoporosis Etiology, Diagnosis and Management*, ed. B. Riggs, and J. Melton. (New York: Raven Press, 1988).

23 Anderson, J. et al., "Diet, athletic performance and bone mineral measurements of post-menopausal vegetarian and omnivorous women." "Endocrine control of bone and calcium metabolism." International Congress, Series 635 *Excerpta Medica*, 1987: 306–309.

24 Halle, J.S., et al., "Relationship between trunk muscle torque and bone mineral content of the lumbar spine and hip in healthy postmenopausal women," *Phys Ther* 70.11 (1990): 690–9.

25 Becker, R., and G. Selden, *The Body Electric: Electromagnetism and the Foundation of Life*, (New York: William Morrow & Co., 1985).

26 Nilsson, B.E., et al., "Bone Density in Athletes," *Clinical Orthop* 71 (1971): 179.

27 Jacobson, P.C., et al., "Bone density in women: college athletes and older athletic women," *J Orthop Res* 2 (1984): 328–332.

28 Dalsky, G., "Exercise: Its Effects on Bone Mineral Content," *Clinical Obstetrics and Gynecology* 30.4 (1987): 820–832.

29 Cavanaugh, DJ, and CE Cann, "Brisk walking does not stop bone loss in postmenopausal women," *Bone* 9. 4 (1988): 201–204.

30 Nelson, Miriam, et al., "Effects of High-Intensity Strength Training on Multiple Risk Factors for Osteoporotic Fractures: A Randomized Controlled Trial," *JAMA* 272.24 (1994): 1909–1914.

31 Anon, "Jumping can strengthen bone, reduce fractures," *Medical Tribune* November 25, 1993:

32 Elias, Marilyn, "Fewer teens exercise their workout option," *USA Today* November 8 1994:

33 Mead, Nathaniel, "Kids and Fat," *Natural Health* 1992: 101.

34 Hellmich, Nanci, "Today's Kids Weigh In Heavier," *USA Today* September 25 1992:

35 Drinkwater, Barbara L, et al., "Menstrual History as a Determinant of Current Bone Density in Young Athletes," *JAMA* 263.4 (1990): 545–548.

36 Cann, C., et al., "Spinal Mineral Loss in Oophorectomized Women," *J Am Med Assoc* 244 (1980): 2056–2059.

37 Dugowson, C. F., "Nontraumatic femur fracture in an oligamenorrheic female," *Medicine & Science in Sports & Exercise* 23.12 (1991): 1323–5.

Chapter 7

Other Bone-Robbing Lifestyle Factors

❖ TOBACCO HARMS BONE

*T*obacco use is closely associated with the development of osteoporosis.[1-3] Women who smoke one pack a day during adulthood have 5 to 10 percent less bone mass at the age of menopause than do nonsmokers.[4] Swedish studies report that the bone density of a 70-year-old woman who smokes is equivalent to an 80-year-old nonsmoker.[5] Men who smoke a pack a day over 16 years have twice the bone loss and average 5.8 percent less bone mineral density than nonsmokers. Everyone who smokes doubles their risk of osteoporotic fractures.[6,7] Noted osteoporosis expert, Dr. John Aloia, suggests that 10 to 20 percent of all hip fractures in women are attributable to smoking.[8] Smokers are also very much more likely to suffer vertebral fractures and even ex-smokers show an increased risk over women who have never smoked.[5,9]

Overall, patients with osteoporotic fractures are twice as

likely to smoke than are those who do not suffer fractures.[10] Smoking also hinders bone self-repair and when injured the bones of smokers heal more slowly than nonsmokers.

Smoking Damages Bone in Many Ways

Smoking inflicts its damage in many ways. First, it toxifies the liver which can in turn contribute to poor vitamin D activation and decreased blood levels of free estrogen. This anti-estrogenic effect of smoking is quite interesting. Some researchers suggest that smoking is sufficiently anti-estrogenic to cancel the beneficial effects of estrogen therapy. Thus women who smoke cannot expect to reduce their risk of hip fractures by using estrogen drugs. Likewise, smoking is also associated with lower testosterone levels in males. Lowered levels of both estrogen and testosterone increase the risk of osteoporosis. Smoking also depletes the body of certain nutrients, especially vitamin C, which are essential for bone building. In addition, smoking increases the body's toxic burden of cadmium, lead, nicotine and dozens of other toxic substances which interfere with calcium absorption and directly damage bone.[11,12]

Roughly one-third of all Americans over 21 years of age smoke and smoking is the leading cause of premature deaths in the United States.[17] In addition, an estimated 22 million people in the United States use smokeless tobacco. A figure of concern is the increased incidence of smoking among women ages 20 to 24. Each year tobacco use costs the nation over $52 billion in health care expenses and productivity losses.[13-15]

❖ ALCOHOL ROBS BONE

As of the mid-1980s each person in this country, on a yearly basis, consumed an average of 28 gallons of beverages containing alcohol.[14] About that same time, average annual water consumption was 39 gallons.[16] Authorities estimate that there are over 25 million alcoholics in the United States today and alcoholism is one of the most expensive health problems in the country today with a projected annual cost to the nation of $160 billion in 1995. Alcohol is a substance toxic to the human body which produces wide-ranging negative effects. It's not surprising, therefore, to find that alcohol also damages bone. It has been noted for some time that alcoholics are more likely to suffer from osteoporosis than the population at large.[2, 17] Chronic alcoholism may be five to ten times more frequent among patients with fractures than among those without fractures.

How Does Alcohol Cause Bone Loss?

Alcohol use damages bone in many ways. First, those who consume high amounts of alcohol tend to be malnourished and frequently underconsume calcium, magnesium, protein, vitamin C and other essential bone-building nutrients.[18] To make this situation worse, alcohol consumption both inhibits absorption and increases excretion of important bone-building nutrients like calcium, magnesium, vitamin C, zinc and copper.[19] Alcohol also appears to inhibit vitamin B_6 functioning. In addition, alcohol damages the liver, an organ very important in vitamin D metabolism and bone health. It is also directly toxic to bone cells, causing a decrease in spongy inner trabecular bone.[20] If all this is not enough, both short- and long-term ingestion of alcohol reduces blood testosterone concentration in men. Finally, chronic alcohol intake is often combined with the long-term use of aluminum-containing antacids, which are also devastating to bone. This exposure to aluminum worsens bone loss by disrupting the body's phosphorus balance, causing considerable loss of calcium when large amounts of aluminum are consumed.

Whatever its varied actions, research now confirms that those who consume large amounts of alcohol run a greater risk of cumulative, unnatural bone loss leading to osteoporotic fractures.[21-24]

Is Moderate Drinking a Problem for Bone Health?

Some, but not all, studies suggest that alcohol abusers may not be the only ones at risk for alcohol-induced bone loss. A few researchers report that even a few drinks a day could be detrimental to bone. In one study of social drinkers, men who drank alcoholic beverages ran nearly two-and-a-half times the risk of osteoporosis as nondrinkers.[2] In another study women who drank in moderation, consuming just under one ounce of alcohol per day, had over two times the risk of hip fracture as compared with women who did not consume alcohol.[25]

❖ Under-Nutrition, Dieting and Anorexia Accelerate Bone Loss

The Dieting-Osteoporosis Link

It is now clear that the nutrition and exercise patterns of our youth are strong determinants of bone health in old age. If during the "growing" years we give our body all the nutrient building blocks it needs, and if we get plenty of physical activity, our adult bones will be dense and strong. If young people are poorly nourished, and tend to be "couch potatoes," they will not fulfill their genetic potential for peak bone mass. Their bones will be thin and less strong as they move into adulthood. If one has a low bone density at the beginning of adult life, one is much more likely to develop osteoporosis as one ages.[26]

The generalized poor nutrient intake of many Americans is made worse by the large scale tendency towards dieting and worse yet, crash dieting. Many women, and some men, spend much of their lives alternating between binge eating and semi-starvation diets attempting to be fashionably thin. Patterns of self-imposed under-nourishment often begin early in life as adolescents become weight conscious. For example, essential bone building nutrients like vitamin B_6, A, iron, calcium, zinc, copper and magnesium are those most commonly deficient in the diets of adolescent girls and dieting makes things worse.[28]

The most consistent finding among the hundreds of osteoporosis studies I have read is the link between osteoporosis and low body weight. Researchers find body weight to be one of the best predicators of bone mineral density. Thin women have thin bones.[29-32] This is eminently logical. Under-weight persons do not consume enough calories to maintain their weight and right along with low calorie consumption goes low nutrient consumption. Lifelong low nutrient intake guarantees low bone mass.

Anorexia Debilitates Bone

At the extreme end of the current "thinness mania" we find anorexia. Anorexia is a form of self-imposed starvation, which is all too frequent in our culture. It is estimated that nearly one million people in America are victims of anorexia and 15 percent, that is 150,000 people, mostly women, are dying of it.[33] Excessive bone loss is one of the many health problems stemming from anorexia. Adult women with an-orexia were found to have 30 percent less bone density than those without the disorder. Worse yet, teenagers whose menstrual periods ceased as a result of anorexia had bones that were even 20 percent weaker than adult anorexics.[34] Anorexic women frequently show a three percent per year loss of trabecular bone. During periods of hospitalization and tube-feeding, bone loss is even greater, so that one year after hospitalization a woman might lose a total of 17 per-cent of her pretreatment trabecular bone. Such rapid bone loss can cause osteoporosis within a few years.[35] We need not go to the extreme of anorexia, however, to see the impact of under-eating and under-nourishment on bone health. Every single day our body requires that we consume sig-nificant quantities of over 40 essential nutrients. If we do not consume these nutrients, we do not provide our body with the basic building blocks it needs for growing and maintaining health. "A house built on a weak foundation will not stand," so goes the old saying. Nowhere is this more true than in the area of bone health. The strong foundation for lifelong healthy bones must be built in youth and maintained in adulthood. Under-eating and crash dieting damages bone. Half of all American women consume less than 1493 calories per day, a level where it is next to impossible to create meals which provide the RDA for the main nutrients required for optimum bone health.[36]

The negative impact of under-eating frequently manifests itself among female athletes. Many consume too few calories, and this is directly linked to osteoporosis. Athletes who weigh less than 75 percent of their ideal weight suffer many more stress fractures that those with an ideal weight. Further, excessive weight and body fat loss can cause a cessation of menstrual periods. With the loss of menstrual periods comes premature and often excessive bone loss. Young, apparently healthy, female athletes are becoming osteoporotic, suffering needless fractures and jeopardizing skeletal integrity by indulging in under-nutrition.

❖ Many Medications Cause Osteoporosis

A variety of medications can directly cause unusual and excessive bone loss. These include: corticosteroids, thyroid hormones, aluminum containing antacids, some diuretics, anti-convulsant therapy and antibiotics. Other medications like tranquilizers, sedatives and antidepressants increase the risk of osteoporotic fracture by increasing the risk of falling. For example, in this country each year 32,000 hip fractures (over 11 percent of all hip fractures) are attributed to prescription drugs that leave the elderly sedated or imbalanced.[37]

Corticosteroids

Adrenal cortical steroid drugs are given to treat inflammatory conditions allergies, collagen disorders such as
lupus, arthritis and other diseases. Cortisone and prednisone
are two of the most commonly prescribed corticosteroids.
Extended corticosteroid use has long been associated with
osteoporotic fractures[42, 44] and an estimated 20 percent of the
patients on long-term corticosteroid therapy suffer osteoporotic fractures. Among patients on steroid treatment for
rheumatoid arthritis, the figure rises to 40 percent. Looking
at it another way, patients with fractures have been reported
to be 5 to 10 times more likely to be on appreciable amounts
of corticosteroid drugs than others not suffering fractures.[38]

Just how much steroid medication can be taken before
bones begin to fracture? While not a well studied question,
a recent analysis of vertebral collapse in those with juvenile
chronic arthritis reported that no patients sustained vertebral
collapse until they had received a cumulative dose of at least
five grams of prednisone. These researchers concluded that
the ideal dose of prednisone should not exceed five mg per
day, probably best given as 10 mg on alternate days.[41] Endo-
crinologist Drs. Adler and Rosen suggest that patients who
receive glucocorticoid therapy for more than a few weeks
are clearly at risk of osteoporosis.[42] Preliminary investigation
suggests that high dose use of steroid inhalers is also linked
to bone loss.[43] Steroid hormones damage bone in many
ways. They decrease the synthesis of collagen and protogly-
can. Steroids also appear to increase parathyroid hormone,
inhibit calcium absorption, increase urinary loss of calcium,
lower estrogen levels, impair bone buildup and increase
bone breakdown.[44, 45]

Preliminary research suggests that the consumption of supplemental nutrients can limit bone loss induced by steroid medications. The nutritional substances used with greatest effect include a specially processed bone product called microcrystalline hydroxyapatite (MCHC), calcium and vitamin D. Particularly interesting results have been shown with MCHC. In several studies, six to eight grams of MCHC daily were found to dramatically reduce skeletal pain and bring about favorable bone changes in patients on prednisone therapy. Steroid-induced bone loss was reduced or halted and at times bone density was even increased on this therapy.[46-48] So striking were the study results that one set of British scientists concluded their study on rheumatoid arthritis with the recommendation that the MCHC should be started right along with the corticosteroid rather than waiting for osteoporosis to develop.[48] Equally, preliminary studies showed steroid-induced bone loss to be slowed and fracture incidence decreased with the use of 500 mg calcium twice a day along with the prescription drug Calcitrol, an active metabolite of vitamin D.

Thyroid Hormones

The thyroid is a tiny paired gland which regulates countless aspects of our metabolism. An excess of thyroid hormone from thyroid medication can result in excessively active metabolism and subsequent bone loss. Some, but not all, researchers suggest that overprescription of thyroid medication can contribute significantly to an increased incidence of osteoporosis. Many, but not all studies, suggest that supplemental thyroid hormone, especially in high doses, causes bone loss. Other studies, however, report little or no link between thyroid supplementation and bone loss. If you use thyroid hormones, it would be wise to have your hormone levels carefully monitored and to take only the minimum necessary amount.[50-53] A few researchers suggest that such loss is reported to occur even if the patient exhibits no clinical or biological signs of excessive thyroid replacement therapy.

Aluminum-Containing Antacids

Many popular antacids contain aluminum in the form of aluminum hydroxide. Aluminum is toxic to bone, inhibits calcium absorption, interferes with mineralization and collagen production and thus contributes to excessive bone loss.[54-57] Aluminum-containing antacids include Rolaids, Maalox, Mylanta, Di-Gel and Gelusil. On a diet low in calcium, even small doses of aluminum-containing antacids can cause a loss of calcium from the body. The lower a person's calcium intake the greater risk that aluminum-containing antacids will cause bone loss.[58]

Diuretics

Selected diuretics such as Lasix, Edecrin, Diamox, Aldactazide or Aldactone and Dyazide have been shown to significantly increase urinary calcium excretion. These drugs encourage bone loss.[59]

Antibiotics

While in many ways antibiotics are the "miracle drugs" of the 20th century, they also bring with them varied detrimental effects. Most notably antibiotics kill off health-promoting friendly bacteria in the process of destroying the targeted harmful bacteria. These friendly bacteria aid in digestion and themselves actually manufacture at least seven essential nutrients including vitamins B_2, B_6, B_{12} and K. Antibiotics upset the intestinal bacterial balance which can result in weakened digestion and decreased nutrient absorption as well as Candida (yeast) overgrowth. Decreased absorption can lead to malnourishment. Yeast infections cause a whole series of health problems recognized as the "Candida Syndrome."[60-62] Because of all of these processes, antibiotics indirectly hamper bone health. In addition, tetracycline directly threatens bone by decreasing calcium absorption. Those interested in natural alternatives to antibiotics will find valuable information in *Beyond Antibiotics* by Drs. Lendon Smith and Michael Schmidt.

Unfortunately, you do not have to take antibiotics to be exposed to them. Approximately half of all antibiotics manufactured in the United States are given to animals raised for food. According to 1979 figures from the Office of Technology Assessment, 99 percent of all poultry, 90 percent of swine and 70 percent of cattle are routinely given antibiotics.

Other Medications

Other medications known to cause bone loss include drugs for tuberculosis (para-amino salicylic acid), some chemotherapeutic agents such as methotrexate and anticonvulsants such as Dilantin. Foremost osteoporosis researcher Dr. Steven Cummings has found that older women taking anti-convulsants are at especially high risk for hip fracture.[63] Long term anticonvulsant use, for example, can create a vitamin D deficiency which leads to bone loss. In these cases, treatment with vitamin D and calcium may help. New research, however, suggests that the increased risk for anticonvulsant drugs might be due to impairments of neuromuscular function rather than bone loss *per se*.[30]

The use of the injectable contraceptive depo medroxy-progesterone (DMPA), which reduces ovarian estrogen production, is also associated with a loss of bone density. Current users of DMPA with a minimum of five years previous use were found to have 7.5 percent less spinal bone mass and 6.6 percent less hip bone density than similar women not on the drug.[64] This finding from New Zealand is very important as DMPA is being widely promoted within developing countries.

Finally, the use of psychotrophic drugs for depression and mental illness have been found to increase one's risk of suffering an osteoporotic fracture. The sedative effects of these drugs increase one's risk of falling which in turn increases the likelihood of fracture. A recent epidemiological study of persons 65 years and older showed that current users of long half-life psychotrophic benzodiazepines, such as Valium and Librium, ran a 70 to 80 percent greater risk of hip fracture than persons not using psychotrophic drugs.[65] Again, this link between tranquilizers and hip fractures was recently confirmed by the large scale 1995 Cummings study.[66]

❖ Toxic Metal Exposure Damages Bone

Toxic metals including lead, mercury, cadmium, aluminum and tin are not easily excreted and can accumulate in the body. Each is damaging to bone and contributes to bone loss.

Lead inhibits activation of vitamin D and limits calcium intake. Humans suffering from chronic lead poisoning exhibit bone abnormalities and animals injected with lead exhibit bone loss in all parts of the skeleton.[67, 68] A special risk for postmenopausal women, lead can be stored in bone displacing calcium; it can later being returned to the blood as the bone is demineralized.[69] Studies on American women have shown a significant increase in blood lead levels during menopause as a result of bone breakdown freeing stored lead. This circulating lead can in turn aggravate osteoporosis by inhibiting vitamin D activation and calcium uptake.[69]

Dr. Alan Gaby in his comprehensive review of toxic metals and osteoporosis points to an interesting additional way in which lead might contribute to osteoporosis. This involves lead's interference with the hormone progesterone. In one study the administration of 0.5 percent lead in the diet of pregnant mice prevented the rise in plasma progesterone that normally occurs during pregnancy.[70, 71] As we shall see in the next chapter, progesterone deficiency has been linked to the development of osteoporosis among young women. The obvious question is, "What causes progesterone deficiency?" Lead exposure might be a part of the answer.

Widespread lead poisoning is well documented and a major public health problem within the United States. Unacceptably high levels of lead are found in our air, water, food and soils. Sources of lead exposure include drinking water, auto exhaust, industrial processes, lead-based paints, dust in and around homes and buildings, leaded glass, leaded gasoline, pottery glaze, hair dyes and rinses, pesticides, newsprint, solder, batteries, inks, lead-soldered food cans, tobacco smoke, waste incineration and land fills.[70, 72]

Cadmium has a damaging effect on the kidneys and alters calcium metabolism. This toxic metal can be found in cigarette smoke (smokers have twice the body burden of cadmium as nonsmokers) paints, metal plating, colored plastics, fertilizers and fungicides, antiseptics, solder, batteries, gasoline, soil and air around cities and industrialized areas, land fills, sewage sludge and waste incineration.[72]

Aluminum, as already mentioned, also damages bone. It interferes with the mineralization process and modifies collagen production and bone formation in addition to lessening calcium absorption. Even small quantities of aluminum such as from aluminum-containing antacids can lead to negative calcium balance. Unlike our ancestors, we today are exposed to unprecedented amounts of aluminum. As Dr. Alan Gaby in his review of the topic summarizes, aluminum is everywhere.[70] This toxic metal along with a host of other environmental pollutants make an undeniable and significant contribution to the development of osteoporosis and the full array of the diseases of civilization.

The major sources of aluminum exposure are aluminum-containing antacids, aluminum cookware, aluminum foils, aluminum-containing antiperspirants, tin cans, baking powders, food additives, soft water and aluminosilicates from aerosol contaminants.[54-57, 72]

❖ Stress is an Unsuspected Bone Killer

Believe it or not, stress also contributes to osteoporosis. Stress imbalances endocrine gland functioning and can lead to an excretion of calcium and other nutrients into the urine. For example, under stress the adrenal gland produces cortisol, a hormone which mobilizes calcium from the bone and increases urinary calcium loss. As one calcium researcher reports, "If we have a bad marriage, we are probably spilling calcium. If we are having a row with the neighbors, we are probably spilling calcium."[73] Also depression, another stress related condition, has recently been linked to excessive bone loss by German researchers.

The thoughts we think and the way we respond to stress have a great deal to do with our health, even with bone health. Undesirable stress comes in many packages: accidents, emotional and economic difficulties, life crises, health problems and so on. For prevention of osteoporosis and many other ills, it is important that we seek ways to minimize our exposure to stress, as well as seeking ways to limit the negative impact of stress on our health. Physical exercise and relaxing hobbies, for example, have long been known to combat stress.

Meditation is another extremely successful means of nurturing the nervous system and building the body's resistance to stress. I have practiced Transcendental Meditation for many years because it helps me feel relaxed and more productive even in the face of stress. Scientific studies now document that meditation can lower production of the stress hormones including cortisol, while increasing the adrenal youth hormone DHEA-S.[74, 75] Meditation is also a powerful way to contact and enliven that innate intelligence and organizing power within our magical bodies. More on the "how-to's" of strengthening the adrenal glands and building resistance to stress in Chapter 16.

❖ WEAK DIGESTION LIMITS BONE HEALTH

Strong digestion and good assimilation are essential for proper nutrient utilization, and in no case is this more true than with mineral metabolism. When we speak of calcium intake and calcium requirements, for example, we must remember that only a portion of the calcium we ingest is absorbed; the rest is excreted in the feces, urine and sweat. Adults absorb anywhere between 15 to 30 percent of the calcium they ingest, depending on age, need, digestion, endocrine health and other factors. Premature infants, on the other hand, absorb 80 percent of all calcium they consume, while full term infants absorb 52 to 63 percent of the calcium ingested.[76] At the other extreme, elderly people absorb even less calcium than the average young adult. Anything which limits the absorption of calcium or any other mineral is detrimental to bone. Anything which works to increase mineral absorption benefits bone and calcium is not the only mineral of importance. Proper vitamin absorption is also essential. For example, poor B_{12} absorption appears to play a role in bone health. Mayo Clinic researchers report that those with pernicious anemia have reduced bone mineral density and increased bone fracture incidence in comparison with the general community. Patients with pernicious anemia were found to have a double incidence of hip and spinal fractures and nearly a three-fold increase in wrist fractures.[77] Numerous studies now point to the bone-building value of strong digestion and good absorption.

Various osteoporosis researchers, in fact, now propose that malabsorption of calcium (and I would add other minerals as well) is often a major cause of thin, weak bones. One very important digestive weakness that hinders calcium absorption is low stomach hydrochloric acid (HCL). Without adequate stomach acid, our food is poorly digested and absorption of many nutrients, including calcium iron, folic acid, vitamins B_6 and B_{12} is limited. Calcium, for example, must be in a soluble ionized form for absorption. This requires an acidic environment within the stomach, provided by adequate HCL. Dr. Jonathan Wright, a well known author and practicing physician, reports that the majority of his patients with osteoporosis suffer from insufficient HCL.[78] Other research supports this finding. As early as 1941 people suffering jawbone loss were found to have one-half the HCL level of those without jawbone loss. In another study from 1963 investigators reported that 40 percent of postmenopausal women had no basal gastric acid secretion.[79] Since exhaustion of HCL-producing cells within the stomach occurs with prolonged stress, it is likely that more HCL deficiency exists today than ever before.

A common hydrochloric acid deficiency might help explain the conflicting data around calcium supplementation and osteoporosis prevention. The confusion and controversy might well center around the issue of poor calcium absorption due to low hydrochloric acid. Most studies which show no beneficial effect of added calcium used calcium supplements in the form of calcium carbonate. Calcium carbonate is poorly digested without adequate hydrochloric acid and thus of little use to those with weak digestion. When the more absorbable forms of calcium are administered, such as calcium citrate, beneficial results are generally reported.[80] The Better Bones, Better Body Program in Chapter 11 updates you on the best forms of calcium to use.

Food intolerances and food allergies can also weaken bones. For example, the inability to digest milk causes gastrointestinal distress which weakens digestion as well as limiting calcium absorption. Not only do those intolerant of milk tend to consume less calcium-rich dairy foods, but they also tend to have poorer overall digestion, especially if they persist in using dairy products.[81, 82] Dairy intolerance can be caused by either an allergic reaction to the protein in milk or by an inability to digest lactose, the sugar in milk. The latter is known as "lactose intolerance" While no one has yet studied those with milk allergies, it is known that lactose intolerance occurs much more frequently in those with osteoporosis than in those free from the disease.[82] To date no one has looked to see if an allergy to milk protein is linked to osteoporosis. The problem of dairy intolerance is especially important in the United States, as some researchers suggest that even one-half the population might be allergic or sensitive to dairy products.[78] Other factors that can severely limit the proper digestion and assimilation of nutrients include constipation, diarrhea, pancreatic enzyme deficiency, yeast overgrowth (Candidiasis), bacterial pathogens and parasites.

Ongoing problems with intestinal gas, cramping, bloating, stomach pain, acid indigestion, diarrhea and constipation all signal some problem with digestion which is likely causing suboptimal nutrient absorption. If such symptoms persist, you should consult your health care professional. A comprehensive 10 step approach to stronger digestion is provided within the Better Bones, Better Body Program in Chapter 12.

❖ OUR INDOOR EXISTENCE LIMITS BONE HEALTH

The detrimental effects of our sedentary lifestyle are compounded by the increasing amount of time we spend indoors without adequate exposure to sunlight. Humans evolved living outdoors, and sunlight is "nutritious" even though it never reaches the stomach. For one thing, the "sunshine vitamin" stimulates our body to produce an essential hormone we call vitamin D. Vitamin D is required for many phases of bone health and maintenance. Lack of sunlight exposure for only five to six weeks leads to depletion of vitamin D stores sufficient to cause inadequate absorption of calcium.[83] Television, computers and heavy office work schedules combined with modern conveniences help keep us indoors most of the time. As one workaholic friend recently said, now that she has an electric garage door opener and parks in a garage attached to her office building, she can spend a full work week without ever going outdoors! On top of all this, a growing fear of skin cancer has many of us concerned about the safety of any exposure to sunlight.

Researchers looking into the growing problem of low vitamin D status among those with osteoporosis remind us about the universal importance of getting adequate sunlight exposure. In the summer, 15 minutes of midday sunlight exposure is reportedly sufficient for generating vitamin D in light skinned people, while dark skinned people are reported to need more than this exposure. In the winter, 30 minutes of sunshine exposure is more appropriate if one relies on sunlight for vitamin D. Researchers at Tufts University suggest that exposing the face, arms and legs to the sun for 30 minutes a day may achieve the same benefit as increasing vitamin D from the current daily average of 100 IU per day to 400 IU per day.[84] Without adequate sunlight exposure, old and young alike can become deficient in vitamin D. Moderate exposure to the sun year round promotes better bones, better body and better health. Combining exposure to sunlight with a period of physical activity is a winning combination.

❖ References

[1] Daniell, H., "Smoking, Bones and Tooth Loss," *Complementary Medicine.* May/June (1986): 25.

[2] Seeman, E., et al., "Risk Factors for Spinal Osteoporosis in Men," *Am J Med* 75 (1983): 977–983.

[3] Slemenda, Charles, and et al, "Cigarettes and the Skeleton," *The New England Journal of Medicine* 330.6 (1994): 430.

[4] Hopper, J.L., et al., "The Bone Density of Female Twins Discordant for Tobacco Use," *The New England Journal of Medicine* 330.6 (1994): 387–392.

[5] Mellstrom, Dan, "Epidemiological Aspects," *Osteoporosis: Pharmacological Treatment and Prophylaxis*, ed. Kjell Strandberg, et al. (Uppsala, Sweden: National Board of Health and Welfare Drug Information Committee, 1989) 7–21.

[6] Slemenda, Charles W., and Conrad C. Johnston, "Epidemiology of Osteoporosis," *Treatment of the Postmenopausal Woman*, ed. Rogerio A. Lobo. (New York: Raven Press, 1994) 161–168.

[7] Nguyen, T.V., et al., "Bone loss and lifestyle factors," *Journal of Bone and Mineral Research* 9.9 (1994): 1339–1345.

[8] Aloia, John, *Osteoporosis: A Guide to Prevention and Treatment*, (Champagne, IL: Human Kinetics, 1989).

[9] Coney, Sandra, *The Menopause Industry*, (Emeryville, CA: Publishers Group West, 1994) 369.

10 Notelovitz, M., and M. Ware, *Stand Tall: The Informed Women's Guide to Preventing Osteoporosis*, (Gainesville, Florida: Traid Publishing Company, 1982).

11 Michnovicz, J., "Increased 2-Hydroxylation of Estradiol as a Possible Mechanism for the Anti-Estrogenic Effect of Cigarette Smoking," *N Engl J Med* 315.21 (1986): 1305–1309.

12 Briggs, M., "Cigarette Smoking and Infertility in Men (letter)," *Med J* 1 (1973): 616–617.

13 Fielding, J., "Smoking: Health Effects and Control," *Medical Progress* 313.8 (1985): 491–498.

14 Bureau of Census, *Statistical Abstract of the United States*, (Washington, D.C.: U.S. Department of Commerce, 1988).

15 Gross, J., et al., "Smokeless Tobacco: Health Hazard on the Rise," *Southern Medical Journal* 81.9 (1988): 1089–1091.

16 Anon., "Soft Drink Consumption Surpasses Water," *Food Engineering* 58.8 (1986): 21.

17 Heaney, R., "Nutritional Factors in Postmenopausal Osteoporosis," *Roche Seminars on Aging* 5 (1981): 1–11.

18 Cohen, L., A. Laor, and R. Kitzes, "Lymphocyte and Bone Magnesium in Alcohol-Associated Osteoporosis," *Magnesium* 4.2/3 (1985): 148–152.

19 Laitinen, K, et al., "Alcohol and Bone," *Calcif Tissue Int* 49 (1991): s70–3.

20 Baran, D., et al., "Effect of Alcohol Ingestion on Bone and Mineral Metabolism in Rats," *Am J Physiol* 238 (1980): E507–510.

21 Giovetti, A., and R. Russell, "Effect of Ethanol Ingestion on Serum and Urine Zinc and Serum Copper in Chronic Alcoholics," *Clin Res* 27 (1979): 232 A.

22 World, M., "Alcoholic Malnutrition and the Small Intestine," *Alcohol Alcoholism* 20 (1985): 89–124.

23 Middleton, H., "Intestinal Hydrolysis of Pyridoxal 5-Phosphate in Vitro and in Vivo in the Rat: Effect of Ethanol," *Am J Clin Nutr* 43 (1986): 374–381.

24 Krishnamra, N., and P. Boonpimol, "Acute Effect of Ethanol on Intestinal Calcium Transport," *J Nutr Sc V* 32 (1986): 229–236.

25 Hernandez-Avila, Mauricio, et al., "Caffeine, moderate alcohol intake, and risk of fractures of the hip and forearm in middle-aged women," *Am J Clin Nutr* 54 (1991): 157–63.

26 Kriska, A., et al., "The Assessment of Historical Physical Activity and its Relation to Adult Bone Parameters," *Am J Epidemiol* 127.5 (1988): 1053–1063.

27 National Osteoporosis Foundation, Audrey Singer, "Personal Communication (October 20, 1995).

28 Morgan, K., M. Zabik, and G. Stampley, "Breakfast Consumption of U.S. Children and Adolescents," *Nutr Res* 6 (1986): 635–646.

29 Kin, K., et al., "Bone Mineral Density of the Spine in Normal Japanese Subjects Using Dual-Energy X-Ray Absorptiometry: Effect of Obesity and Menopausal Status," *Calcified Tissue International* 49 (1991): 101–106.

30 Cummings, Steven, et al., "Risk Factors For Hip Fracture in White Women," *The New England Journal of Medicine* 332.12 (1995): 767–774.

31 Reid, I.R., et al., "Determinants of total body and regional bone mineral density in normal postmenopausal women—a key role for fat mass," *J Clin Endocrinol Metab* 75.1 (1992): 45–51.

32 Lloyd, T., et al., "Determinants of bone density in young women. I. Relationships among pubertal development, total body bone mass, and total body bone density in premenarchal females," *J Clin Endocrinol Metab* 75.2 (1992): 383–7.

33 Kinoy, B., J. Atchley, and E. Miller, *When Will We Laugh Again: Living and Dealing with Anorexia Nervosa and Bulimia*, (New York: Columbia University Press, 1984).

34 Kilbanski, "Weak Bones Linked to Anorexia," *New York Times* April 18, 1989.

35 Ruegsegger, P., et al., "Bone Loss in Female Patients with Anorexia Nervosa," *Schweiz Med Wochenschr* 118.7 (1988): 233–238.

36 Krehl, "Vitamin Supplementation," *The Nutrition Report*. May (1985): 36.

37 Anon, "Prescribing Harm," *USA Today* July 27, 1994

38 Eufemio, M., "Advances in the Therapy of Osteoporosis. Part V," *Geriatric Medicine Today*, vol. 9, no. 2, February 1990: 41–57.

39 Albanese, A., *Bone Loss: Causes, Detection and Therapy*, (New York: Alan Liss, 1977).

40 Melton, L., and B. Riggs, "Epidemiology of Age-Related Fractures," *The Osteoporotic Syndrome: Detection, Prevention and Treatment*, ed. L. Avioli. (New York: Grune and Stratton, 1983) 45–72.

41 Varonos, S., et al., "Vertebral Collapse in Juvenile Chronic Arthritis: Its Relationship with Glucocorticoid Therapy," *Calcif Tissue Int* 41 (1987): 75–78.

42 Adler, Robert A., and et al, "Glucocorticoids and osteoporosis," *Cushing's Syndrome* 23 (1994): 641–650.

43 Puolijoki, H., et al., "Inhaled beclomethasone decreases serum osteoclacin in postmenopausal asthmatic women," *Bone* 13.4 (1992): 285–8.

44 Hodgson, S.F., "Corticosteroid-induced osteoporosis," *Endocrinol-Metab-Clin-North-Am* 19.1 (1990): 95–111.

45 Cutler, W., *Hysterectomy: Before & After*, (New York: Harper & Row, 1988).

46 Pines, A., et al., "Clinical Trial of Microcrystalline Hydroxyapatite Compound (MCHC) in the Prevention of Osteoporosis Due to Corticosteroid Therapy," *Curr Med Res Opin.* 8.734 (1984).

47 Stellon, A., A. Webb, and R. Williams, "Microcrystalline Hydroxyapatite Compound in Prevention of Bone Loss in Corticosteroid-treated Patients with Chronic Active Hepatitis," *Postgrad Med J* 61 (1985): 791.

48 Nileen, E.M., M.I.V. Hayson, and A.S.J. Dixon, "Microcrystalline Hydroxyapatite Compound in Corticosteroid-treated Rheumatoid Patients; A Controlled Study," *Brit Med J* 2 (1978): 1124.

49 Sambrook, et al., "Prevention of corticosteroid osteoporosis," *New England Journal of Medicine* 328.24 (1993): 1747–1752.

50 Coindre, J., et al., "Bone Loss in Hypothyroidism with Hormone Replacement. A Histomorphometric Study," *Arch Intern Med* 146.1 (1986): 48–53.

51 Lehmke, J., et al., "Determination of bone mineral density by quantitative computed tomography and single photon absorptiopmetry in subclinical hyperthyroidism: a risk of early osteopaenia in postmenopausal women," *Clin Endocrinol* 36.5 (1992): 511–7.

52 Baker, Barbara, "Suppressive Thyroxine Doses May Have Harmful Effects on Bone," *Family Practice News* January 15, 1994: 23.

53 Paul, T.L., et al., "Long-term L-thyroxine therapy is associated with decreased hip bone density in premenopausal women," *JAMA* 259 (1988): 3137–3141.

54 Adler, A., et al., "Aluminum absorption and intestinal vitamin D-dependent Ca binding protein," *Kidney Int* 37 (1990).

55 Goodman, William G., "Aluminum Metabolism and the Uremic Patient," *Nutrition and Bone Development*, (New York: Oxford University, 1990).

56 Eastwood, J. B., et al., "Aluminum deposition in bone after contamination of drinking water supply," *The Lancet* 336 (1990).

57 Ikeda, K., "Inhibition of in vitro mineralization by aluminum in a clonal osteoblast like line," *Calcif Tissue Int* 39 (1986).

58 Spencer, H., et al., "Effect of Small Doses of Aluminum-Containing Antacids on Calcium and Phosphorus Metabolism," *American Journal of Clinical Nutrition* 36 (1982): 32–40.

59 Roe, D., *Drug-Induced Nutritional Deficiencies*, (Westport, Conn: The Avi Publishing Co., Inc., 1976).

60 Remington, D. W., *Back to Health: Yeast Control*, (Provo, Utah: Vitality House International, 1986).

61 Trowbridge, J., and M. Walker, *The Yeast Syndrome*, (New York: Bantam Books, 1986).

62 Crook, William G., *The Yeast Connection and the Woman*, (Jackson, Tennessee: Professional Books, 1995).

63 Cummings, S., et al., "Epidemiology of Osteoporosis and Osteoporotic Fractures," *Epidemiol Rev* 7 (1985): 178–208.

64 Cundy, Tim, et al., "Bone density in women receiving depot medroxyprogesterone acetate for contraception," *BMJ* 303 (1991): 13–6.

65 Ray, W., et al., "Psychotropic Drug Use and the Risk of Hip Fracture," *N Engl J Med* 316 (1987): 363–9.

66 Cummings, Steven R., "Appendicular Bone Density and Age Predict Hip Fracture in Women," *JAMA* 263.5 (1990): 665–668.

67 Mongelli Sciannameo, N., "Radiologic observations on the skeletal apparatus of young persons affected by chronic lead poisoning," *Biological aspects of lead: An annotated bibliography*, ed. I.R. Campbell, and E.G. Mergard. (Washington: US Environmental Protection Agency, 1972) Abstract 1355: 260.

68 Hancox, N., *The Biochemistry and Physiology of Bone*, ed. G.H. Bourne (New York: Academic Press, 1956).

69 Silbergeld, E.K., et al., "Lead and osteoporosis: mobilization of lead from bone in postmenopausal women," *Environmental Research* 47.1 (1988): 79–94.

70 Gaby, Alan R. Ph.D., *Preventing and Reversing Osteoporosis*, (Rocklin: Prima Publishing, 1994) 304.

71 Jacquet, P., et al., "Plasma hormone levels in normal and lead-treated pregnant mice," *Experientia* 33 (1977): 1375–1377.

72 Serammune Physicians Lab, *Description of Items Tested*, (Reston, Va.: Serammune Physicians Lab, 1995).

73 Fisher, W.H., "The Dentist Examines Bone Loss," *Complementary Medicine*. May/June (1986): 17–21.

74 Chopra, Deepak, *Creating Affluence Wealth Consciousness in the Field of All Possibilities*, (San Rafael, CA: New World Library, 1993).

75 Mullenneaux, Lisa, "Ayurveda: Restoring the Balance," *Yoga Journal* May/June (1988): 66–71.

76 Ehrenkranz, R., et al., "Absorption of Calcium in Premature Infants as Measured With a Stable Isotope 46Ca Extrinsic Tag," *Pediatr Res* 19.2 (1985): 178–184.

77 Melton, L.J., "Risk of Fractures in Patients with Pernicious Anemia," *Journal of Bone and Mineral Research* 7.5 (1992): 573–9.

78 Wright, J., and A. Gaby, "Nutrition Seminar," Omega Institute, (1988).

79 Grossman, M., J. Kirsner, and I. Gillespie, "Basal and Histalog-stimulated Gastric Secretion in Control Subjects and in Patients With Peptic Ulcer or Gastric Cancer," *Gastroenterology* 45 (1963): 15–26.

80 Reid, Ian R., et al., "Effect Of Calcium Supplementation On Bone Loss in Postmenopausal Women," *The New England Journal Of Medicine* 328.7 (1993): 460–464.

81 Abraham, G., "The Calcium Controversy," *Journal of Applied Nutrition* 34.2 (1982).

82 Birge, S., et al., "Osteoporosis, Intestinal Lactase Deficiency and Low Dietary Calcium Intake," *The New England Journal of Medicine* 276.8 (1967): 445–447.

83 Davies, R., and S. Subrata, "Osteoporosis," *American Family Practice* 32.5 (1985): 107–117.

84 Anon., "Daily Vitamin D Can Reduce Fracture Risk," *Medical Tribune* August 20 1992: 25.

Chapter 8

Bone-Robbing Endocrine Imbalance

- THE PARATHYROID • THE THYROID

- THE ADRENALS • THE OVARIES • THE KIDNEYS

❖ THE ENDOCRINE–BONE LINK

*T*he endocrine glands are the glands which produce hormones, chemical messengers which direct many of the body's countless biochemical processes. Released directly into the bloodstream, hormones travel to the cells that have receptors for that particular hormone. The hormone slips into its receptor site on the cell membrane, much as a key slips into a lock and delivers its message. Once attached to its receptor the hormone delivers its biochemical message.

All hormones deliver messages to stop or start a multitude of biochemical reactions. Generally short-lived, hormones are deactivated, excreted or recycled after their message is delivered. Some are rather magically transformed into other, even opposite-acting hormones. For example, testosterone can be converted into the estrogen known as estradiol; the adrenal hormone androstenedione can become either testosterone or the estrogen known as estrone; estrone and estradiol can be transformed one into the other.[1] Minute by minute the correct type and amount of hormones are produced to meet the ever changing needs of an ever changing body.

All of the endocrine glands, and most notably the pituitary, thyroid, parathyroid, adrenals, ovaries/testes, liver and pancreas produce hormones related to bone health. If any of these glands are functioning poorly, or worse yet, if they have been surgically removed, bone health suffers.

❖ THE PARATHYROID GLAND

The parathyroid is composed of small glands in the neck near the thyroid. They produce and secrete parathyroid hormone (PTH). Working as a team with the thyroid hormone calcitonin, PTH helps regulate the balance between calcium in the blood, calcium in the bone and calcium excreted in the urine or feces. Calcitonin adds calcium to the bones in response to high blood calcium, whereas PTH does just the opposite. PTH takes calcium from the bone and moves it into the blood in response to low blood calcium.

As discussed in Chapter 1, parathyroid hormone produced by the parathyroid gland is brought into play when blood calcium levels fall. Parathyroid hormone travels through the blood to its target cells and delivers the message to "turn on" several biological activities which work to raise the blood calcium level. The body is told to mobilize calcium from the bones, to increase intestinal calcium absorption, synthesize vitamin D and so on. When blood calcium rises adequately, other hormones signal to reverse the actions and to halt the process. The removal of calcium from the bone is halted; more calcium is allowed to be excreted in the urine.

An Overactive Parathyroid Causes Bone Loss

In hyperparathyroidism, excessive parathyroid hormone (PTH) is produced and excess PTH causes a withdrawal of calcium from the bones. A diet high in phosphorus while low in calcium is documented to induce hyperparathyroidism, that is, overactivity of the parathyroid gland. Scientists have long noted this bone-depleting process in seniors. As we move into old age, most of us experience an increase in PTH associated with a vitamin D deficiency and low calcium intakes. This age-dependent increase of PTH seen in the United States further reduces bone density. Studies now document that in many cases this age-related increase in PTH can be corrected, hip fractures prevented and lost bone even somewhat rebuilt, with simple calcium and vitamin D supplementation.[2, 3]

Diet-induced hyperparathyroidism has now been documented in healthy young women as well. Recently researchers at the Mayo Clinic presented data suggesting that young women consuming diets providing calcium and phosphorus intakes which parallel our national consumption patterns show increased parathyroid hormone activity and may be at greater risk for increased bone loss. This secondary hyperparathyroidism and increased bone breakdown was caused by a diet containing 500 mg calcium and 1,500 mg phosphorus.[4]

❖ THE THYROID GLAND

The paired thyroid gland lies in the neck near the parathyroid glands. This gland produces various bone-regulating hormones, notably thyroxin and calcitonin.

Thyroxin Level is Critical

Thyroxin regulates the rate of metabolism in all cells throughout the body, including bone cells. The production of too much or too little thyroxin is known to cause bone loss. Overactivity of the thyroid results in excessive production of thyroxin, which increases metabolic rates in all cells. The net result of this on bone is increased bone breakdown and increased risk of osteoporotic fracture.[5] The same thing occurs with too much thyroid medication, as discussed in Chapter 7. It might be supposed that if too much thyroxin results in an undesirable condition, too little thyroxin might be a good situation. However, too little thyroxin causes a decrease in calcium absorption and can lead to a negative calcium balance in the body. This too leads to a loss in bone mass. Delicate balance is the key.

Calcitonin Counterbalances Parathyroid Hormone

Calcitonin is another thyroid hormone important to bone health. It is secreted in response to high blood calcium levels and brings about a lowering of calcium and phosphorus levels in the blood. Calcitonin appears to stimulate the kidneys to increase their absorption of calcium and phosphorus from the blood and to stimulate the bones to increase mineralization. Calcitonin acts to oppose and counterbalance parathyroid hormone to retard bone loss, and thus preserve bone. Calcitonin moves calcium from the blood back into the bones. Parathyroid hormone takes calcium from the bone and moves it back into the blood. One hormone counterbalances the other. The two hormones working together maintain blood calcium levels within an optimal range.

❖ THE ADRENAL GLANDS

The adrenals are the most underrated and overlooked of all bone-regulating endocrine glands. Western medicine largely ignores the essential role they play in maintaining bone health. Particularly overlooked is their role in postmenopausal bone health.

The adrenals are two tiny endocrine glands that sit on top of the kidneys. Although small, these complex and dynamic glands produce dozens of hormones. With elegant precision adrenal hormonal secretions fluctuate from minute to minute in response to bodily stresses. Among other things, adrenal hormones contribute to the control of blood pressure; blood sugar and carbohydrate metabolism; protein synthesis; potassium, sodium and magnesium excretion; DNA synthesis; gastric secretion; anti-inflammatory reactions including response to allergens; and regulation of the immune and reproductive systems. Glucocorticoids, mineral corticoids, estrogen, androgens and progesterone are among the hormones produced by the adrenals. The importance of these tiny glands is reflected in the fact that the entire outer part of the adrenal cortex can be regenerated from only a few cells left after surgical adrenal removal.[6]

Suboptimal Adrenal Functioning as a Cause of Osteoporosis

Considering its range of actions, it should be no surprise that our adrenals are a key player in bone health maintenance. Overactivity of the adrenals, known as hyperadrenalism, leaves the body with excessively high levels of glucocorticosterioid stress hormones. Cortisol is one of these stress hormones. These hormones are secreted in response to all types of stress. They prepare the body for the 'fight or flight' mode of action. While their occasional presence can be life-saving in the face of a true emergency, prolonged exposure to these hormones damage the body in many ways. Prolonged high levels of these hormones can cause bone thinning, and as such are frequently associated with osteoporosis. The glucocorticoid hormones attach to bone cells and direct the withdrawal of calcium from the bones. They also reduce intestinal absorption of calcium, which in turn leads to increased withdrawal of calcium from the bone. Thus, glucocorticoids also directly inhibit new bone development.[7]

As previously discussed, drug therapy with cortisone, prednisone and other corticosteroids can cause excess adrenal hormone levels. The most common causes of adrenal overactivity, however, are chronic stress and/or abusive and poor nutritional patterns. Initially stress causes overactivity of the adrenal glands. Prolonged consistent stress exhausts them. Both processes contribute to excessive bone loss.

In addition to the glucocorticoids, another set of adrenal hormones, known as the adrenal androgens, play an even more important role in bone health. These androgens, or "male-type" sex hormones of adrenal origin, include androstenedione, testosterone, dehydroepiandrosterone (DHEA) and dehydroepiandrosterone sulfate (DHEA-S). Depending on the body's needs, these adrenal hormones can be converted into estrogen by subcutaneous fat cells, hair follicles, mammary adipose tissue and probably many other tissues. In fact, postmenopausally the vast majority of a woman's estrogen is derived from these adrenal hormones. Thus, postmenopausal estrogen status depends upon adrenal status.[6, 8] Even though a women's estrogen production might drop by some 75 percent at menopause,[9] she need not suffer from estrogen deficiency symptoms if her adrenals are functioning optimally. In healthy women with full adrenal function, estrogen production is lowered enough to halt menstrual periods, but not enough to cause unwarranted bone loss, hot flashes, vaginal dryness or other signs of excessive estrogen deprivation.[6, 10]

Low postmenopausal levels of the adrenal hormones androstenedione and DHEA are known risk factors for osteoporosis.[11, 12] Several studies have documented the correlation between high DHEA and DHEA-S levels and greater bone mineral content.[11-13] This appears partly due to the conversion of adrenal hormones into estrogen. These adrenal hormones, however, also appear to have direct bone-building effects all on their own.[12]

In fact, neither excessive bone loss nor the menopausal symptoms many Western women experience around menopause are natural or universal. They both are linked to suboptimal adrenal functioning. When the ovaries go into what I call "semi-retirement," the adrenals should take over. Often, however, the adrenals are not healthy enough to do the full job. The obvious implication is that we should learn how to better care for our adrenals. How to do this is detailed in Chapter 16.

❖ THE OVARIES

The ovaries, paired glands that lie on either side of the uterus, are the major glands regulating female reproduction. The ovarian hormone estrogen has been widely studied. It serves many functions and plays various roles aimed at maximizing female reproductive potential. Estrogen stimulates growth of the ovaries, follicles and external genitals. It also initiates breast development, increases fat deposits in breasts, hips and thighs and causes fluid retention. Somewhat less studied is progesterone, another ovarian hormone. While estrogen is produced in high quantities during the first half of the menstrual cycle, progesterone production dominates in the second half of the cycle. Progesterone is essential for ovulation and successful pregnancy. Production of progesterone rises dramatically during pregnancy. Smaller amounts of this hormone are also produced by the adrenal glands in both sexes and by the testes in males. Adrenal progesterone is the precursor of other adrenal steroid hormones.[14]

Estrogen Promotes Bone Health

One of the many actions of estrogen is to conserve calcium within the body. It does this is by increasing calcium absorption and inhibiting the loss of calcium from bones. Estrogen also has an inhibiting effect on parathyroid hormone, which as you will recall is a bone breakdown hormone. Thus estrogen promotes bone building and maintenance in various ways. From an evolutionary point of view, estrogen's ability to conserve calcium allows women to nourish the fetus and breastfeed the infant, both requiring high amounts of calcium, even in the face of low calcium intakes.

Progesterone Promotes Bone Health

Recently it has become clear that the ovarian hormone progesterone also promotes bone health. The bone-building cells (osteoblasts) contain progesterone receptors and this hormone appears to directly encourage the building of bone. During the reproductive years, progesterone works along with estrogen to conserve calcium within the body and limit the withdrawal of calcium from the bones. Progesterone deficiency in young women has been linked to osteoporosis by Dr. Jerilynn Prior in British Colombia. In studying athletes she inadvertently discovered that many "normal" healthy young women had abnormal menstrual periods and an absence of ovulation due to progesterone deficiency. This hormone deficiency, in turn, was linked to excessive bone loss. Supplementation with progesterone, Dr. Prior found, resolved the menstrual irregularities and appeared capable of correcting the excessive bone loss.[15] In postmenopausal women with osteoporosis, progesterone supplementation, particularly natural progesterone, has been shown to rebuild substantial amounts of lost bone.[1, 16] More about natural progesterone in Chapter 17.

Other Ovarian Hormones are Also Important

In addition to estrogen and progesterone the ovaries produce other hormones which are important in bone health. These ovarian hormones are other "male-type" hormones known as androgens. The androgens or male sex hormones produced by the ovaries take on special importance after menopause when ovarian production of estrogen nearly ceases and their progesterone production totally ceases. The ovarian androgens, testosterone and androstenedione, along with the hormones produced by the adrenals, are converted by the body into estrogen. Even after menopause 50 percent of the plasma testosterone and 30 percent of the androstenedione are produced by the ovaries. Even after menopause the ovaries produce hormones which end up as estrogen. Obviously, a woman's ovaries were meant to serve an entire lifetime, not just during the reproductive years.

Ovary Malfunction and Ovary Removal Jeopardize Bone

Improper ovarian functioning and/or cessation of menstrual periods leads to reduced bone mass. For example, women who always had regular menstrual cycles were found to have greater spinal bone density than women who experienced frequent irregularities in their periods. Women who never had regular cycles had the lowest bone density. The women at greatest risk were those with severe menstrual irregularities and low body weight.[17] That female athletes who lose their periods experience rapid bone loss is well documented. Bone loss of three percent per year is frequently reported in these cases. Fortunately, this galloping bone loss can be reversed if the woman's periods are restored within the first two to three years after their cessation.[18]

If suboptimal ovarian functioning pushes a woman towards osteoporosis, ovary removal catapults her in that direction. Each year well over half a million women in the United States undergo surgical ovary removal. Without hormone replacement, most young women who lose their ovaries will begin to show signs of osteoporosis within four years of surgery.[9] Furthermore, as mentioned earlier, even uterus removal, which leaves the ovaries intact, can result in cessation of ovarian functioning and its associated increased risk of bone loss. Up to one-half of all the 650,000 women who undergo a hysterectomy each year in the United States could experience subsequent ovarian failure.[19-22]

Male Sex Hormones and Male Bone Health

Men also face a similar problem in that a low level of the male sex hormone, testosterone, is also associated with the development of osteoporosis. This is even true to the extent that men who experience delayed puberty, that is an onset of puberty beyond 13.5 years of age, are less likely to achieve their peak bone mass, and thus, more likely to suffer from osteoporotic fractures as they age.[23] Furthermore, having a vasectomy also appears to increase a man's risk of osteoporosis and this likely has to do with altered testosterone levels. The testes and the sex hormones they produce are just as important to bone health in the male as are the ovaries and their hormones are in the female.

❖ THE KIDNEYS

The kidneys are paired organs located on either side of the spine, toward the lower back. We most commonly recognize them as organs of excretion and blood purification. As the central part of our urinary system, each day our kidneys filter from 158 to 190 quarts of fluid, sorting out the waste material from that which can be recycled and reused. Only a tiny proportion of this fluid, around 1.5 quarts, leaves the body as urine. The rest is cleaned and recycled. Equally, the kidneys filter our blood, removing the waste by-products of the body's innumerable chemical reactions and excess water. The kidneys, however, serve many other functions including regulation of bodily fluids and acid-base balance.

The Kidney-Bone Link

In Oriental medicine the kidneys take on additional importance beyond the functions mentioned above. To the Chinese, the "kidney system" includes the adrenals, the tiny glands that sit on top of the kidneys, as well as the kidneys themselves. Bones, bone marrow and the teeth are all regulated by the kidney-adrenal system. To understand this it is helpful to recall that a major function of the kidneys is to filter the blood, excreting waste substances while retaining minerals and other substances in the blood. For example, from the near 200 quarts of liquid processed by the kidneys each day some 7,000 plus milligrams of calcium are filtered with only 150 to 300 mg lost in the urine; the rest is recycled. Excessive urinary loss, or "leaking" of minerals from the kidneys, leads to bone loss. While Western medicine offers few methods of enhancing kidney health, the treatment for bone demineralization and osteoporosis in traditional Chinese medicine includes acupuncture and herbal combinations aimed at strengthening the kidney-adrenal system.

While Western medicine does not consider the kidneys as important as does Oriental medicine, our science does recognize the kidneys' role in vitamin D metabolism. Vitamin D, in turn, is seen as essential for bone metabolism. Dietary vitamin D is absorbed in the intestine and transported to the liver where it undergoes a chemical transformation to a substance known as 25-hydroxyvitamin D_3. This substance is then transported to the kidney where it undergoes another essential transformation to the active form of vitamin D, known as 1,25 (OH2D3). Equally, vitamin D production within the body upon exposure to sunlight must also be transformed into the active metabolite by the kidneys. It is this active form of vitamin D which regulates calcium and phosphorus absorption. Because of its role in vitamin D production and its role in mineral recycling, Western medicine recognizes that disease or even weakness of the kidneys can cause osteoporosis. In Oriental medicine, however, the kidney-adrenal role in bone health is much more defined and prominent.

❖ References

1 Lee, John R., *Natural Progesterone*, third ed. (Sebastopol, CA: BLL Publishing, 1994) 99.

2 Chapuy, Marie C., et al., "Vitamin D$_3$ and Calcium to Prevent Hip Fractures in Elderly Women.," *New England Journal of Medicine* 328.23 (1992): 1637–1642.

3 Meunier, P.J., and M.C.. Chapuy, "Calcium and Vitamin D Supplementation For Preventing Hip Fractures in the Elderly," *Challenges of Modern Medicine* 7 (1995): 22–227.

4 Calvo, M., and H. Heath, "High-Phosphorus, Low-Calcium Diets, Typical of National Survey Trends, Induce Secondary Hyperparathyroidism (2 HPT) in Normal Young Adults," *Fed Proc* 45 (1986): 3214.

5 Cummings, Steven, et al., "Risk Factors For Hip Fracture In White Women," *The New England Journal Of Medicine* 332.12 (1995): 767–774.

6 Bondy, P., "Disorders of the Adrenal Cortex," *Williams Textbook of Endocrinology*, ed. J. Wilson, and D. Foster. 7 ed. (Philadelphia: Saunders Co., 1985).

7 Kaplan, F., "Osteoporosis," *Clinical Symposia* 35.5 (1983): 2–32.

8 Crilly, R., R. Francis, and B. Nordin, "Steroid Hormones, Aging and Bone," 10 (1981): 115–139.

9 Cutler, W., C. Garcia, and D. Edwards, *Menopause: A Guide for Women and the Men Who Love Them*, (New York/London: W. W. Norton & Company, 1983).

10 Marshall, D., R. Crilly, and B. Nordin, "Plasma Androstenedione and Oestrone Levels in Normal and Osteoporotic Postmenopausal Women," *Br Med J* 2 (1977): 1177–1179.

11 Spector, T.D., et al., "The relationship between sex steroids and bone mineral content in women soon after the menopause," *Clin Endocrinol* 34.1 (1991): 37–41.

12 Taelman, P., et al., "Persistence of increased bone resorption and possible role of dehydroepiandrosterone as a bone metabolism determinant in osteoporotic women in late postmenopause," *Maturitas* 11 (1989): 65–73.

13 Wild, R.A., et al., "Declining adrenal androgens: an association with bone loss in aging women," *Proceedings of the society for experimental biology and medicine* 186 (1987): 355–360.

14 Lee, John, "Progesterone Therapy," *Townsend Newsletter*. August/September (1994).

15 Prior, Jerilynn C., "Progesterone and the prevention of osteoporosis," *The Canadian Journal of Ob/Gyn & Women's Health Care* 3.4 (1991): 178–184.

16 Gaby, Alan R. Ph.D., *Preventing and Reversing Osteoporosis*, (Rocklin: Prima Publishing, 1994) 304.

17 Drinkwater, Barbara L., et al., "Menstrual History as a Determinant of Current Bone Density in Young Athletes," *JAMA* 263.4 (1990): 545–548.

18 Drinkwater, B., K. Nilson, and C. Chesnut, "Bone Mineral Content of Amenorrheic and Eumenorrheic Athletes," *N Engl J Med* 311 (1984): 277–281.

19 Cutler, W., *Hysterectomy: Before & After*, (New York: Harper & Row, 1988).

20 Siddle, N., P. Sarrel, and M. Whitehead, "The Effect of Hysterectomy on the Age at Ovarian Failure: Identification of a Subgroup of Women With Premature Loss of Ovarian Function and Literature Review," *Fertil Steril* 47.1 (1987): 94–100.

21 Garcia, C., and W.B. Cutler, "Preservation of the Ovary: A Reevaluation," *Fertil Steril* 42.4 (1984): 510–514.

22 Ranney, B., and S. Abu-Ghazaleth, "The Future Function and Control of Ovarian Tissue Which is Retained in Vivo During Hysterectomy," *Am J Obstet Gynecol* 128 (1977): 626–634.

23 Finkelstein, Joel, et al. "Osteopenia in men with a history of delayed puberty," *The New England Journal of Medicine* 326.9 (1992): 600–604.

PART THREE

❖ Regaining Bone Health

Chapter *9*
················

Determining Your Risk of Developing Osteoporotic Fractures

*R*egardless of your current bone health or osteoporosis fracture risk, you will benefit from implementing the Better Bones, Better Body Program. If you are at low risk this health-enhancing program will help keep you that way while also helping to prevent other degenerative diseases. If you are at high risk, do not be discouraged. There is a wide variety of proven and available options to help regenerate bone and avoid fractures. You might interpret a high risk status as simply a strong push from nature encouraging you to help yourself now. No matter what your current bone health, implementation of these lifestyle practices will bring bone-building results.

Any program to estimate risks of suffering an osteoporotic fracture should start with a thorough individual history. Such a history includes:

1. An assessment of your personal history and the bone-depleting lifestyle factors commonly associated with an increased risk of osteoporosis, and

2. A review of the actual signs and symptoms of bone loss you are now experiencing.

Take a moment to fill out this checklist.

Illustration 9.1

OSTEOPOROSIS FRACTURE RISK ASSESSMENT: YOUR PERSONAL CHECKLIST

	Yes	No
I am 65 years of age or older.	___	___
I am Caucasian or Asian living in the U.S.	___	___
✦ I am underweight or have lost weight since age 25.	___	___
I am physically inactive and rarely exercise.	___	___
✦ I am weak; for example I cannot rise from a chair without using my arms.	___	___
✦ I rank my overall health as poor.	___	___
I was taller than my peers at age 25.	___	___
I spend less than 30 minutes three times a week outdoors in the sunshine.	___	___
My resting pulse is 80 beats or more per minute.	___	___
I generally do not consume milk, yogurt or cheese every day.	___	___
I generally consume less than one serving per day of green leafy vegetables (collards, kale, broccoli, bok choy; dandelion greens, etc.)	___	___
I eat meat, fish or other flesh foods more than once a day.	___	___
I regularly add salt to my food.	___	___
I use canned or packaged foods more than twice a day.	___	___
I use sugar or have sweetened foods more than twice a day.	___	___
I drink two or more cups of coffee, or four or more cups of tea or chocolate daily.	___	___

I consume two or more colas or soft drinks daily. _____ _____
I eat fast foods two or more times a week. _____ _____
✦ I presently smoke. _____ _____
I used to smoke. _____ _____
I have two or more alcoholic drinks per day. _____ _____
✦ I regularly use or have regularly used over long periods of _____ _____
   time glucocorticoids such as Prednisone.
✦ I use anti-convulsant drugs such as Dilantin. _____ _____
✦ I use tranquilizers and mood-altering drugs. _____ _____
I used Depo Provera for several years. _____ _____
I use aluminum-containing antacids on a daily basis (e.g. _____ _____
   Rolaids, Maalox, Mylanta, Gelusil).
✦ One of my parents fractured a hip. _____ _____
✦ I have documented low bone density (2 1/2 standard devi- _____ _____
   ations or more below young normal values).
✦ I experienced a fracture after age 50. _____ _____
I have receding gums or periodontal disease. _____ _____
I have false teeth. _____ _____
I have thin, transparent skin. _____ _____
I have little muscular development. _____ _____
I have weak, brittle fingernails. _____ _____
I suffer frequent indigestion, gas, bloating, belching or _____ _____
   diarrhea.
I have regular nocturnal leg cramps. _____ _____
I have undergone intestinal or stomach surgery. _____ _____
I have an overactive thyroid. _____ _____
I am lactose intolerant or allergic to dairy products. _____ _____
I frequently feel light-headed if I stand up quickly. _____ _____
✦ There were times when my period stopped for many _____ _____
   months (not including pregnancy, lactation or
   menopause).
Menopause was naturally early (before age 43). _____ _____
Menopause was surgically induced by ovary removal. _____ _____
                                                 Total _____ _____

    Each of these factors listed above may well be associated with the development of osteoporosis and an increased risk of osteoporotic fracture. The greater your number of *yes* answers, the more reason for you to begin a serious osteoporosis-prevention and bone-rebuilding program now.[1] If you answered *yes* to four or more of the bulleted items, or had a total of 10 or more *yes* answers overall, you are likely at high risk for an osteoporotic fracture at some point in the future. Even a total score of 8 or more *yes* answers likely indicates an above average risk.

Also remember that the "average risk" for a Caucasian woman in the U.S. is thought to be roughly a 50 percent chance that she will experience some form of osteoporotic fracture within her lifetime. Thus, ideally one would like to be at a lower than average risk. Although you cannot change the genetic or medical history factors on this checklist, many of the other bone-depleting factors reflect lifestyle patterns you can modify. Look at the list again and note how many factors are directly under your control.

If you answered *yes* to 10 or more questions, you might also want to consider a professional osteoporosis risk assessment. Such an assessment would most likely include either a bone density measurement and/or one of the new urine tests for bone resorption described on page 213. Keep in mind that low bone density alone will not necessarily result in an osteoporotic fracture. Low bone density *combined with multiple risk factors* is shown to be much more predictive of future fracture.[1]

There will be more about modifying these bone breakers in the next section of the book. For now let's review your body's tell-tale signs of bone loss.

❖ Tell-Tale Signs of Bone Loss

The next self-help step for judging the strength of your bones involves taking a hard look at the tell-tale signs of bone loss. Our bodies give us various signs and signals which can reveal information about the strength of our bones. Any individual tell-tale sign need not be a strong indicator of accelerated bone loss, *but a cluster* of these signs should encourage you to pay attention.

Jawbone Loss as a Sign of Overall Bone Loss

Did you know that your dentist can tell you something about the condition of your bones? The jawbone, known as the alveolar bone, is often the first place to look for signs of declining bone mass. Receding gums, that is the shrinking of the gums, indicate that the jawbone is eroding due to mineral loss.[2-4] As the gums recede, the roots of the teeth become visible. Healthy gums do not recede because "we brush too vigorously" or because "the teeth grew longer." Gums recede due to demineralization and subsequent loss of alveolar bone.

Noticeable jawbone loss occurs as early as 35 years of age in most American women. By age 60, nearly 40 percent of all women in this country have lost all their teeth. This loss of teeth is due largely to gum problems, not tooth problems.[5] Next time you visit your dentist ask about the condition of your gums. Are they receding? Do you have periodontal disease, a condition where infection develops in a weakened jaw bone? These dental problems may suggest that you are beginning to lose bone in other parts of the body.

You might well be asking just why early osteoporosis can be detected in the jaw. The jawbone contains a high proportion of spongy trabecular bone. This spongy bone is very active metabolically and has a much higher turnover rate than denser cortical bone. As such it is this spongy bone which supplies mobile calcium for transfer to the blood when blood calcium drops. Its high trabecular content, combined with the fact that the jawbone is the most visible of all bones, makes it an early detection site for excessive bone loss.

Healthy gums and teeth are a reasonable indicator of healthy bones and the loss of teeth in postmenopausal women has been linked with systemic osteoporosis. Overall, those who have lost their teeth are more likely to be suffering from osteoporosis than those who still have them. Shifting dental plates could also signal osteoporosis. A set of false teeth that fit when they are made but no longer fit after a while probably reflect a further erosion of the jawbone due to osteoporosis.[6-9]

How Strong Are Your Muscles?

Strong bones are usually attached to strong, well developed muscles. Our bones, in fact, weaken and thin at about the same rate as our muscles atrophy. Good muscle mass indicates that we are putting stress on the bones, and our bones grow strong in response to the stress we put on them. In several studies lean body mass, or muscle, was found to be the best single indicator of bone density.

Looking at the spine in particular, researchers at the Mayo Clinic have found that the strength of the back extensor muscles correlates well with lumbar spine bone mineral density. The back extensors are those muscles along both sides of the spine. The women in the Mayo Clinic study had back extensor strength which ranged from 37 to 145 pounds.

Those with a greater back muscle strength had greater spinal bone density.[11] Other studies have reported similar findings.[12] Interestingly enough, some researchers suggest that the low incidence of osteoporosis among Afro-Americans is at least in part due to their greater muscle mass.[13]

How Fit Are You?

Just as muscle strength is linked with bone strength so is overall fitness. Numerous studies have shown that persons with greater aerobic capacity, that is greater oxygen uptake from the lungs, have greater bone density. From our holistic perspective this makes good sense. Greater aerobic capacity implies a history of greater physical exertion which is inevitably linked to stronger bones. As emphasized earlier, no part of the body is isolated and osteoporosis does not stand alone. All things being equal, fit individuals have fit bones. The highest hip fracture rate, for example, is found among the least fit elderly.

Are You Shorter Than You Were?

Everyone knows an elderly person who has shrunk with age. Indeed, as our bones get thinner, we become especially susceptible to spinal fractures. As one spinal micro-fracture adds to the next, eventually an individual vertebra becomes so weak it collapses. With accumulated vertebral deformity and collapse there develops a curvature of the spine and a subsequent loss in height. In cases where this spinal fracturing is advanced, a hump in the upper back, known as the "dowager's hump" becomes obvious.

A simple indicator of existing osteoporosis is a loss in height. Unfortunately, a considerable degree of spinal bone loss has already occurred by the time a person can see that she or he is losing height. Nonetheless, spinal bone loss occurs long before the hipbones undergo life-threatening loss of substance. There is still time to prevent further bone loss, time to stop hipbone loss and prevent hip fractures even if you are already losing height. There is also a great need to halt this bone loss. While spinal fractures are not life-threatening, the latter occurring hip fractures can be. Consider measuring your height annually to see if you are losing height. If so, you might want to seek professional help in developing a personalized bone-building program in addition to the Better Bones, Better Body Program which follows in the next chapter.

Do You Have Transparent Skin?

Clinician and osteoporosis researcher Dr. Morris Notelovitz notes that there is very likely a link between thin, transparent skin and thin, weak bones. The transparency of skin, he explains, is due to a lack of the collagen in the skin's outer layers. Since collagen is also a major component of bone, the link between collagen deficient skin and weak bones is reasonable. While skin thickness and transparency is far from being a accurate predictor of excessively thin bone, it is a likely tell-tale sign to keep in mind. Dr. Notelovitz says you can detect transparent skin by looking at the back of your hand. If the skin is loose and lacks pigmentation and if you can see the edges of both the large and small veins, then you have transparent skin.[14]

Signs of Nutrient Inadequacy

While not true indicators of osteoporosis, nutrient deficiencies can lead to fragile bones and, as such, they can warn of a problem in the making. Let's look at few key bone-building nutrients and review the tell-tale signs of their deficiency.

Tell-tale signs of calcium deficiency include fingernails that are brittle or break easily; a tendency to leg or toe cramps, especially at night; the formation of plaque or calculus on the teeth; receding gums and/or periodontal (gum) disease; shifting teeth or ill-fitting dentures; joint tenderness or inflammation and lower back pain. If you seem to have a cluster of these signs the next step is to ask yourself, "Do I consume adequate calcium each day?" You can estimate your calcium intake using the table "Calcium: Your Best Wholesome Food Sources" in Appendix 3. A more accurate evaluation is available through a computerized diet analysis as offered by the Nutrition Education and Consulting Service (Appendix 2). If you feel you consume adequate calcium, yet still experience signs of calcium deficiency, you may not be absorbing your calcium. In this case, you would want to pay special attention to Chapter 12's Ten Steps To Stronger Digestion.

Zinc is another nutrient essential to bone health. Signs of zinc insufficiency can include a loss of taste, wounds that heal slowly, poor night vision and white spots on the fingernails. Magnesium is commonly deficient in the American diet, and it is very important for bone maintenance. Signs of possible magnesium insufficiency include muscle cramps, muscle spasms, twitches, irregular heart beat, asthma and premenstrual syndrome. Using the nutrient food source tables in Appendix 3 you can estimate your zinc and magnesium intakes. Finally, vitamin C is another bone-building nutrient with clear tell-tale signs of insufficiency. Bleeding gums and a tendency for black-and-blue marks tell us we should increase our vitamin C intake.

If you scored high on the osteoporosis risk checklist, or if you show many tell-tale signs of bone loss, the next step is to learn how medicine measures osteoporosis risk and to evaluate your need for such testing. The medical tests currently available include direct bone density measurements and indirect biochemical markers.

❖ How Medicine Measures Osteoporosis Risk

Bone Density Measurements

Bone density can be measured directly by bone biopsies and by various types of bone scans. Bone biopsy, while accurate, is very invasive and not widely used. Bone scanning techniques involve a sort of advanced x-ray technology, but they are far more sophisticated than conventional x-rays. While some 30 percent of bone mineral must be gone before bone loss can be seen on a standard x-ray, these new scanning techniques can detect small changes in bone density.

The simplest scan is known as the single photon absorptiometry and is used to measure the density of the "appendicular skeleton" (bones such as wrist and heel). In this, as in the other scanning tests, a radioactive material emits photons and the density of bone is calculated based on the number of photons absorbed as compared to those that pass through the bone. The greater the absorption, the greater the bone mineral content. This single photon test cannot be used to measure density of the "center bones" of the body, such as the spine or the hip. These "central" bones can be measured by more sophisticated scanning techniques including dual photon absorptiometry, dual energy x-ray absorptiometry and quantitative computed tomography.[14, 15]

The dual photon absorptiometry (DPA) test is similar to the single photon, but here the radioactive material emits photons with two effective energies. DPA can measure the central skeleton, but cannot differentiate between cortical and trabecular bone.[15]

The dual x-ray absorptiometry test (DEXA) is the upgraded version of the DPA. Here the radioactive material has been replaced by a stable x-ray tube. With the DEXA test the examination time is less and reproductibility of measurements improved over the DPA.[15] Today this is the preferred test for osteoporosis screening.

The QCT or Quantitative Computed Tomography is a modified CAT scan. QCT exposes both bones and internal organs to relatively high amounts of radiation up to 100 times the radiation dose of the DEXA scan. All of these scanning techniques, however, involve some radiation exposure.

Limitations of Bone Density Measurements

An important limitation of bone scans is that half of the people who are shown to have low bone density on these tests will never suffer an osteoporotic fracture.[16-18] For example, in one study Mayo Clinic researchers found that by age 65 half of the normal (fracture-free) women had vertebral bone mineral densities similar to that of women who had suffered vertebral fractures. By age 85 virtually all women had densities within the fracture group range.[18] As mentioned earlier, osteoporosis, or low bone density alone, does not cause osteoporotic fractures.

These scans can detect if your bone density is lower than that of other individuals of the same age and sex, but they cannot really predict if you will suffer a fracture.[19, 20] Those with lower bone density are more likely to suffer fractures, although they will not necessarily do so. The highest risk of hip fracture is experienced by those in the lowest 10 percent of hip femoral neck bone density. The highest risk of spinal fracture is seen in women in the lowest 30 percent of spine density. Bone density is a better predictor of spinal fracture than hip fracture, but in both cases those with the greatest bone loss are at greatest risk. Specifically, in this country the threshold below which the risk for non-traumatic vertebral factures increases is reportedly a spinal bone mineral density of 0.83 to 0.96 grams/cm.^{2} The femoral-neck-hipbone density value among those who suffer hip fractures has been estimated to be 0.55 to 0.65.[18, 21] These values are some 2 to 3.5 standard deviations below bone mineral values in normal premenopausal women. Remember that while those experiencing an osteoporotic fracture often have bone density within or below these thresholds, many women with these low bone density values never experience any osteoporotic fracture at all.

If you have a bone density measurement, remember that your density is likely being compared to that of "normal young women" and as such the results can be needlessly frightening. As nearly all women in the United States lose significant bone density as they age, when compared to young women most older women have significantly less bone density. In fact, osteoporosis authority Dr. Lawrence Melton of the Mayo Clinic suggests that about 45 percent of all normal Caucasian postmenopausal women have a bone density more than two standard deviations below that of young normal women at one or more sites in the hip, spine or forearm. Specifically his studies found 32 percent of postmenopausal Caucasian women had this low a bone density in their lumber spine; 29 percent in the hip, and 26 percent in the forearm.[23] Until recently, United States scientists have defined osteoporosis as bone mass more than two standard deviations below that of normal young women. By this definition, by age 50 many women, and a few decades later most older women in this country would be considered to have osteoporosis. Only 16 to 17 percent of all Caucasian women in the United States, however, will suffer a hip fracture at any point in their life.

It is interesting to note that the World Health Organization has recently redefined osteoporosis as bone mass 2.5 standard deviations below the normal youth level.[24] By the new definition the number of Americans with osteoporosis has dropped significantly from some 25 million to seven or eight million.

Overcoming the Limitations of Bone Density Measurements

As highlighted by the National Women's Health Network, a more realistic bone density evaluation might be obtained comparing a women's bone density to that of other healthy, fracture-free women of her age.[25] Furthermore, once low bone density for the age group was determined the next step would be to assess a person's fracture risk factors. It is now clear that bone density alone is a rather poor predicator of fracture. On the other hand, the likelihood of fracture is better predicted by a combination of bone density and personal risk factor assessment.

Groundbreaking research by Dr. Steven Cummings and associates at the University of California, San Francisco recently verified that low bone density combined with a high number of known osteoporosis risk factors is the best predictor of osteoporotic fracture. In a very sophisticated study they analyzed the risk factors for hip fracture among 9516 Caucasian women aged 65 and over. The research project lasted four years and sought to judge the importance of hip fracture risk factors other than low bone density. Interestingly enough they found nearly two dozen factors important for predicting the risk of hip fracture. A full 16 of these risk factors were independent of bone density; that is the existence of any of these 16 risk factors in themselves significantly increased a woman's risk of hip fracture, regardless of the woman's bone density.[1] So, these researchers found that bone density and 16 other risk factors all by themselves are especially meaningful indicators of osteoporosis hip fracture risk. For example, a woman whose mother had a hip fracture is at least twice as likely to fracture her hip as a woman without such a maternal history. Most of the 17 independent risk factors increased a woman's chance of breaking a hip by 50 to 100 percent. These total 17 independent risk factors are listed on the next page.

Forty-seven percent of 9,516 women studied had two or fewer of the first 17 factors not including low bone density. Their incidence of hip fracture was only 1.1 per 1,000 woman-years. Fifteen percent of the women had five or more of the risk factors listed not including low bone den-

Illustration 9.2

THE 17 INDEPENDENT RISK FACTORS FOR HIP FRACTURE[1]

1. Current use of anti-convulsant drugs.
2. The inability to rise from a chair without using one's arms.
3. A history of maternal hip fracture (especially if the mother fractured a hip before age 80).
4. Previous hyperthyroidism.
5. Current use of long-acting benzodiazepines (tranquilizers and mood altering drugs).
6. A resting pulse of 80 beats or more per minute.
7. Poor overall self-rated health.
8. Tendency to stand on feet less than four hours a day.
9. Advancing age.
10. Any fracture since age 50.
11. Weighing less than you did at age 25.
12. Current caffeine intake.
13. Poor distant depth perception.
14. Low-frequency contrast sensitivity (impaired vision).
15. Being taller at age 25.
16. Lack of exercise, as in not walking for exercise.
17. Low bone density.

Other less significant risk factors identified in this study included:
   Current smoking (versus never having smoked).
   Current thyroid medication.
   Having fallen in previous year (versus no falls).
   Poor neuromuscular function (as gait speed and coordination).
   Low body weight.
   Poor functional-status score (low functioning in general).

sity. Their incidence of hip fracture was 19 per 1,000 woman-years. Most strikingly, the six percent of women who had five or more risk factors and bone density in the lowest third for their age had an incidence of hip fracture of 27 per 1,000 woman-years. This represents nearly a 27-fold difference from the women with two or fewer risk factors. Even more, this latter group accounted for a full 32 percent of all hip fractures reported.[1]

The conclusion of this important study was that a small number of women with multiple risk factors and low bone density have an especially high risk of hip fracture. This small high risk group accounts for a large proportion of all hip fractures and should be the focus of intensive efforts to prevent them.[1]

In summary, not every older women is at high risk and not even every older woman with low bone density is at high risk. The women with lowest bone density in their age group and the most risk factors are at the greatest risk. Bone density measurement can provide useful information in deciding how much of a bone-building program is necessary, but such tests should be interpreted hand in hand with your personal risk factors.

Follow-up bone density measurements help assess the success of your bone-building program. Remember, however, it takes a few years to see changes in bone density. Generally the only change detectable within a year or less is unusually rapid bone loss.[25-29] The new urine tests described on the next page probably can better help you assess the short term progress of your bone-building program.

Finally, remember that if you are concerned about hip fractures you should have a direct measurement of the hip bone density and likewise for the spine or any other bone. Measurement of the spine or forearm, for example, will not accurately reveal hip density or vise versa.[30, 31]

❖ THE NEW URINE TESTS FOR BONE RESORPTION

Needless to say, it would be safer and less expensive if we were able to detect excessive bone loss and predict fracture likelihood with simple blood or urine tests. Indeed, researchers have been looking for such a test or series of tests. It now appears likely that selected biochemical markers found in the urine can help predict one's likelihood of developing osteoporosis. Currently at least two urine tests aimed at detection of excessive bone breakdown are commercially available.

When properly used, the direct bone measurements discussed above can help identify those at immediate risk of osteoporotic fracture due to excessively low bone density. These new urine tests, on the other hand, have the potential to address future risk. Even if your bone density is within the acceptable range now, if you are currently losing bone rapidly you are more like to suffer excessive cumulative bone loss in the future than is someone experiencing a slow current rate of bone loss. Also these non-invasive, inexpensive tests can help assess the success of your prevention and treatment program.

Both of these new tests look at the urinary excretion of bone breakdown by-products. Bone tissue is constantly broken down and replaced. With each cycle of breakdown and replacement, however, a bit more bone is broken down than is replaced. Thus a high rate of breakdown likely translates into greater bone loss over time.

The first test looks at the excretion of Type 1 collagen, a protein found in bone. Active bone loss, known as resorption, requires a breakdown of this protein. Thus the more of these protein fragments found in the urine, the more bone breakdown. The secondary urinary test for bone resorption involves the measurement of the collagen crosslinks, pyridinium and deoxypyridinium. Bone collagen contains both these substances and as bone breaks down they are released in the urine. The presence of higher than normal levels of pyridinium and deoxyprinidium crosslinks in the urine indicates an increased rate of bone breakdown. These urine tests appear to provide an accurate, inexpensive and non-invasive means of uncovering rapid bone loss in the process. Such early warning could serve as a stimulus for implementing a personal bone-building program as well as providing a means of assessing its success.[32-38]

As with bone density measurements the question of what "normal" values the laboratories choose to use is important. Again it appears that the standard used is normal young premenopausal women. For example, national studies of Type 1 collagen excretion suggest that some 65 percent of postmenopausal women have urinary levels higher than the upper limit of the normal range for premenopausal women.[36] As most Western women appear to undergo accelerated bone loss for a few years around menopause, this sounds reasonable.

While these new urine tests for bone breakdown look promising, many questions remain. For example, what is the cut-off point that distinguishes rapid peri- or postmenopausal bone losers from the more normal slower rates of bone loss? As women move a few years beyond menopause any stage of the more rapid bone loss that did develop around menopause tends to halt giving way to a much slower more typical rate of loss. What are the standards for this age bracket and how can a woman distinguish if she is continuing to lose excessive bone or if she has moved into the more common next stage of limited bone loss? Will a decrease in bone breakdown actually translate into greater bone density and fewer osteoporotic fractures?

While potentially very useful, these tests will require some refinement including the development of normal and ideal values for each stage of life. In the worst scenario, loosely interpreted tests could lead to massive and needless medication of older women. Ideally these tests will serve to distinguish the true rapid bone losers at any life stage and women will be given a full range of options for halting the excessive bone resorption rate. Also tests of bone resorption do not identify the causes of excessive bone breakdown. The underlying causes are often detected through careful risk-factor analysis and the sought-for corrections gained through risk-factor modification. A list of laboratories offering these simple and relatively inexpensive urine tests is given in Appendix 4.

Hopefully the information gained from both bone density measurements and the new urine tests for bone resorption will be used to encourage full development of life-supporting bone-building programs such as the one that follows. Hopefully they will not be used as a rationale for the mass medication of older women. Women's health advocacy groups like the National Women's Health Network and my Osteoporosis Education Project will be evaluating the implementation of these tests and assessing their usefulness.

❖ References

1 Cummings, Steven, et al., "Risk Factors For Hip Fracture In White Women," *The New England Journal of Medicine* 332.12 (1995): 767–774.

2 Alpan, J., "Preventive Dentistry," *Let's Live* Nov. (1983): 99.

3 Krook, L., et al., "Human Periodontal Disease and Osteoporosis," *Cornell Vet* 62.3 (1972): 371–391.

4 Mohammad, Abdel Rahim, et al., "Osteoporosis and Periodontal Disease: A Review," *California Dental Association Journal* March (1994): 69–74.

5 Albanese, Anthony A., "Diet and Bone Fractures," *The Nutrition Report* November 1986: 84–85.

6 Alpan, J., "Denture Fit—Preventive Dentistry," *Let's Live* Feb (1986): 61.

7 Daniell, H., "Postmenopausal Tooth Loss: Contributions to Edentulism by Osteoporosis and Cigarette Smoking," *Arch Intern Med* 143 (1983): 1678–1682.

8 Renner, R., "Osteoporosis in Postmenopausal Women," *The Journal of Prosthetic Dentistry* 52.4 (1984).

9 Wical, K., and C. Swoope, "Studies of Residual Ridge Resorption. Part II: The Relationship of Dietary Calcium and Phosphorus to Resorption," *J Prosthet Dent* 13 (1974): 13–22.

10 Anderson, J., F. Tylavsky, and P. Jacobsen, "Aging and Clinical Problems in Calcium Regulation Hormones," ed. E. Ogata, and H. Orimo. (Amsterdam: Excerpta Medica Publishers, 1984).

11 Sinaki M., et al., "Relationship Between Bone Mineral Density of Spine and Strength of Back Extensors in Healthy Postmenopausal Women," *Mayo Clinic Proceedings* 61.2 (1986): 116–122.

12 Halle, J. S., et al., "Relationship between trunk muscle torque and bone mineral content of the lumbar spine and hip in healthy postmenopausal women," *Phys Ther* 70.11 (1990): 690–9.

13 Pollitzer, William S., and John J.B. Anderson, "Ethnic and genetic differences in bone mass: a review with a hereditary vs. environmental perspective," *Am J Clin Nutr* 50 (1989): 1244–59.

14 Notelovitz, M., and M. Ware, *Stand Tall: The Informed Women's Guide to Preventing Osteoporosis*, (Gainesville, Florida: Traid Publishing Company, 1982).

15 Kuijk, Cornelius Van, and Harry K. Genant, "Detection of Osteopenia and Osteoporosis," *Treatment of the Postmenpausal Woman*, ed. Rogerio A. Lobo. (New York: Raven Press, 1994) 169–174.

16 Mazess, R., "Personal Communication," Continuing Education Course on Osteoporosis: Harvard University, 1987.

17 Stevenson, J.C., "Pathogenesis, prevention, and treatment of osteoporosis," *Obstet Gynecol* 75.528 (1990): 368–418.

18 Riggs, B.L., "Differential Changes in Bone Mineral Density of the Appendicular and Axial Skeleton with Aging Relationship to Spinal Osteoporosis," *J Clin Invest* 67 (1981): 328–35.

19 Melton, L., "Epidemiology of Fractures," *Osteoporosis Etiology, Diagnosis and Management*, ed. B. Riggs, and L. Melton. (New York: Raven Press, 1988) 133–154.

20 Raisz, L., and J. Smith, "Osteoporosis," *Clinical Endocrinology of Calcium Metabolism*, ed. J. Martin, and L. Raisz. (New York: Marcel Dekker, 1987).

21 Mazess, Richard B., "Fracture Risk: A Role for Compact Bone," *Calcified Tissue International* 47 (1990): 191–193.

22 Cummings, S.R., et al., "Bone density at various sites for prediction of hip fractures," *Lancet* 341 (1993): 72.

23 Melton, L., et al., "How many women have osteoporosis?," *J Bone Miner Res.* 7 (1992): 1005–1010.

24 National Osteoporosis Foundation, Audrey Singer, personal communication (October 20, 1995.)

25 Network, National Women's Health, "Osteoporosis Fact Sheet," National Women's Health Network, 1995.

26 Davis, J.W., et al., "Long-term Precision of Bone Loss Rate Measurements among Postmenopausal Women," *Calcified Tissue International* 48 (1991): 311–318.

27 Slemenda, Charles, and C. Conrad Johnston Jr., "Osteoporotic Fractures," *Nutrition and Bone Development*, ed. David Jason Simmons. (New York: Oxford University Press, 1990) 131–147.

28 Parfitt, A., "Metabolic Bone Disease After Intestinal Bypass For Treatment of Obesity," *Ann Intern Med* 89 (1978): 193–199.

29 Dalsky, G., "Exercise: Its Effects on Bone Mineral Content," *Clinical Obstetrics and Gynecology* 30.4 (1987): 820–832.

30 Mazess, Richard B., "Bone Density in Diagnosis of Osteoporosis: Thresholds and Breakpoints," *Calcif Tissue Int* 41 (1987): 117–118.

31 Carter, M.D., et al., "Bone mineral content at three sites in normal perimenopausal women," *Clin Orthop* 266 (1991): 295–300.

32 Bonde, Martin, et al., "Immunoassay for Quantifying Type I Collogen Degradation Products in Urine Evaluated," *Clin. Chem.* 40.11 (1994): 2022–2025.

33 Delmas, P.D., et al., "Immunoassay of pyridinoline cross-link excretion in normal adults and in Paget's disease," *J Bone Miner Res* 8 (1993): 643–648.

34 Hanson, Dennis A., et al., "A Specific Immunoassay for Monitoring Human Bone Resorption: Quantitation of Type I Collagen Cross-linked N-Telopeptides in Urine," *Journal of Bone and Mineral Research* 7.11 (1992): 1251–1258.

35 Gertz, B.J., et al., "Monitoring Bone Resorption in Early Postmenopausal Women by an Immunoassay for Cross-Linked Collagen Peptides in Urine," *Journal of Bone and Mineral Research* 9.2 (1994): 135–142.

36 Garnero, P., and E. Sornay-Rendu, "Assessment of age-related changes of bone turnover in normal women with new biochemical markers," *J Bone Miner Res* 9.1 (1994): S389.

37 Delmas, P.D., "Biochemical markers of bone turnover for the clinical investigation of osteoporosis." *Osteoporosis Int (1993) Suppl.,* 81–86.

38 Robins, S.P., "Collagen crosslinks in metabolic bone disease." *Acta Orthop. Scand. Suppl. 266* (1995), 66: 171–175.

10

Better Bones, Better Body Program

❖ It Is Never Too Late Or Too Early To Build Bone

*A*s you design your personal bone-building program never forget that osteoporosis is the end result of long-term lifestyle habits and physiological imbalances. Osteoporosis does not occur overnight, nor is it improved overnight. The journey back to good bone health may be long; yet even the longest journey begins with a single step. You can take that step now. Encouraging documentation grows daily that primary osteoporosis is not an inevitable part of aging. It can be prevented, halted and even reversed to some degree at any stage.

No matter where you are on the bone health continuum, no matter what your lifestyle has been, it is never too late to begin building healthy bone. Even the aged confined to wheelchairs have been able to build bone mass with simple exercises and modest nutritional supplementation. Those who have already suffered osteoporotic fractures can build bone density, move to reestablish bone health and thus prevent new fractures. Menopausal women and middle-aged women can regenerate bone and increase bone density instead of losing it. So can men. Adolescents and children have the greatest opportunity because, with proper nutritional and lifestyle modifications, they can achieve their optimal peak bone mass. A high peak bone mass provides the best foundation for ensuring lifelong healthy bones.

In the following chapters you will learn how to develop your own personal bone-building program, no matter what your stage of life. The Better Bones, Better Body Program was designed after careful study of the most successful clinical experiments and trials on osteoporosis. It incorporates the most successful bone-building techniques uncovered by dozens of scientific studies and goes beyond them to include more bone-building approaches than any other program to date.

Current research, although somewhat limited and fragmented, documents that:

1. Young people can build significantly greater bone mass and above average bone strength with simple nutrient supplementation. Adding physical activity provides additional bone-building benefits. The building of strong healthy bones is a natural process. Given adequate nutrients and stimulation in the form of physical activity during one's growing years, bones naturally grow strong and dense. Furthermore, even into the third decade of life it is relatively easy to build bone mass. For example, women aged 25 to 34 were shown to increase spinal bone mass by 10 to 15 percent with regular exercise and calcium supplementation (800–1,000 mg).[1,2]

2. One can halt excessive bone loss once it has begun—
   at any age. This includes halting bone loss and preventing new fractures even if you already have suffered an osteoporotic fracture. So far scientists have
   determined two natural, drug-free ways to stop bone
   loss at any age. One approach is through nutritional
   supplementation. The other is through exercise.

3. Osteoporosis can be overcome and to some degree
   reversed. By combining both nutritional and exercise approaches, researchers have found that lost
   bone density can actually be regained. Exactly how
   much lost bone can be rebuilt is an exciting question still to be answered by future research. Just
   as few people believed individuals could unclog
   blocked arteries and rebuild their own heart health
   until Dr. Dean Ornish proved it with his multifaceted nutrition and lifestyle intervention program[3],
   so few have recognized the potential of a comprehensive bone regeneration program. Only with the
   implementation of such a program can we test the
   limits of human bone regeneration capability.

Halting Bone Loss with Just Nutritional Supplementation

Numerous studies document that in young and old alike,
bone loss can be halted using just a small range of nutritional supplements. To date various combinations of calcium, vitamin D, zinc, manganese and copper have proven
capable of halting bone loss. There is no magic bullet; many

different combinations seem to work. Details about these various simple, successful nutritional programs are given in the following pages.

Some of the most interesting and successful nutritional supplementation studies involve the use of calcium in the form of calcium citrate and calcium citrate-malate along with other trace minerals. This research documents that post-menopausal bone loss can be halted and even minimally reversed, simply by taking daily supplements of calcium, zinc, manganese and copper.[4] This brand new research, using four minerals instead of just calcium, clearly documents that bone loss can be halted without the use of hormone drugs.

Halting Bone Loss with Just Exercise

Another whole set of studies now suggests that one can halt bone loss at any age with a systematic exercise program alone. Various types of exercise programs have been found to halt bone loss and even begin rebuilding bone mass in women of all ages. Illustration 10.1 which follows in a few pages details a sampling of these studies.

Rebuilding Lost Bone with Exercise and Nutritional Supplements

If bone loss can be halted with either exercise or nutritional supplementation, it is logical to expect that both approaches when used together would yield even better results. This is indeed true. One of the most striking combinations of exercise and nutritional supplement studies to date was conducted by Dr. Gail Dalsky at Washington University. In her experiment, outstanding bone regeneration was achieved with a simple program of regular and fairly rigorous exercise combined with calcium and vitamin D supplementation. Bone loss was not just stopped, it was reversed and lost bone was rebuilt. In this study postmenopausal women gained an impressive 6.1 percent in spinal bone mass over the two year program. During that same time period, study controls, that is similar women not doing the exercise and not taking the supplements, lost considerable spinal bone mass.[5] Even elderly nursing home residents were able to build bone mass with exercise and simple calcium and vitamin D supplementation.[6] Isn't it interesting that estrogen drugs, touted to be the best or even the only way to prevent osteoporosis, merely *halt* bone loss and only in some 75 to 80 percent of all women using them.[7]

How Much Bone Regeneration Could Be Achieved if a Comprehensive, Life-Supporting Program Were Implemented?

All this research inevitably leads to one provocative question: How much bone regeneration could be achieved if *all* the bone building nutrients, adequate exercise and bone enhancing lifestyle modifications discussed in this book were implemented to their fullest? Medical researchers have not even begun to ask this question. In fact, their tendency is to go in the opposite direction. For example, as mentioned above, scientists recently found they could halt postmenopausal bone loss and even perhaps begin to rebuild lost bone, using a nutritional supplement containing calcium, zinc, manganese and copper. This is remarkable and their experiments proved that this simple nutritional program is as effective, if not more effective at halting postmenopausal bone loss than estrogen therapy. However, instead of going further to see if using more bone-building nutrients could bring about a significant reversal of osteoporosis, they decided to go in the opposite direction. They began new studies cutting the nutrients one by one to uncover *how few* nutrients they could use and still halt bone loss.

One of the few physicians to move in the direction of seeking optimum bone regeneration is Dr. Guy Abraham, of Torrance, California. While his study did not include an exercise component, it did offer postmenopausal women a broad range of supplemental nutrients with outstanding results. He studied trabecular bone mass changes in two groups of postmenopausal women, both of whom were on estrogen replacement drugs. One group was given nutritional advice for building bone. The other group was given a broad spectrum nutritional supplement containing 26 essential vitamins and minerals which included 500 mg calcium and 600 mg magnesium.

Over the year of study, bone loss was halted but not rebuilt in the estrogen-using women who received dietary advice without supplementation. In contrast, the estrogen-using women who received the broad-spectrum supplement not only halted their bone loss, but gained a whopping 11 percent increase in trabecular bone mass![8] This study clearly documents the reversal of osteoporosis. Not only did women taking the nutritional supplements make unprecedented gains in bone mass, but with such gains, over 50 percent of them moved out of the fracture risk zone. That is, over half of all the women who began the study with bone densities so low that they were at high risk of suffering a fracture gained enough bone mass during the study to move out of the fracture risk zone.

Dr. Ronald Hoffman, director of the Hoffman Holistic Center in New York City, is another physician well experienced in rebuilding bone health through a comprehensive program of nutritional supplementation and lifestyle interventions. To illustrate the bone-building benefits of such an approach he documented for me a typical case of natural bone density regeneration. This case involved a 46-year-old woman who came to him with an average central portion vertebral trabecular bone mineral density of 102.6 mg per cc. This spinal bone density was low enough to put her at an above average risk for osteoporotic fracture. After 17 months on his nutrition, exercise and lifestyle program she was found to have 10.53 percent more bone mineral. This increase raised her vertebral density to 113.13 mg per cc which put her above the fracture risk threshold. The radiologist who measured her bone density was amazed to learn that these gains were made *without* estrogen therapy.[9]

❖ CLINICALLY PROVEN BONE-BUILDING PROGRAMS

All in all, a wide range of exciting studies document our capacity for bone regeneration. An overview of these studies is provided in the illustrations that follow. Remember these four important facts as you plan your Better Bones Program.

1. For every *one percent* increase in bone mass, the risk of a fracture from osteoporosis decreases by *six percent*.[10]
2. A *five percent* to *ten percent* increase in peak bone mass in young adolescents can translate into a *50 percent* reduction in risk of fractures in older years.[11] These reductions can add up to extraordinary financial, emotional and physical savings.
3. Adult Caucasian women in the United States face up to a 17.5 percent lifetime risk of breaking a hip.
4. Most of these devastating hip fractures could be prevented, even by taking action later in life. Moreover, even if you have suffered an osteoporotic fracture you can still prevent further fractures.

There are dozens, if not hundreds, of research studies in the medical literature which illustrate the effectiveness of nutrition supplementation and exercise programs in halting and even reversing osteoporosis. On the next pages, I offer just a sampling of these inspiring research findings in two tables. The first highlights simple programs found to halt and even reverse osteoporosis. The second reviews programs effective in eliminating new fractures in those with osteoporosis.

The research findings on the impact of nutrition and/or exercise on bone health in themselves are quite dramatic. Even more exciting is the fact that these groundbreaking results were achieved with only minimal intervention using only one or two nutrients and/or exercise.

Illustration 10.1

RESEARCH STUDIES ON HOW TO HALT AND REVERSE OSTEOPOROSIS

- ✦ In a Washington University School of Medicine study, postmenopausal women gained a whopping 5.2 percent in spinal bone mass in nine months and 6.1 percent in 22 months on a regular exercise program combined with 1,500 mg total calcium from dietary sources and calcium supplements. Controls not on the program lost spinal mineral during the same periods.[5]
- ✦ A study from the University of California found that postmenopausal women could not only halt spinal bone loss, but actually increase bone density on a nutrient supplement program of calcium (1,000 mg), zinc (15 mg), manganese (5 mg) and copper (2.5 mg). With these four supplements women gained 1.48 percent bone density. Women with no supplements lost over three percent bone mass within the same two year period.[4]
- ✦ In the Netherlands it was found that simple supplementation with 400 IU vitamin D_3 daily produced nearly two percent increase in hipbone density in elderly women.[12]
- ✦ In a Tufts University study 60-year-old women given daily calcium supplementation of 831 mg gained two percent hipbone mass over a one year period. Those without the extra calcium lost 1.1 percent of their hip mass.[13]
- ✦ Over a two year study, postmenopausal women with osteoporosis halted bone loss and even gained one percent trabecular bone density with just magnesium supplementation. The amount of mg used was 250 mg with doses up to 750 mg in the first six months.[14]
- ✦ Early postmenopausal women (average age 53) gained spinal bone density (1.6%) doing an exercise program designed to increase muscle strength. Similar women who did not exercise lost 3.6 percent of their spinal density during the same nine month period. Low intensity resistance exercises were used three times a week for 60 minutes each session.[15]
- ✦ A Canadian study found that women aged 50 to 62 were able to increase total body calcium and bone mass with a program of either aerobic exercises or aerobic exercises and strength training.

Exercises were done three times a week for 45 to 60 minutes. Control subjects who did not exercise lost body calcium.[16]

✦ Nursing home residents, average age of 81, built bone mass doing light exercises and taking 750 mg calcium and 400 IU vitamin D daily. The exercises were done from a chair three days a week for 45 minutes. The elderly on this modest program gained 2.3 percent bone mass while those not on the program lost 3.3 percent bone mass during the same three year period.[6]

✦ Among Boston-area women aged 50 to 70, high-intensity strength training exercises done twice a week for 45 minutes yielded detectable increases in both spinal and hip density while non-exercising controls lost bone from both sites. Muscle mass, muscle strength and dynamic balance also increased in the strength-trained women while these indices declined in controls.[17]

✦ Even older women who had already suffered an osteoporotic fracture increased their spinal density by 3.5 percent after eight months of exercising one hour, twice a week. Similar women who did not exercise lost 2.7 percent of their spinal mass during the same period.[18]

Illustration 10.2

RESEARCH STUDIES ON HOW TO ELIMINATE NEW FRACTURES IN THOSE WITH OSTEOPOROSIS

✦ Mayo Clinic researchers found that simple back strengthening exercises reduced the occurrence of new spinal fractures in osteoporotic women. After several years, only 16 percent of those doing the exercises suffered new spinal fractures, while 67 percent of those doing no exercise had new fractures.[19]

✦ Various combinations of calcium with and without vitamin D halved spinal fractures in osteoporotic women with an average age of 63.[20]

✦ Older French women, average age of 84, gained hip density (2.7 percent) on 1,200 mg tricalcium phosphate and 800 IU of vitamin D3. Controls lost 4.6 percent of their hip mass during the same period. With this simple intervention there were 43 percent fewer hip fractures and 32 percent fewer non-vertebral fractures in the women receiving these two supplements as compared to controls.[21]

✦ A California physician, Dr. Richard Lee, reports reversing osteoporosis using a program of transdermal natural progesterone (progesterone cream), diet, nutritional supplementation and mild exercise. Over the three year study period vertebral bone mass gains averaged 15 percent with no occurrence of new fractures.[22,23]

✦ Women ages 50 to 73 who had already suffered an osteoporotic fracture, increased their lumbar spine density by 3.5 percent after eight months of exercising one hour twice a week. Controls who did not exercise lost 2.7 percent of their lumbar spine during the same period.[24]

❖ GETTING YOUR PERSONAL PROGRAM STARTED: THE FIRST TWO STEPS

The first step in developing your own comprehensive bone-building program involves identifying the factors currently keeping you from perfect bone health.

Step #1 - Identify Your Total Load of Bone Depleting Factors.

Using the camel illustration on the next page, identify your total body burden of bone depleting factors. Circle all the bone-depleting factors you suspect to be significant in your case. Some of these factors, such as acid/alkaline balance and endocrine imbalance will be discussed further in subsequent chapters.

Illustration 10.3

THE TOTAL BODY BURDEN OF BONE DEPLETING FACTORS

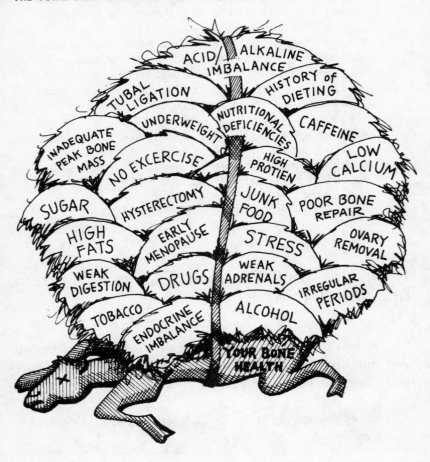

Graphic adapted from: William Crook, THE YEAST CONNECTION
Professional Books, 1986 (with permission)

Step #2 - Prioritize Your Bone-Building Action Program

Now looking at the camel illustration, think about which of your identified bone-burdening factors you would like to modify first. Some, of course, like early menopause or ovary removal, cannot be changed. Make a priority list for yourself of the factors you can change. Put them in order of importance to you. For example, your #1 priority might be to quit smoking, to reduce your meat intake to four ounces a day or to begin an exercise program.

I choose to work on my bone-limiting factors in the following order:

1.	5.
2.	6.
3.	7.
4.	8.

The Better Bones, Better Body Program consists of six key intervention areas.

1. Maximizing Nutrient Intake
2. Building Digestive Strength
3. Minimizing Anti-Nutrient Intake
4. Exercising into Bone Health
5. Developing an Alkaline Diet
6. Promoting Endocrine Vitality

Together these six intervention areas form the strongest, surest program for building and rebuilding bone ever designed. As you read through this book you will have the opportunity to integrate each of these key intervention areas into your personal bone building program. By the end of this book you can be well on your way to building better bones, better body and better health. Now let's work with each of these key intervention areas one at a time in the following chapters.

❖ References

1 Johnston, C., et al., "Calcium Supplementation And Increases In Bone Mineral Density In Children," *The New England Journal of Medicine* 327 (1992): 82–88.

2 Recker, Robert, et al., "Bone Gain in Young Adult Women.," *JAMA* 268.17 (1992): 2403–2408.

3 Ornish, D., *Program For Reversing Heart Disease*, (NY: Ballentine Fawcett, 1995).

4 Saltman, P, and L. Strause, "The Role of Trace Minerals in Osteoporosis," *Journal of the American College of Nutrition* 11.5 (1992): 599.

5 Dalsky, G., et al., "Weight-Bearing Exercise Training and Lumbar Bone Mineral Content in Postmenopausal Women," *Ann Intern Med* 108.6 (1988): 824–828.

6 Smith, E., W. Reddan, and P. Smith, "Physical Activity and Calcium Modalities for Bone Mineral Increase in Aged Women," *Med Sci Sports Exerc* 13.1 (1981): 60–64.

7 Lindsay, R., personal communication, Continuing Education Course on Osteoporosis: Harvard University, 1987.

8 Abraham, Guy E., "The Importance of Magnesium in the Management of Primary Postmenopausal Osteoporosis," *Journal of Nutritional Medicine* 2 (1991): 165–178.

9 Hoffman, Ronald, personal communication, Hoffman Center For Holistic Medicine, New York, NY (1995).

10 Randall, Teri, "Longitudinal Study Pursues Questions of Calcium, Hormones, and Metabolism in Life of Skeleton," *JAMA* 268.17 (1992): 2353–7.

11 Brody, Jane E., "The war on brittle bones must start early in life," *The New York Times* June 15 1994:

12 Ooms, Marcel E., et al., "Prevention of Bone Loss by Vitamin D Supplementation in Elderly Women: A Randomized Double-blind Trial," *J Clin Endocrinal Metab* 80 (1995): 1052–58.

13 Nelson, Miriam, et al., "A 1-year walking program and increased dietary calcium in postmenopausal women: effects on bone," *Am J Clin Nutr* 53 (1991): 1304–11.

14 Stendig-Lindberg, G., R. Tepper, and I. Leichter, "Trabecular bone density in a two-year controlled trial of peroral magnesium in osteoporosis," *Magnesium Res* 6 (1993): 155–63.

15 Pruitt, Leslie A., "Weight-Training Effects on Bone Mineral Density in Early Postmenopausal Women," *Journal of Bone and Mineral Research* 7.2 (1992): 179–185.

16 Chow, Raphael, et al., "Effect of two randomized exercise programmes on bone mass of healthy postmenopausal women," *BMJ* 295 (1987): 231–234.

17 Nelson, Miriam, et al., "Effects of High-Intensity Strength Training on Multiple Risk Factors for Osteoporotic Fractures A Randomized Controlled Trial," *JAMA* 272.24 (1994): 1909–1914.

18 Krolner, B., and B. Toft, "Vertebral Bone Loss: An Unneeded Side Effect of Therapeutic Bed Rest," *Clin Science* 64 (1983): 537–540.

19 Sinaki, M., and B. Mikkelsen, "Postmenopausal Spinal Osteoporosis: Flexion Versus Extension Exercises," *Archives of Physical Medicine and Rehabilitation* 65 (1984): 593–596.

20 Riggs, D. Lawrence, et al., "Effect Of The Fluoride/Calcium Regimen On Vertebral Fracture Occurrence In Postmenopausal Osteoporosis," *The New England Journal of Medicine* 306.8 (1982): 446–450.

21 Chapuy, Marie C., et al., "Vitamin D_3 and Calcium to Prevent Hip Fractures in Elderly Women," *New England Journal of Medicine* 328.23 (1992): 1637–1642.

22 Lee, J.R., "Osteoporosis Reversal. The Role of Progesterone," *Int Clin Nutr Rev* 10.3 (1990):384–91.

23 Lee, J.R., "Is natural progesterone the missing link in osteoporosis prevention and treatment?" *Medical Hypotheses* 35 (1991): 316–18.

24 Krolner, B., et al., "Physical Exercise as Prophylaxis Against Involuntional Vertebral Bone Loss: A Controlled Trial," *Clin Sci* 64 (1983): 541–546.

Chapter **11**

Maximizing Nutrient Intake

❖ How Adequate is Your Diet?

*T*he first step towards increasing your intake of the bone building nutrients is to assess how well your current diet provides you with the essential bone-building nutrients you need. How adequate is your diet?

The 18 key bone-building nutrients described in Chapter Four are listed in the following table. The adult daily recommended intake (RDA) of each nutrient is given along with the more ideal intake level necessary for health optimization along with an estimate of the average American intake. Using the food/nutrient charts in Appendix 3, determine how much of each nutrient you consume. Is your intake even near the ideal level for bone building and maintenance? Is your nutrient intake even near the RDA? Surprisingly, a recent U.S. survey found that not one person out of the 21,000 surveyed consumed the RDA for the ten key nutrients studied.[1]

The most accurate way to assess the adequacy of your diet is with a computerized diet analysis. (See Appendix 2). To analyze your own diet, turn to the tables in Appendix 3 to help you estimate your daily intake of selected key bone building nutrients. To do this write down everything you eat for a week and, using these tables, estimate how much calcium, magnesium, zinc, boron, manganese and vitamin K you consume. Divide by seven to get your average daily intake. If you are consuming the RDA of these selected nutrients, you know you are headed in the right direction. If your consumption of these nutrients is low, it is likely that your consumption of all bone-building nutrients is also inadequate. You can use these same tables to expand your intake of foods high in these key nutrients. Comprehensive wholesome food source tables for all 18 key bone building nutrients are available in the *Nutrition Detective Workbook* as described in Appendix 2.

18 Key Bone Building Nutrients[2-11]

Nutrient	RDA	More Ideal Intake	Average Intake	Your Intake
Calcium	800–1,200 mg	1,000–1,500 mg	400–550 mg. Typical diet is inadequate.	
Phosphorus	800–1,200 mg	800–1,200 mg	Inadequate intake is rare, excessive intake common.	
Magnesium	350 mg adult males, 280 mg adult females.	350–600 mg	Intake generally inadequate: 40% of population, 50% of adolescents consume less than 2/3 the RDA.	
Flourine	No RDA.	unknown	Between 0.2–3.4 mg.	
Silica	No values yet set	100–1,000 mg	Intake is unknown. Silica is the first to go in food processing, current intake is suspected to be low.	
Zinc	12–15 mg adults	15–20 mg	Average intake is 46 to 63% the RDA.	

Nutrient	RDA	More Ideal Intake	Average Intake	Your Intake
Manganese	2.0–5.0 mg adults	5–15 mg	Intakes generally inadequate.	
Copper	2.0–3.0 mg adults	3–4 mg	75% of diets fail to contain the RDA.	
Boron	No RDA.	3–4 mg	1/4 mg intake is common.	
Vitamin D	200 IU adults, 400 IU children	400–800 IU	Deficiency is common among the elderly.	
Vitamin C	60 mg adults	500–3,000 mg	26% of the population consumes less than 70% the RDA.	
Vitamin A	5000 IU adult males, 4000 IU adult females	5,000–10,000 IU	31% consume less than 70% the RDA.	
Vitamin B_6	2.0 mg adult males, 1.6 mg adult females.	5–50 mg	Over one-half consume less than 70% the RDA.	
Vitamin K	70–140 mcg	70–200 mcg	Unknown	
Vitamin B_{12}	2.0 mg adults	10–100 mcg	12% consume less than 70% RDA.	
Folic Acid	400 mcg adults	800–1,000 mcg	Average intake is 50% of the RDA	
Fats	No RDA.	15–25% of total calories.	The average American consumes nearly 40% of his/her calories in fat. The consumption of essential fatty acids, however, is generally deficient.	
Protein	63 grams adult males, 50 grams adult females	50–63 grams	Often approaches 100 grams.	

What Makes A Good Bone-Building Diet?

Even a diet that appears to be well balanced is often still deficient in several key nutrients. For example, let's imagine your daily food intake looked like this:

Breakfast	**Lunch**	**Dinner**
1 cup oatmeal	2 cups homemade lentil	chicken breast, 4 oz. stir-
½ cup 2% milk	soup;	fry vegetables, ½ cup
herb tea	2 cups salad (lettuce,	(with broccoli, carrots,
	carrots, radish, on-	corn and 1 T. olive oil)
	ions, salad dressing)	1 baked potato
	8 wheat thin crackers	2 pats butter
		baked apple
Morning Snack	**Afternoon Snack**	**Evening Snack**
banana	2 rice cakes,	2 chocolate chip cookies
	2 T. peanut butter	

As good as it is, this diet still provides somewhat less than the RDA for three of the 12 key nutrients. It contains only 60 percent of the zinc, 68 percent of the calcium and 75 percent of the B_{12} as analyzed by the Camde Nutri-Calc Plus Program. An additional cup of yogurt, however, would provide the extra calcium, zinc and B_{12} needed to meet the RDA for all of the 12 nutrients analyzed.

My point here is that while building a nutrient-dense diet is essential, it is not easy to obtain all the nutrients we need even from healthy meals. It is clearly impossible if you consume the standard American diet high in sugar, fat and processed foods. Half of all women in the United States consume less than 1500 calories per day and a diet with less than 1800 calories is guaranteed to be seriously deficient in necessary nutrients.[11]

Illustration 11.1

THE BETTER BONES, BETTER BODY EATING GUIDELINES

Whole Grains 1–3 servings at each meal
Brown rice, oats, corn, millet, barley, buckwheat, amaranth, quinoa, whole wheat, teff, triticale, rye, buckwheat, spelt, kamut

Vegetables *Low starch type:* 3 to 4 cups a day
Include 1 cup of high calcium leafy greens such as collards, kale, dandelion, turnip greens or bok choy, Other low starch vegetables include broccoli, carrots, spinach, lettuce, onions, celery, string beans, artichoke, summer squash, endive, cucumbers, asparagus, chard, peppers, parsley, sprouts, tomatoes.

Vegetables *High starch type:* 1 to 2 servings a day
Potatoes, yams, sweet potatoes, parsnips, winter squash, turnips.

Dried Beans 1 or more servings a day
(Legumes) Split peas, lentils, kidney beans, navy beans, chickpeas, aduki beans, black beans, white beans, mung beans, soy beans, tofu.

Flesh Foods Limit to one 4 or 5 oz serving a day. Fish is preferable. Fresh lean meats and poultry acceptable in moderation.

Dairy 0 to 3 servings, as tolerated. Yogurt is the most easily digestible and preferred form of dairy.

Fruits 1 to 3 per day (use fresh fruits in season when possible)

Essential Fats 2 to 3 teaspoons cold-pressed or expeller pressed vegetable oils of flaxseed, canola, safflower, sunflower, sesame.

Nuts and 2 to 3 Tbs. fresh, unsalted nuts and seeds, if desired.
Seeds Home-roasted sunflower, sesame or pumpkin seeds.

Water 8 glasses a day. Purified or spring water is preferred.

❖ EATING FOR BETTER BONES GUIDELINES

By now you might well be asking, "Just what should a good bone-building diet look like?" When considering your food intake keep these three general principles in mind.

> ### Bone-Building Dietary Principle #1:
> **Consume Whole Foods**

Use whole foods rather than processed foods. Vast quantities of nutrients are lost in the processing of foods. For example, in the processing of whole wheat flour to "enriched" white flour you lose more than 80 percent of the vitamin B_6, vitamin E and magnesium; more than 70 percent of the potassium, zinc and fiber; and more than 60 percent of the calcium, folic acid and pantothenic acid.

Using whole foods, for example, would mean consuming whole grains, such as brown rice, millet, barley and quinoa instead of white flour products of bread, pasta and crackers. Also fresh vegetables are used instead of frozen or canned ones. Dried beans, fresh fruits, fresh unroasted nuts and seeds are other nutrient-rich whole foods.

> ### Bone-Building Dietary Principle #2:
> **Keep Balance in Mind**

Consume a balanced diet of these whole foods. For example, a balanced diet would be high in whole grains, vegetables, beans and fresh fruits and low in meats, oils, fats and sugars. In such a balanced bone-building diet some 60 to 65 percent of the calories would come from complex carbohydrates; 8 to 12 percent from protein; 20 to 25 percent from fats and 10 percent from natural sugars.

The Better Bones, Better Body Diet is basically a well-balanced, alkalizing diet rich in vegetables and whole grains with moderate amounts of protein. At first it may seem like you have to make drastic changes in your eating habits, but soon it will feel right to return to fresh whole foods. Also remember that eating patterns are often deeply ingrained and many times deliberate step-by-step changes produce the best long term results.

Bone-Building Dietary Principle #3: Eat A Varied Diet

It is interesting to note that indigenous peoples living traditional lifestyles eat a wide variety of different foods while we tend to consume the same few foods over and over again. While many indigenous peoples consume well over 100 or so different food items from their environment, the average American regularly eats the same 18 or so foods. Variety in the diet is important. Each food has its own nutritional value so all colors, shapes and tastes of food should be consumed. Also consuming the same food over and over again increases the likelihood of developing a food hypersensitivity or allergy. The Japanese Dietary Guidelines for Health Promotion list as their #1 recommendation, "Eat 30 or more different kinds of food daily."[12] We would do well to follow their lead.

Six things I can do this week to move towards The Better Bones Diet:

1. _____

2. _____

3. _____

4. _____

5. _____

6. _____

Specific ways I can modify my very next meal to increase its bone-building value are:

FOR BREAKFAST:

I currently consume: I can modify this to:

FOR LUNCH:

I currently consume: I can modify this to:

FOR DINNER:

I currently consume: I can modify this to:

FOR SNACKS:

I currently consume: I can modify this to:

Your Weight and Your Bone Health

Whether you are overweight or underweight is a significant factor in determining your bone health. Being underweight means you are not eating enough calories, protein and other nutrients to maintain proper tissue and bone. As such, being underweight is one of the greatest risk factors for osteoporosis. Body weight correlates well with bone mass and studies show again and again that underweight persons suffer more osteoporosis than persons of average or above average weight. For example, well known osteoporosis researcher Dr. Ian Reid of New Zealand reported that total body fat was the best predicator of bone strength. Fatter women had stronger bones.[13]

If you are overweight you run less risk of having fragile

bones, but weight alone cannot make up for a low nutrient intake, a lack of exercise or other bone depleting factors. Most often those who are overweight overconsume and are often addicted to empty calorie foods containing high amounts of sugar and fat, but few, if any nutrients. If you are overweight, concentrate on nutrient-dense whole foods and limit empty calorie foods. If you are underweight, it is important you eat more nutritious foods on a regular basis.

Should You Use Supplemental Vitamins and Minerals?

If you tend to consume a low-nutrient diet and find it difficult to eat enough wholesome foods to maintain adequate nutrient intakes, then you might well consider the use of supplemental vitamins and minerals. Having analyzed hundreds of diets, I am convinced that nearly everyone in this country would have stronger bones and the osteoporosis fracture rate would be greatly reduced if everyone were to bring their nutrient intake up to at least the RDA levels. For most folks this would require supplementing their diet with at least a broad spectrum multi-vitamin/mineral tablet. By broad spectrum, I mean one which contains at least some amount of all 40-plus essential nutrients. The idea is to bring your intake of all essential nutrients to at least a minimum adequate level so that you have all the nutrients needed for optimum bone health.

The most successful bone-building programs, in fact, use a wide range of supplemental nutrients, not just calcium. Furthermore, all nutrients are important and should be available together. In fact, taking large amounts of a single nutrient can create imbalance within the body. It can actually be harmful to use nutritional supplements if they are not taken in a balanced way.

Moreover, there is no "one-size fits all" supplement. Some people require more nutrients than others, either because they have lower absorption rates or because they simply have an increased need. Studies on B_6, for example, have pointed to the possibility that some individuals require 40 times the amount of this nutrient than do others.[14] Vitamin E requirements vary at least five-fold in normal adults depending on their lifestyles and dietary habits.[15] Rates of calcium absorption have been found to vary up to three or four-fold. For example, two normal children living in the same environment were found to vary greatly in their calcium absorption. On the same diet, one retained an average of 264 mg calcium per day over the 45 day study period, but the other retained 469 mg per day, 78 percent more.[16,17]

At the very least, everyone would do well to know the exact nutrient content of their diet and to use nutritional supplements to bring their nutrient intake up to at least the minimal RDA levels if not to a more optimum, health promoting level. If you suspect special nutrient needs or inadequacies, you should consider consulting a nutritionist for the development of a personalized nutrition supplement program. In the meantime, a full-spectrum vitamin/mineral supplement would certainly do no harm.

Don't Take Calcium Without Companion Nutrients

Each bone-building nutrient is important and each has a certain relationship, a balance, with all others. If we consume high levels of one nutrient and low levels of the rest, we run the risk of disrupting the balance among all nutrients.

The risks of high level calcium supplementation deserve special attention given the current media push for increasing calcium intake. Over and over we are told to consume adequate calcium. What we are not told however, is that we also need all 17 other bone-building nutrients. They also forget to tell us that it can actually be harmful to consume high levels of calcium without its companion nutrients. Among other things, high and imbalanced calcium intake can:

✦ Block uptake of manganese.
✦ Interfere with absorption of magnesium.
✦ Decrease iron absorption leading at times to iron deficiency anemia.
✦ Interfere with vitamin K synthesis.
✦ Increase fecal phosphorus excretion.

Furthermore, using high doses of calcium in the face of magnesium deficiency can contribute to a depositing of calcium in the joints promoting arthritis, in the kidney contributing to kidney stones or in the arteries contributing to vascular and heart disease. This is a very important consideration as magnesium deficiency is very common in the United States. Additionally, very high doses of calcium carbonate (4 to 5 grams per day) have been documented to cause a serious, kidney damaging disorder called "milk alkali syndrome."

❖ BONE IS BUILT BEST WHEN ALL BONE-BUILDING NUTRIENTS ARE CONSUMED IN ADEQUATE SUPPLY

Science now verifies what common sense would dictate: we can build bone best when we supply our body not just with calcium, but with all the necessary bone-building nutrients. Nearly a decade ago, Dr. Anthony Albanese of White

Plains, New York found significantly greater increases in bone density resulted when a whole series of nutrients were given along with the calcium.[18] Recent research by Dr. Guy Abraham documented the same effect, as mentioned earlier in this chapter. Dr. Abraham supplemented postmenopausal women on estrogen therapy with a broad range of nutrients, including twice the RDA for magnesium and obtained an 11 percent increase in trabecular bone.[19]

Other scientists have supplemented postmenopausal women not on estrogen therapy with a smaller number of bone-building nutrients and found they can easily halt bone loss. In their breakthrough study Dr. Saltman and associates gave one group of postmenopausal women a placebo, that is a sugar pill. A second group was given just calcium citrate-malate (1,000 mg). A third group was given three bone-building trace minerals: zinc (15 mg), manganese (5 mg) and copper (2.5 mg). The fourth group was given the more complete program of the same three trace minerals (zinc, manganese and copper) along with 1,000 mg calcium in the form of citrate-malate. Women receiving the most complete supplemental program gained a significant amount of bone mass while those on just calcium remained the same. The women in the placebo group and the group with just the trace minerals without calcium suffered significant bone loss.[20] It is now clear postmenopausal bone loss can be halted without estrogen drugs by simply supplementing the diet with four minerals.

All these groundbreaking studies move *beyond calcium and beyond estrogen*. They represent the first steps of the medical establishment's slow move toward a more comprehensive approach to osteoporosis and bone regeneration. Over time, medical researchers will come to realize that all bone building nutrients should be used together and in balanced fashion. One day this holistic approach to preventing osteoporosis and regenerating lost bone will be standard medical practice.

❖ Designing Your Own Bone Building Supplement Program

There are countless vitamin/mineral products on the market and numerous special bone-building formulas. Given this wide range of products you may have difficulty choosing the best supplements for your needs. Let me share with you the guidelines I use in developing bone-building supplement programs for my clients.

Bone-Building Nutritional Supplement Programs:
The Better Bones Four Step Program

Step #1: Begin with a combination multi-vitamin/mineral supplement.

Step #2: Add as necessary a special calcium-centered bone building formula.

Step #3: Add as necessary other important bone-building nutrients not provided in the above preparations. Silicon, boron, adrenal glandulars and extra vitamin C are nutrients commonly added at this stage.

Step #4: Add nutritional digestive aids and self-help programs to enhance digestion as necessary.

Let's look at each of these four steps in detail.

Step #1 Selecting Your Multi-vitamin/Multi-mineral

Multi-Vitamin/Mineral Selection Guidelines

✦ The product should be broad spectrum. It should contain some amount of the 40-plus known essential nutrients.

✦ It should provide for balanced bone-building nutritional needs. For example, I like to see at least half as much magnesium as calcium. For those with arthritis, I prefer a formula that has equal magnesium to calcium. Although bone is high in phosphorus, I generally avoid high levels of phosphorus supplementation, as most of us get plenty in our diet.

✦ I personally favor formulas that are higher in the protective antioxidants (vitamin C, E, A, zinc and selenium).

✦ The forms of each nutrient in the formula should be of the highest quality and those most easily absorbed. For example, I look for calcium citrate, instead of calcium carbonate. I prefer multi-vitamin/ minerals without iron for several reasons. One is that iron and calcium compete for absorption and calcium wins, so calcium should be taken separately from iron. The second is that iron tends to oxidize and damage other nutrients in the supplement. The third is that iron can accumulate in the body and should only be taken if one is actually deficient in the mineral. When an iron supplement is called for, I recommend iron in the form of ferrous fumerate or ferrous gluconate. I avoid iron in the form of ferrous sulfate.

✦ Many higher quality formulas will contain substances to aid in the digestion and assimilation of the nutrients, e.g. betaine hydrochloric acid, pepsin or amylase.

✦ I recommend "hypoallergenic" formulas. These products are labeled as such and contain no artificial colors, flavors or other ingredients that may cause a reaction such as yeast, wheat, corn, phenol, sugar, etc.

The range of nutrients you will find in a good quality broad spectrum multiple/vitamin and mineral product are illustrated in the following table. Also you might find the

"Adult Guidelines For Total Nutrient Intake From Combined Food and Supplement Sources" helpful which is found in Appendix 1. This chart allows you to compare the RDA levels with a reasonable dietary intake level. In addition it lists a standard treatment level dosage for each nutrient.

In addition to your multivitamin/mineral formula, you might also need extra calcium and magnesium. This is especially true if both your multiple vitamin/mineral formula and diet are both below the RDA in these minerals.

Step #2 Selecting Your Source of Additional Calcium and Magnesium

My guidelines for selecting a calcium-based bone-building product to supplement the multiple vitamin/mineral are as follows:

Calcium-Based Bone-Building Formula Selection Guidelines

✦ Not all calcium supplements are the same. The key issue is which form of the nutrient is the most easily absorbed and assimilated. For absorption and bioavailability, the best calcium compounds known to date are: calcium citrate, calcium citrate-malate, mixes of calcium ascorbate, fumerate, pantothenate, malate, succinate, tartrate and microcrystalline hydroxyapatite.

✦ Calcium citrate, and its relative, calcium citrate-malate (CCM), are sources of calcium that do not require stomach hydrochloric acid for absorption, thus they are more bio-available. Calcium in the form of calcium citrate also appears to play a protective role against the formation of kidney stones and does not appear to interfere with iron absorption.[21]

Illustration 11.2

NUTRIENT CONTENT OF A BROAD SPECTRUM MULTI-VITAMIN/MINERAL SUPPLEMENT

Vitamins	Dose Range
Vitamin A	5,000 to 10,000 IU
Beta Carotene	5,000 to 15,000 IU
Vitamin D_3	30 to 400 IU
Vitamin E	100 to 400 IU
Vitamin C	100 to 1,200 mg
Vitamin B_1 (Thiamin)	15 to 100 mg
Vitamin B_2 (Riboflavin)	15 to 50 mg
Vitamin B_6 (Pyridoxine)	25 to 70 mg
Vitamin B_{12}	25 to 100 mcg
Niacin	25 to 50 mg
Niacinamide	25 to 150 mg
Pantothenic Acid	50 to 500 mg
Folic Acid	400 to 800 mcg
Biotin	100 to 500 mcg
Choline	50 to 150 mg
Inositol	50 to 100 mg
Bioflavonoid Complex	50 to 100 mg
PABA	20 to 50 mg
Minerals	
Calcium	50 to 500 mg
Magnesium	50 to 500 mg
Zinc	15 to 30 mg
Manganese	5 to 20 mg
Copper	1 to 2 mg
Chromium	50 to 200 mcg
Selenium	50 to 200 mcg
Molybdenum	25 to 100 mcg
Vanadium	25 to 50 mcg
Boron	1 to 3 mg
Digestive Aids	
L-Cysteine HCL	100 to 200 mg
Glutamic Acid HCL	10 to 25 mg
Betaine HCL	50 to 150 mg

✦ Microcrystalline hydroxyapatite (MCHC) is a specially processed whole bone extract. It contains all the minerals found in bone in the normal physiological proportions. The calcium and other nutrients in MCHC are very well absorbed. MCHC is widely used in Europe for the treatment of osteoporosis and has even been shown capable of slowing or halting bone loss induced by steroid treatment. Furthermore, it has been documented to help restore bone loss in cases of bilary cirrhosis where osteoporosis always occurs.[24-27]

✦ Calcium supplementation should always be balanced with magnesium supplementation. Some scientists such as Dr. Russell Jaffe, director of Serammune Physicians Lab and clinician, Dr. Guy Abraham of Torrance, California, favor magnesium-centered formulas with equal or slightly more magnesium than calcium. For details on enhancing magnesium absorption, see Appendix 4. As a rule of thumb I recommend at least one half as much magnesium as calcium. However, persons with osteoarthritis may want to use equal amounts of magnesium and calcium.

Many United States experts now suggest that the ideal calcium intake from all sources, food and supplements would range from 1,000 to 1,500 mg.[28-30.] See page 82 for the 1994 NIH Calcium Intake Recommendations.

An ideal magnesium intake would be higher than the current RDA and provide between 300 and 600 mg for both adolescents and adults and 100 to 200 mg for children. Once again, remember that anyone with kidney disease or other special health problems should consult her physician before taking supplemental magnesium or other minerals.

Step #3 Adding Other Bone-Building Nutrients

Using the supplements suggested in Steps 1 and 2, you should obtain a basic level of most bone-building nutrients. There are some nutrients I believe require higher doses than generally provided in Steps 1 and 2, and there are a few others that are not generally found in the first two steps. These nutrients include vitamins D and C and minerals like silicon and boron in addition to glandulars.

First, consider your vitamin D intake. The vitamin/mineral products and special bone-building products from Steps 1 and 2 are likely to contain some vitamin D_3. The RDA for vitamin D is 400 IU for ages 1 to 24 and 200 IU for those 25 and older. Interestingly enough, the RDA for vitamin D is lower for older people than for the young. Yet today our need for this nutrient appears to increase with age. Recent research at Tufts University found that 200 IU of vitamin D is not sufficient to halt the loss of bones from the hips of women in their mid-60s. These researchers suggest that somewhere between 700 and 800 IU daily is necessary to reduce hip loss for women living at Boston's latitude. So, an older person who gets little sunlight exposure would likely do well on 800 IU vitamin D_3[31] or even more, if directed by her physician. Remember, however, vitamin D is one of those fat-soluble vitamins that can accumulate in the liver and cause toxicity. Your total vitamin D intake should not exceed 800 IU unless recommended and supervised by your health professional.

Next, I often recommend using from 1,000 to 3,000 mg of vitamin C on a regular basis. For some people, 1,000 mg may be sufficient. If you suffer from signs of likely vitamin C deficiency (e.g. bleeding gums, periodontal disease or a tendency to black and blue easily) 2,000 to 3,000 mg per day is preferable. Also, for those with severe allergy, infection or immune compromise, I recommend vitamin C to bowel tolerance. Two self-tests to measure vitamin C adequacy are printed in Appendix 2. The form of vitamin C I prefer is fully buffered, alkalizing vitamin C powder (See Appendix 2). Pantothenic acid (vitamin B_5) is a companion adrenal-building nutrient which I often use along with vitamin C. You will learn more about this important nutrient in the next chapter. I recommend using 100 to 500 mg of pantothenic acid if one is under a lot of stress or has a tendency towards hypoglycemia.

The mineral boron is a hot new nutrient on the bone-building scene. It appears to help mineral metabolism in various ways. Scientists are just exploring the bone enhancing effects of boron and the ideal intake has yet to be established. Vegetarians and those on diets high in fruits and vegetables can consume 6–8 mg of boron daily, while the United States population as a whole might obtain less than one mg. Boron researchers suggest that a minimum intake of two to three mg might be more appropriate than the commonly consumed one milligram. Research on the use of boron as a supplement, however, has just begun and its safety as a supplement has yet to be documented. Going back to the table of wholesome food sources of boron given in Appendix 3, you can estimate your average boron intake and increase your consumption of foods high in this mineral. Also, there may be some boron in your multivitamin/mineral and/or in your calcium-centered bone-building formula. Given the limited experimentation with this "new" nutrient, it is wise to limit boron supplementation to three mg per day. Boron from food sources need not be limited.

Silica is another nutrient of importance to bone which you might want to add at this time. It is especially recommended in cases of serious bone loss or for those trying to heal fractures. The form to be used is organic silica from springtime horsetail grass in doses ranging from one to three tablets per day.

Vitamin K_1 is another nutrient essential to bone found only in selected nutritional supplements. Vitamin K_1 is produced by plants and is found in certain vegetables as listed in the table on Vitamin K sources. A diet high in green vegetables is the best way to ensure adequate Vitamin K intake.

Finally, I find that individuals with a tendency towards low blood sugar (hypoglycemia), allergies or those who are excessively fatigued most frequently benefit from adrenal glandular products. One or two capsules can be taken with each meal. I recommend a freeze dried adrenal which contains whole adrenal with a little adrenal cortex and licorice, Siberian ginseng, vitamin C, pantothenic acid and zinc. See Appendix 4.

Is the timing of vitamin and mineral use important?"

As supplements to our food intake, vitamins and minerals are generally best taken with meals. In this fashion, they are digested with the food. Also, many people will experience an upset stomach if they take supplements without food. It is wise to spread your supplements out over the day, taking some with each meal. Remember to save some of your calcium and magnesium supplements for use before bed. Many people note that these nutrients have a calming effect and promote better sleep. Postmenopausal women in particular experience increased calcium excretion overnight, which might be reduced by calcium intake around bedtime.[32] Finally, it is important to note that some nutrients are best taken apart from one another. Specifically, studies document that calcium and iron compete for absorption and that calcium wins. So if you need iron and want good iron absorption, as in the case of anemia, take your iron supplement at a different time of day than your calcium.

Step #4 Deciding on Aids to Enhance Digestion

Consuming adequate nutrients is one thing, absorbing and assimilating them is another. Good digestion and assimilation are essential for optimal bone health. Signs that your digestion might be weak include intestinal gas, cramps, bloating, diarrhea or constipation, stomach problems or deficiency syndromes like anemia, malabsorption and fatigue. The Better Bones approach to enhancing digestion is detailed in the next chapter.

❖ SPECIAL NOTES ON MAXIMIZING NUTRIENT INTAKE FOR THOSE WITH OSTEOPOROSIS

If you have dangerously low bone density or have suffered an osteoporotic fracture, take heart. There is much you can do to limit any further bone loss, avoid future fractures and even rebuild lost bone. The basic nutrition guidelines to consider are:

1. **Consume more nutrient-dense foods including more fresh vegetables, fruits, grains, beans, fish and perhaps even meat if you do not consume one serving a day.**

    The need to eat more is especially true if you are underweight. If you are overweight, cut out the empty calories and low nutrient foods like sugared foods, desserts, commercial breads, pastas, processed snacks and fried foods of all sorts. Use instead the fresh, whole foods as close to their natural state as possible. If your appetite is poor, you may well be suffering from a zinc deficiency. Inadequate zinc intake is especially common among elderly folks in this country. Ask your physician to run a red blood cell zinc test. In the meantime, begin taking 15 to 20 mg zinc in supplemental form. It is also possible you need to consume more protein. While most Americans consume too much protein, many elders consume too little. Unless you use whole grains and dried beans daily, you should eat at least one serving of animal protein each day. Protein malnutrition is a well documented risk factor of osteoporosis among the aged and protein supplementation along with vitamin and mineral supplementation has been shown to accelerate fracture healing.

2. **Use nutritional supplements to increase your intake of all essential bone-building nutrients.**

If you have osteoporosis, it would be wise to use a broad spectrum multivitamin/mineral supplement containing all essential nutrients. In addition, you should use supplements as necessary to bring your intake of all the key bone-building nutrients to optimum levels. Key nutrients and their reasonable intake levels are calcium (1,500 mg), magnesium (600–800 mg), zinc (15–20 mg), manganese (5 mg), copper (2 mg) and vitamin C (500–3,000 mg). Additionally, you may well need extra vitamin D. While the RDA for persons 25 years of age and older is only 200 IU, those with osteoporosis and especially older persons probably need much more. With age we lose about half of our ability to produce the active form of vitamin D from sunlight. Thus growing older, our need for dietary vitamin D greatly increases. Recently, a French team found they could reduce the hip fracture incidence in women with osteoporosis by about one half simply by adding a daily dose of 800 IU of over-the-counter vitamin D_3 and 1,200 mg calcium in the form of calcium triphosphate. This simple dietary intervention also lowered the number of wrist and forearm fractures in these women with osteoporosis while building their bone mass.[33]

Hip fractures are the greatest problem caused by osteoporosis. They bring the greatest loss of function and crippling, the greatest cost of care and the greatest loss of life. Scientists find that with proper nutritional supplementation, hip fractures can be prevented or at least delayed even if osteoporosis is established. While this is good news for individual women it is great news for society as a whole. As experts report, if we could simply delay the occurrence of hip fractures in the elderly by five to six years, we could reduce by half the total number of hip fractures.[34]

Finally, remember it is never too late to use nutritional supplementation to build bone health. Studies now document more rapid healing and dramatically better outcome in hip fracture patients given vitamin/mineral and protein supplements as opposed to those not given nutritional supplementation.[35]

3. Reduce Anti-Nutrients

Take a look at your consumption of sugar and sweets and cut these back to one serving or less a day. Avoid the salt shaker and minimize the use of processed foods. Eliminate caffeine totally or reduce your intake to just one caffeinated beverage per day. Alcohol consumption should also be restricted. Also remember medications can rob nutrients, decrease your agility and increase your chance of falling. Long-acting mood altering and sedative drugs significantly increase the risk of hip fracture and the latest recommendation is that older women avoid these drugs.[36] If your medications make you sleepy or less alert, ask your physician if the medication can be changed to one that would leave you more alert and less likely to fall.

4. Develop an Alkaline Diet
The development and maintenance of an alkalizing diet as described in Chapter 14, is one of the most important things you can do to reduce your risk of osteoporotic fracture.

❖ Special Notes on Maximizing Nutrient Intake for Perimenopausal Women

Studies have shown that many, but not all women in the United States lose a significant amount of bone around menopause. This period of accelerated bone loss occurs a few years before and a few years after the last period. Apparently bone is lost as the body readjusts to the tapering off of ovarian estrogen and progesterone. A likely possibility is that women in Western cultures like ours have higher estrogen levels during their reproductive years than women in traditional cultures. Because of this, Western women experience a more dramatic drop in estrogen at menopause. This in turn is associated with more dramatic menopausal

symptoms and perhaps greater bone loss during this perimenopausal period.

Little research attention has been given to how one can
naturally halt or reverse this phase of accelerated loss. Most
of the research attention has focused on estrogen drugs. Estrogens do tend to reduce the rate of bone loss in a majority
of women at this time. Also it is likely that natural progesterone creams will also halt perimenopausal bone loss. When
either the estrogen or progesterone supplements are with-
drawn, however, rapid bone loss begins anew.

Although not yet proven, I also suspect that a well developed program combining vigorous exercise and appropriate
nutritional supplementation along with an alkalizing diet
and adrenal enhancement would allow women to halt and
perhaps even build bone rather than lose it during this tran-
sitional period. The addition of abundant foods and herbs
containing phytoestrogens and phytoprogesterones is also
advisable. Foods and herbs containing compounds with
estrogen-like activity include soy foods such as tofu and
tempeh, fennel, nuts, whole grains, apples, alfalfa, red clover, dong quai, licorice root, and black cohosh root. Those
with progesterone-like activity include beans, wild yam,
chastetree berries (vitex), sarsparilla root, yarrow flowers
and leaves.[37,39]

Supplements with optimum levels of nutrients and herbs
that tonify the adrenals are vitamin C and pantothenic acid.
Ginseng is also useful as is the incorporation of nutrients
which extend the half-life of our natural estrogen such as
PABA, and those that seem to mimic estrogen, like the bioflavanoids and boron. There are several excellent books
which detail these and other ways to naturally raise hormone levels and smooth the menopausal transition. For further information see Appendix 5.

Also it is now clear that accelerated perimenopausal bone

loss need not be associated with increased osteoporotic fracture rates. The Mayan Indians of Mexico, for example, undergo a rate of perimenopausal bone loss similar to ours and their postmenopausal estrogen levels are even lower than ours. Yet osteoporotic fractures have not been seen nor could researchers even find any evidence of height loss among aging Mayan women. Interestingly, researchers also found no incidence of menopausal hot flashes among the Mayan women![40,41] Their diet is likely to be on the alkaline side and rich in phytohormones. Junk foods are uncommon in this culture and the lifestyle is rugged.

In Japan, the situation is somewhat similar in that postmenopausal women have lower bone density than their American counterparts, yet suffer many fewer fractures. Again an alkaline diet high in phyto-hormones and an active lifestyle combine to illustrate that thinner bone density does not necessarily mean more fractures.

For American women, the period around menopause is an important time to fortify one's health building program. Since certain women can lose an excessive amount of bone during these years, those at high risk would do well to consider the new urinary test for detecting bone breakdown discussed in Chapter 9. Then you will know if you are in fact losing bone at a troublesome rate and need to step up your bone-building program.

Menopause is a big business in the United States so you will be hearing a lot from your doctor, the media and the pharmaceutical companies about your need for hormone replacement, bone density measurements, calcium supplements, osteoporosis drugs, antidepressants, sleeping pills and the like. Underneath the uproar of this push for the medicalization of menopause, remember that the transition out of our reproductive years is as natural as the transition into them. In our culture puberty has it ups and downs. So might menopause. Yet menopause represents a simple, natural transition which women have experienced for millions of years without mass medication.

❖ SPECIAL NOTES ON MAXIMIZING NUTRIENT INTAKE FOR YOUTH STILL IN THEIR GROWING YEARS

Clearly the best way to prevent osteoporosis is to build strong, dense bones during the growing years. Around ten years of age a growth spurt occurs. The entire body, including the skeleton, undergoes rapid growth at this time. New bone is laid down at an accelerated rate. This is the time when one can most easily accumulate bone density. Almost all osteoporotic fractures could be prevented if individuals fulfilled their optimum peak bone mass in youth. Young people have a great opportunity to free themselves forever from this growing degenerative plague.

A nutrient dense diet is the place to begin. Many authorities now recommend that adolescents consume 1,500 mg of calcium, rather than the RDA of 1,200 mg for children ages 11 to 14.[19] In addition it is important that intake of all other nutrients reach at least the RDA level for their age. For example, adolescents would do well to consume daily 400 mg of magnesium, 15 mg zinc, 5 mg manganese and 2 to 3 mg copper in addition to their calcium. While adolescence produces dramatic nutrient needs, don't wait until then to enhance your child's nutrition program.

Most young people consume nowhere near adequate levels of the key bone-building minerals. Using the nutrient food source tables provided in Appendix 3 you can make dietary changes to increase intake of these minerals. Vitamin and essential fatty acid adequacy is also important. These nutrients can be obtained from the regular consumption of fresh fruits, vegetables, nuts and seeds as outlined in The Better Bones, Better Body Eating Guidelines (Illustration 11.1). Supplementation with a broad spectrum multivitamin and mineral will also help bring up vitamin levels while a few teaspoons of flaxseed oil will provide adequate essential fatty acids.

Finally, remember that diet alone will not ensure peak bone mass fulfillment. Physical activity is also essential. All children should engage in regular and vigorous exercise.

❖ References

1 Kanig, Joseph L., "Filling the Nutrition Gap," *Nutrition News* 12.9 (1989).

2 NIH, "Consensus Development Conference on Osteoporosis," (Washington, D.C.: National Institute on Aging, 1984).

3 Morgan, K., "Magnesium and Calcium," *J American College Nutrition* 4.2 (1985): 195–206.

4 Heaney, Robert P., "Prevention of Osteoporotic Fracture in Women," *The Osteoporotic Syndrome*, (New York: Wiley-Liss, Inc., 1993) 89–107.

5 Lakshmanan, F., "Calcium and Phosphorus Intakes, Balances, and Blood Levels of Adults Consuming Self-Selected Diets," *The Amer Jrnl of Clinical Nutrition* 40 (1984): 1368–1379.

6 Pennington, J., et al., "Mineral Content of Food and Total Diets: The Selected Minerals in Foods Survey, 1982 to 1984," *J Am Diet Assoc* 86 (1986): 876–891.

7 Freeland-Graves, J., "Manganese: An Essential Nutrient For Humans," *Nutrition Today* Nov/Dec (1988): 13–19.

8 Klevay, L., "Evidence of Dietary Copper and Zinc Deficiencies," *JAMA* 241 (1979): 1917–1918.

9 Nielsen, F., C. Hunt, and L. Mullen, "Effect of Dietary Boron on Mineral, Estrogen, and Testosterone Metabolism in Postmenopausal Women," *FASEB J* 1 (1987): 394–397.

10 Pao, E., and S. Mickle, "Problem Nutrients in the United States," *Food Technology* Sept. (1981): 58–64.

11 Krehl, "Vitamin Supplementation," *The Nutrition Report.* May (1985): 36.

12 Anon., "Japanese Guidelines," *Currents* 2 (1986): 17.

13 Reid, Ian, "Determinants of Bone Density in Postmenopausal Women," (Paper at a meeting of the Auckland Medical Research Society February 11, 1991).

14 Serfontein, W.J., et al., "Vitamin B⁶ revisited," *SA Medical Journal* 66 (1984): 437–40.

15 Anon., "An Overview of Vitamin E Efficacy in Humans: Part I," *The Nutrition Report* 11.3 (1993): 1–24.

16 Macy, I., *Nutrition and Chemical Growth in Childhood I*, (Springfield, III.: Charles C. Thomas, 1942).

17 Randall, Teri, "Longitudinal Study Pursues Questions of Calcium, Hormones, and Metabolism in Life of Skeleton," *JAMA* 268.17 (1992): 2353–7.

18 Albanese, A., "Effects of Calcium and Micronutrients on Bone Loss of Pre- and Postmenopausal Women," Paper presented at American Medical Association Meeting, 1981.

19 Abraham, Guy E., "The Importance of Magnesium in the Management of Primary Postmenopausal Osteoporosis," *Journal of Nutritional Medicine* 2 (1991): 165–178.

20 Saltman, P., and L. Strause, "The Role of Trace Minerals in Osteoporosis," *Journal of the American College of Nutrition* 11.5 (1992): 599.

21 Wabner, C., and C. Pak, "Modification by food of the calcium absorbability and physiochemical effects of calcium citrate," *J Am Col Nutr* 11 (1992): 548–552.

22 Grossman, M., J. Kirsner, and I. Gillespie, "Basal and Histalog-Stimulated Gastric Secretion in Control Subjects and in Patients With Peptic Ulcer or Gastric Cancer," *Gastroenterology* 45 (1963): 15–26.

23 Eufemio, Michael, "Advances in the Therapy of Osteoporosis-Part VIII," *Geriatric Medicine Today* 9.11 (1990): 37–49.

24 Dixon, A., "Non-Hormonal Treatment of Osteoporosis," *Br. Med J.* 286.6370 (1983): 999–1000.

25 Nileen, E.M. et al., "Microcrystalline hydroxyapatite compound in corticosteroid treated rheumatoid patients: a controlled study," *Brit Med J* 2 (1978): 1124.

26 Pines, A., et al., "Clinical Trial of Microcrystalline Hydroxyapatite Compound (MCHC) in the Prevention of Osteoporosis Due to Corticosteroid Therapy," *Curr Med Res Opin.* 8.734 (1984).

27 Epstein, O., et al., "Vitamin D, Hydroxyapatite, and Calcium Gluconate in Treatment of Cortical Bone Thinning in Postmenopausal Women With Primary Biliary Cirrhosis," *Am J Clin Nutr* 36 (1982): 426.

28 National Osteoporosis Foundation, *Physician's Resource Manual On Osteoporosis*, (Washington D.C.: National Osteoporosis Foundation, 1991).

29 NIH, "Optimal Calcium Intake," *National Institutes of Health* 12.4 (1994): 1–24.

30 NIH, Consensus Development Panel, "Optimal Calcium Intake," *JAMA* 272.24 (1994): 1942–1948.

31 Dawson-Hughes, et al., "Rates of Bone Loss In Postmenopausal Women Randomly Assigned to One of Two Dosages of Vitamin D," *Am J Clin Nutr* 61 (1995): 1140–1145.

32 Blumsohn, A., et al., "The Effect of Calcium Supplementation on the Circadian Rhythm of Bone Resorption," *Journal of Clinical Endocrinology and Metabolism* 79.3 (1994):730–5.

33 Chapuy, Marie C., et al., "Vitamin D_3 and Calcium to Prevent Hip Fractures in Elderly Women," *New England Journal of Medicine* 328.23 (1992): 1637–1642.

34 Farmer, M., et al., "Race and Sex Differences in Hip Fracture Incidence," *Am J Public Health* 74 (1984): 1374–1380.

35 Delmi, M., et al., "Dietary supplementation in elderly patients with fractured neck of the femur," *Lancet* 335 (1990): 1013–16.

36 Cummings, Steven, et al., "Risk Factors For Hip Fracture In White Women," *The New England Journal Of Medicine* 332.12 (1995): 767–774.

37 Lee, John R., *Natural Progesterone. The Multiple Roles Of A Remarkable Hormone*, (Sebastopol, CA: BLL Publishing, 1995) 105.

38 Fujita, T., and M. Fukase, "Comparison of osteoporosis and calcium intake between Japan and the United States," *Proceedings of the Society for Experimental Biology & Medicine* 200.2 (1992): 149–152.

39 Weed, Susan W., *Menopausal Years*, (Woodstock: Ash Tree Publishing, 1992) 199.

40 Martin, Mary C., et al., "Menopause without symptoms: The endocrinology of menopause among rural Mayan Indians," *Am J Obstet Gynecol* 168 (1993): 1839–45.

41 Beyene, Y., "Cultural significance and physiological manifestations of menopause," *Culture, Medicine & Psychiatry* 10.1 (1986): 47–71.

12

Building Digestive Strength

❖ Digestion and Your Magical Body

*D*id you ever stop to ponder just how your body transforms the foods you eat into blood, liver, heart, lung, bone and all your bodily tissues? How do we make all these varied tissues from hamburger, tofu, broccoli or carrots? Digestion and assimilation, the transformation of food into our fuel and our physical being, is "alchemy" at its best and indeed a magical feat of our magical body.

Many circumstances, imbalances and diseases can disrupt digestion and assimilation and less than ideal digestion and assimilation means less than ideal nutrient uptake. My grandmother, who broke her hip at the age of 101, suffered from poor digestion as a result of stomach ulcer surgery. Since that operation in later mid-life she ate a more restricted diet and absorbed less of what she did eat. All this contributed to the development of osteoporosis. At times I wonder if she would have lived out her full 120-year genetic potential lifespan had she not experienced this limitation in digestion and assimilation.

As an anthropologist, I am struck by the care that other traditional cultures give to the processes of food preparation and eating. In many cultures, foods are combined carefully at each meal to produce a variety of tastes and colors. Indian cuisine, for example, recognizes the therapeutic value of each taste and provides all five tastes (sweet, sour, bitter, astringent and salty) at each meal. The Japanese pay considerable attention to the appearance of food, knowing that an attractive plate of food opens the appetite and stimulates digestion. Equally, spices are used all over the world to enhance digestion, be they chilies in Mexico, curry in India or pickled radish in Japan.

In traditional cultures which maintain the wisdom of their ancestors over the generations, the creation of a peaceful environment for eating is also commonplace. Frequently children eat before the adults and while growing up, youngsters are taught the importance of sitting peacefully and quietly while eating. The importance of chewing one's food is also emphasized. In these cultures eating has a special time and place all its own. A priority is given to sitting down to eat at the same time each day. Children's recreational schedules do not override the regularity of meals, as occurs in our culture. So many of my clients report that their family hardly ever sits down together for a regular meal. The parents, it appears, spend more time chauffeuring for their children than cooking for them.

Furthermore, eating in traditional cultures is not accompanied by business talk, arguments, decision making, reading the paper or anything else. Eating is a time for eating, as I was informed by a Dominican peasant when I sat down to ask him some questions at dinner, "He who eats, eats," he said. Needless to say the questions were saved for later.

Traditional cultures respect the magical nature of digestion and assimilation more than we do and they set the stage for its success.

Digestion is indeed the hub of our physical existence and the improvement of any condition from bone health to psoriasis should begin with a program to enhance digestion. The Ten Steps To Stronger Digestion listed on the next page are simple recommendations I developed several years ago for my clients who were experiencing intestinal gas, bloating, loose stool and diarrhea or other signs of weak digestion. Time and time again they find that making these simple changes strengthens their digestion and alleviates their symptoms. It is no surprise that these simple guidelines should help for they are time-tested eating behaviors and patterns of traditional cultures around the world. In fact, when people from traditional cultures come to our country they are amazed by our careless and chaotic eating patterns.

I will never forget a brief conversation I had with a Chinese mechanic in the Los Angeles Chinatown. Stopping for gas, I asked the man if he knew of a good doctor of Traditional Chinese Medicine in Los Angeles, explaining that I thought Chinese medicine could help me. His reply was immediate. He looked at me and asked, "Why do you Americans want to see Chinese doctor? What do you expect for health when you drive around eating a hamburger?" Quite unsolicited, he made a few unforgettable points—and I was not even eating in the car when I spoke to him!

I now know that all of us living fast-paced contemporary American lives would do well to spice our eating with old fashioned wisdom. Consider implementing the following Ten Steps To Stronger Digestion. You might want to practice one step at a time. After following any given behavior for a few weeks it will become second nature. With each step you will note an improvement in your digestion.

❖ Ten Steps to Stronger Digestion

1. **Eat warm, cooked foods instead of cold or raw foods.** As traditional Eastern medicine explains, food must be "burned" in the fire of digestion. Cold and raw foods must be "heated-up" more than cooked foods and as such, they dampen and weaken the fire of digestion. Persons with weak digestion would do well to eat little or no raw or cold food or drinks. This means favoring cooked vegetables and fruits over raw ones and using hot soups, casseroles or grain and bean dishes instead of sandwiches or snack type meals. It also means drinking hot drinks. Ice water taken with meals weakens digestion.

2. **Chew your food well and eat at a moderate pace.** Ideally we should chew each mouthful some 30 times, breaking the food into small particles and allowing the salivary enzymes to begin their work digesting the food. Putting the fork down between each mouthful and swallowing one bite before taking another also helps.

3. **Eat in a peaceful and relaxed environment.** If you do a little comparative test, you will note that you feel better and your digestion is smoother when you eat in a quiet and peaceful environment. Avoid watching television, reading, working or arguing with others when you eat. You will see the difference.

4. **Eat simply.** Mixing many different types of foods taxes the digestive system. Experiment with simple meals of just two or three different foods.

5. **Eat fruit between meals and favor cooked fruit over raw fruit.** Raw fruits dampen the digestive

fire, especially during the winter when we are already cold. As such, those with weak digestion might find the ingestion of raw fruits with meals causes intestinal gas and bloating. Cooked fruit is a fine dessert, but keep the raw fruit for snacks. Even then raw fruit might be a problem if your digestive fire is smoldering rather than blazing.

6. **Drink hot water and hot herb teas.** Hot water is an excellent way to detoxify the body and build digestive strength. Simmering a few slices of ginger root in boiling water makes a ginger root tea that stimulates digestion. Ginger in food has the same effect, as does candied ginger root taken after meals.

7. **Eat freshly cooked foods.** Freshly cooked foods are most nourishing and free of molds or staleness. Better to eat a freshly cooked simple meal than a complicated one made of leftovers.

8. **Avoid overeating.** Excessive intake of food greatly burdens the entire digestive system. Ancient Ayurveda medicine recommends consuming the amount of food that will fit into two cupped hands. Practice moving away from the table while you are still a bit hungry.

9. **Sit still and relax a few minutes after eating.** Digestion is an amazing process; it turns tofu enchiladas into blood and cells. Resting a few minutes after eating gets this very complicated process off to a good start.

10. **Use supplemental digestive aids as necessary.** If you suffer from an "acid stomach," bloating or excessive flatulence which are not easily corrected by the above steps, you might want to try a few of the other self-help approaches listed below.

❖ Increasing Hydrochloric Acid Production

Many American suffer a significant decrease in stomach acid as they age. This translates into reduced digestive strength. It also means a reduced capacity to "sterilize" the contents of the stomach by the action of HCL killing off any unwanted bacteria, parasites or other pathogens that we are exposed to through eating and drinking.

Many people with common gas, bloating and even acid indigestion actually suffer from a lack of hydrochloric acid and/or low pancreatic enzymes. While your doctor can perform tests of such deficiencies, there are a few home tests and self-help remedies you can try. For example when you feel acid distress or reflux, try taking a glass of warm water with one tablespoon of apple cider vinegar. If your stomach feels better it is likely your indigestion was related to low stomach hydrochloric acid. If the vinegar water makes the situation worse, then you might really have an excess of acid. Many people with this problem, however, actually lack stomach acid.

There are various natural approaches to raising HCL. An old Vermont home remedy to naturally raise stomach acid production is to take one tablespoon of apple cider vinegar with a teaspoon of unrefined honey in a small glass of water before each meal. If you are severely diabetic or hypoglycemic you can omit the honey. Try this for three weeks and see how things go.

The Ayurvedic combination of ginger, ghee and brown sugar also stimulates digestion naturally. Also the use of bitters before a meal will enhance HCl production. In many cultures the use of herbal bitters or a salad of bitter greens such as escarole, artichokes, dandelion and mustard greens is taken for this purpose at the beginning of a meal. Alcoholic bitters such as the Italian aperitif Campari can serve the same purpose. Herbalist Susun Weed suggests drinking lemon juice in water with or after meals and/or adding 10 to 15 drops of dandelion root tincture to several ounces of water about 15 minutes before you eat.[1] Although it does not directly increase HCL, aloe vera drink is also excellent for the digestion and you might try taking one ounce after meals.

Dr. Russell Jaffe recommends using miso and other broths as well as bitters to begin meals as a way of enhancing HCL production. He also suggests using vitamin B_{12} in three divided doses, two mg each dose, three times a day plus the amino acid L-histidine. Histidine should be taken on an empty stomach, 600 mg four times per day.

If these home remedies are not sufficient, talk with your health professional about the use of digestive enzymes and/or additional medical testing. Always remember that none of these self-help suggestions are meant to replace standard medical care. If you suffer from any significant digestive or other health problem, be sure to consult with your health practitioner.

❖ THE RIGHT FOOD MIGHT BE WRONG FOR YOU: FOOD ALLERGIES AND OSTEOPOROSIS PREVENTION

Over my many years of practicing clinical nutrition I have come to appreciate the fact that food allergies and hypersensitivities are an underlying precipitating factor for many health complaints including digestive disorders. I have found that the vast majority of all those who seek my services have one or more immediate or delayed food allergies or sensitivities. Immediate food sensitivities are usually easily detected because reactions are immediate and occur shortly after ingestion of the food. Delayed allergies and hypersensitivities are more difficult to uncover because these reactions can take from five hours to five days to manifest. Any food reaction, be it immediate or delayed, represents a challenge to both the digestive and immune system and can have widespread consequences.

It is obvious that the true extent of food allergy and hypersensitivity has been seriously overlooked by the medical community at large. In my daily practice I see chronic symptoms ranging from heartburn and irritable bowel to sinusitis and headaches that are corrected once the offending foods are identified. Dr. James Breneman, a past president of the American Academy of Allergy, estimates that up to 60 percent of all Americans have food allergies or intolerances that are overlooked by the individual's physician.[2] A good part of the reason why food reactions are so often overlooked is because some 80 percent of these reactions are of the delayed type.

While no one to date has tried to establish a link between food allergies and osteoporosis, such a connection is likely. Healthy bone requires healthy digestion and full assimilation, while food allergies indicate breakdown in both digestion and assimilation. Also the chemical nature of the allergic response adds to the acid load. Increased acid load means a greater potential for bone loss. Should you suspect you have a food sensitivity or should you have symptoms commonly seen with allergies, I suggest you look into the food allergy connection.

As mentioned, immediate food allergies are easy to detect. You eat chocolate and get hives, a headache or diarrhea immediately or within a few hours. Signs of a delayed allergy or hypersensitivity, however, can take days to occur and they are hard to detect. If you get joint pain two days after eating wheat you probably would not connect the pain to the ingestion of wheat. Because of this, delayed reactions are often "hidden." While most immediate food reactions can be uncovered with a trial elimination diet as described below, the identification of delayed reactions requires sophisticated testing. Consult a doctor who specializes in food sensitivities or see Appendix 4 for details on how to obtain information on the Elisa/Act™ Test offered by Serrammune Physicians lab.

Immediate reactions can often be detected through a self-help elimination diet. The basic idea of an elimination diet is to remove from your diet the most common foods known to cause allergy problems. The most common food allergens include our most commonly used foods such as wheat and wheat products, milk and all dairy products, soy and soy products, corn and corn products, chocolate, peanuts, eggs, sugar, yeast or yeasted foods and additives and preservatives. So to begin a multiple elimination diet, you omit all of these from your diet for four or five days. You then reintroduce the food items one by one having it the first thing in the morning on an empty stomach. Also have the food in its simplest form. For example, when testing wheat, you might have plain spaghetti which is pure wheat and not bread which probably has yeast, sugar, additives and the like. Frequently symptoms will disappear during the elimination period and then reappear as the offending foods are introduced. For further information on developing a trial elimination diet, see Appendix 2.

Early in this century, the old school of healers and herbalists were fond of saying that "death begins in the colon." Interestingly enough, now as we move into the next century, intestinal health is once again finding a place on center stage. Again today there is a growing awareness that intestinal health is essential to wellbeing and that imbalances within the gut and a loss of gut integrity contribute to many chronic diseases.

❖ References

1 Weed, Susun W., *Menopausal Years*, (Woodstock: Ash Tree Publishing, 1992) 199.

2 Breneman, J.C., *Basics of Food Allergy*, (Springfield, IL: C. Thomas, 1978).

Chapter **13**

Minimizing Anti-Nutrient Intake

*A*nti-nutrients are substances which work against good nutrition. They rob nutrients and rob bone. Caffeine, alcohol and tobacco are anti-nutrients. Also certain food substances including protein, sugar, fat and salt taken in excess can act as anti-nutrients. Anti-nutrients are often addictive substances which we use in excess as stimulants. As addictions, they may take some time to kick. Take one step at a time, but be persistent.

❖ CUTTING EXCESSIVE PROTEIN INTAKE

While we all think of protein as "healthy" and necessary, few of us realize that the protein intake of persons living in the United States is generally much too high. The adult RDA for protein averages 50 grams for females and 63 grams for males. Many of us consume upwards of 100 grams of protein per day. High protein consumption contributes to a host of health problems including constipation, colon cancer, heart disease and osteoporosis.[1] High protein intake can cause a significant loss of calcium from bones. This is especially true if a high-protein diet is combined with a low-calcium intake.

Using the table below and the chart on the next page, estimate your daily protein intake. For a more exact calculation, consider obtaining a computerized diet analysis.

Most of the concentrated protein we consume comes from animal products. Cutting your intake of meat is by far the best way to reduce excessive protein intake. Switching some of your diet away from animal protein to vegetable protein is also wise. Protein from vegetable sources causes less urinary calcium loss than does flesh food proteins.[4]

The recommended daily protein intake is 50 grams for adult females and 63 grams for adult males.

I consume _____ servings of meat, chicken or fish each day and I estimate my total protein intake at _____ grams.

I can reduce my protein intake by making the following changes:

1.

2.

3.

4.

Remember, dried beans (e.g. kidney beans, lentils, split peas, chick peas or soybeans, as in tofu) make an excellent meat substitute. Combinations of vegetable foods, such as beans and grains, yield very usable, high quality protein.

BETTER BONES, BETTER BODY

Illustration 13.1

PROTEIN CONTENT OF SELECTED FOODS[2,3]

Flesh Foods	Serving Size	Grams of Protein
Turkey	4 oz	33
Fish	4 oz	25–30
Beef	4 oz	33
Chicken	4 oz	33
Eggs	1	6.2
Dairy		
Yogurt	1 cup	11
Milk	1 cup	8
Cheese	1 oz	7
Beans and legumes, cooked		
Soy beans	½ cup	9.9
Tofu	½ cup	9.8
Chick peas	½ cup	8.4
Lentil, kidney and lima beans	½ cup	7.8
Peanut butter	1 Tbs	3.9
Grains		
Oatmeal, cooked	1 cup	6.0
Bread	1 slice	2.0
Rice	½ cup	2.2
Vegetables		
Not a good source of protein		
Nuts/Seeds		
Almonds	¼ cup	7
Cashews	¼ cup	7
Peanuts	¼ cup	9
Walnuts	¼ cup	7

❖ REDUCING YOUR CAFFEINE COUNT

As already mentioned, as little as 300 mg of caffeine can cause a considerable loss of calcium from the body. Using the following illustration, calculate how much caffeine you currently consume.

Illustration 13.2

THE CAFFEINE COUNT

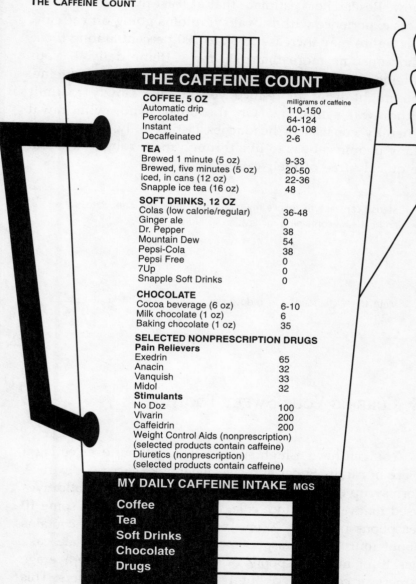

THE CAFFEINE COUNT

COFFEE, 5 OZ — milligrams of caffeine
Automatic drip	110-150
Percolated	64-124
Instant	40-108
Decaffeinated	2-6

TEA
Brewed 1 minute (5 oz)	9-33
Brewed, five minutes (5 oz)	20-50
iced, in cans (12 oz)	22-36
Snapple ice tea (16 oz)	48

SOFT DRINKS, 12 OZ
Colas (low calorie/regular)	36-48
Ginger ale	0
Dr. Pepper	38
Mountain Dew	54
Pepsi-Cola	38
Pepsi Free	0
7Up	0
Snapple Soft Drinks	0

CHOCOLATE
Cocoa beverage (6 oz)	6-10
Milk chocolate (1 oz)	6
Baking chocolate (1 oz)	35

SELECTED NONPRESCRIPTION DRUGS
Pain Relievers
Exedrin	65
Anacin	32
Vanquish	33
Midol	32

Stimulants
No Doz	100
Vivarin	200
Caffeidrin	200

Weight Control Aids (nonprescription)
(selected products contain caffeine)
Diuretics (nonprescription)
(selected products contain caffeine)

MY DAILY CAFFEINE INTAKE MGS

Coffee	
Tea	
Soft Drinks	
Chocolate	
Drugs	
TOTAL	

Caffeine is very addictive, as many coffee drinkers know. Researchers estimate that at least five percent of all users experience withdrawal symptoms going off caffeine. This figure may increase to 82 to 100 percent among those who consume more than 600 mg caffeine daily. If your caffeine intake is high or if you are sensitive to caffeine, you might want to reduce your intake slowly to limit withdrawal symptoms. On the other hand, withdrawal generally consists of headaches lasting only a few days. Many people choose to live through these rough days and be quickly free of their caffeine addiction.

Steps I can take to reduce my intake of coffee, tea, chocolate, colas and caffeine-containing medication include:

1.   3.

2.   4.

With these changes I can reduce my daily caffeine intake to _____ mg.

❖ CURBING YOUR SWEET TOOTH

You can have a high sugar intake without ever eating a piece of candy. Sugar and sweeteners like sucrose, dextrose, corn syrup and fructose are the most popular food additives used today. A 10-ounce cola, for example, contains some 10 teaspoons of sugar. A one-ounce serving of jelly contains about four to six teaspoons and a piece of chocolate cake has 10 or more teaspoons of sugar. Each year, the average American consumes about 140 pounds of sweeteners. This works out to be the equivalent of one-half cup of sugar per day. The sugar content of various foods is listed in the following table.

Illustration 13.3

SUGAR CONTENT OF SELECTED FOODS

Food	Amount	Tsp. Sugar
Soft Drinks		
Cola drinks	12 oz.	10
Ginger ale, 7-Up	12 oz.	7
Cider	8 oz.	6
Desserts		
Angel food cake	1 piece	7
Chocolate cake, iced	1 piece	15
Cupcake	1	6
Fig newton	1	5
Macaroons	1	6
Donut, glazed	1	6
Candies		
Fudge	1 oz.	4.5
Gum drop	1	2
Chocolate bar	1.5 oz.	2.5
Peanut brittle	1 oz.	3.5
Jams and Jellies		
Jelly, marmalade, jam	1 oz.	4–6

The high sugar foods I consume include:

1.	4.
2.	5.
3.	6.

I can cut down or eliminate my consumption of processed sugar and sweeteners by making the following changes:

1.	4.
2.	5.
3.	6.

Remember, a strong craving for sweets indicates nutrient deficiencies and imbalances. An intractable sweet tooth can be corrected with appropriate nutrient and herbal supplementation, along with simple dietary modifications. If you find it difficult to resist sweets, try the following program.

FIVE STEPS FOR CORRECTING YOUR SWEET TOOTH

1. Avoid all sugars and sweeteners; substitute fresh fruits. Warmed apple cider with the juice of one half a lemon and a bit of honey can help cut cravings.
2. Elimiate caffeine, alcohol and other stimulants which tend to lower blood sugar and produce an artificial hunger for sweets.
3. Use supplemental chromium. Chromium is a mineral needed by your body to produce "glucose tolerance factor," a factor which helps stabilize blood sugar and eliminate cravings. Generally 200 mcg is enough to do the trick. If not try 400 mcg for a few weeks.
4. Supplements of adrenal glandular tissue are also helpful, especially if you have a tendency towards hypoglycemia.
5. If you are still having trouble with sweets you can add an herbal supplement called *"Sweet Tooth Blues"* produced by the Medicine Wheel Company and available in most health food stores. This is a licorice/dandelion formula which works well to reduce the sweet craving and to build adrenal, spleen and pancreas strength. This herbal formula however should not be used by those with high blood pressure as licorice has been known to raise blood pressure.

❖ TRIMMING EXCESSIVE FAT

As a group, Americans currently consume roughly 40 percent of their total calories from fat. In contrast, the typical Oriental diet is 10 to 15 percent fat. Cutting fat helps to build bone as well as reduce the risk of cardiovascular disease, many cancers, diabetes, stroke, obesity, hypertension and numerous other disorders.

The following table lists the fat content and percent of total calories in fat of selected foods. The average woman would do well to limit her fat intake to roughly 35 to 45 grams of fat per day and a man, perhaps 45 to 55 grams. Those desiring to lose weight will find it much easier to do so if they limit their daily fat intake to 30 grams or less.

Illustration 13.4

FAT CONTENT OF SELECTED FOODS

Flesh Foods	Serving Size	Grams Fat	% Calories from Fat
Turkey, dark meat w/skin	4 oz	8	35%
Turkey breast, no skin	4 oz	2	11%
Chicken, light meat w/skin	4 oz	12.3	44%
Chicken breast, w/o skin	4 oz	4.13	20%
Fish, flounder	4 oz	1.4	8%
Beef, roast, no visible fat	4 oz	14.6	48%
Beef, roast, w/visible fat	4 oz	51.2	88%
Beef, ground	4 oz	17.7	53%
Ham, smoked, w/o fat	4 oz	10	42%
Tuna in water	4 oz	0.93	6%
Fish, haddock	4 oz	1	9%
Eggs	1	6	65%

Dairy

Yogurt, plain whole milk	1 cup	7.4	48%
Yogurt, plain lowfat	1 cup	3.5	22%
Yogurt, fruit lowfat	1 cup	2.5	10%
Milk, skim	1 cup	0.4	4%
Milk, whole	1 cup	8.1	49%
Swiss cheese	1 oz	7.8	66%
Cheddar cheese	1 oz	9.4	74%
American cheese	1 oz	8.9	76%

Beans and Legumes

Soy beans, cooked	½ cup	5.1	39%
Tofu	½ cup	5.4	54%
Chick peas, cooked	½ cup	2.4	16%
Lentils, cooked	½ cup	Trace	0%
Kidney beans, cooked	½ cup	0.5	4%
Lima beans, cooked	½ cup	0.2	2%
Peanut butter	1 Tbs	7.4	77%

Grains

Oatmeal	1 cup	2	12%
Bread, wheat/white	1 slice	1	14%
Croissant	1	12	46%
Rice, brown	½ cup	0.5	5%

Vegetables

Plain vegetables have small or
negligible amounts of fat

Other

Apple pie	1 piece	18	40%
Doughnut	1	12	51%
Frosted chocolate cake	1 piece	21	49%
All oils	1 Tbs.	14	100%
Butter	1 Tbs.	11	99%
Margarine	1 Tbs.	11	100%

I calculate my current fat intake to be roughly _____ grams per day. I can reduce my fat intake by making the following dietary modifications

1.   5.

2.   4.

3.   6.

❖ Setting Aside Salt

We consume too much salt and this can cause a loss of calcium and other minerals from the body. Most of the salt we consume does not come directly from our salt shakers, but is added to the food we eat during food processing. Did you ever notice you were thirsty after eating? This is a sure signal that your body found the food too salty.
To reduce your intake of salt:

1. Cook with only a small amount of salt.
2. Avoid processed foods especially canned foods and fast foods.
3. Check labels for sodium content, if you use packaged foods.

Remember, our government recommends that we limit daily sodium intake to 2,000 mg (about 1 teaspoon) or less and if you keep your salt down to that level, you will be more likely to retain calcium. Our Paleolithic ancestors of the Stone Age consumed only 700 mg per day. What is your sodium intake?

Illustration 13.5

SODIUM CONTENT OF SELECTED FOODS

Dairy Foods	Amount	Mg Sodium
Milk, whole or skim	1 cup	120–125
Swiss cheese	1 oz	74
Cottage cheese	4 oz	457
American cheese	1 oz	406
Roquefort cheese	1 oz	513
Pizza	1 slice	600
Flesh Foods		
Shrimp, raw	3 oz	137
Shrimp, canned	3 oz	1,955
Tuna, fresh	3 oz	50
Tuna, canned	3 oz	384
Tuna pot pie	1	715
Smoked fish	3 oz	500 to 5000
Beef, fresh	3 oz	55
Jumbo burger, fast food	1	990 to 1510
Beef, corned	1 oz	487
Beef broth	1 cup	782
Bologna	1 slice	220
Hot dog	1	639
Corned beef hash	1 cup	1520
Chicken, roasted	½ breast	69
Chicken pot pie	1	907
Chicken fast food dinner	1	2,243
Pork, fresh	3 oz	59
Bacon	4 slices	548
Ham	3 oz	1,114
Vegetables and Beans		
Potato, baked	1	6
Potato chips,	10	200
Potato, instant mashed	1 cup	485
Vegetables, fresh steamed	1 serving	1 to 24
Vegetables, canned	1 serving	326 to 584
Tomato, fresh	1	1 to 14
Tomato soup, canned	1 cup	932

Tomato sauce	1 cup	1498
Corn, fresh off ear	1 cup	trace
Corn flakes	1 cup	256
Corn, canned	1 cup	384
Peas, fresh cooked	1 cup	trace
Peas, canned	1 cup	493
Split pea soup, canned	1 cup	1956
Beans, dried and cooked without salt	1 cup	13
Pork and beans, canned	1 cup	2130
Soy beans, cooked	½ cup	2
Grains		
Rice, brown (and most other grains)	1 cup	trace
Rice, beef flavored, Uncle Ben's	1 cup	1284
Macaroni, cooked without salt	1 cup	2
Macaroni and cheese, packaged	1 cup	574 to 1086
Oatmeal, regular, no salt	¾ cup	trace
Oatmeal, instant	¾ cup	255
Fruits		
Fresh, most all	1	trace
Fruit pie,	1 piece	605
Seasoning		
Salt	1 tsp	2,132
Soy sauce	1 Tbs	440

❖ Avoiding Tobacco and Alcohol

Smoking is one of our cultural habits and lifestyle factors most damaging to bone. In a recent study of nearly 10,000 women aged 65 and over, current smoking was associated with a double risk of hip fracture as compared to non-smokers and former smokers. In this study, the qualities of smokers that contributed to this increased risk of hip fracture included the fact that they had gained less weight, or lost more, than nonsmokers; had poorer health in general; had more difficulty rising from a chair; spent fewer hours on their feet; were less likely to walk for exercise; and had faster heart rates.[5] It is never too late to stop smoking. It will not only lower your risk of dying of heart disease or cancer, but it also will reduce your risk of hip fracture.[5,6]

My favorite approach to smoking cessation is the "Smoking Awareness" technique taught by Deepak Chopra. This approach uses our awareness to awaken our body's natural intelligence. The suggestion is that when one smokes, one should put his or her full attention on smoking. Go to a special place to have a cigarette, sit down and do nothing else but smoke. Do not read, drink coffee or partake in any other activity. So many times smoking is a habitual response to something else like reaching for a cigarette each time you drink coffee, when you take a break or when you answer a stressful telephone call. In opposition to this habitual almost unconscious smoking, the goal here is to put one's full attention on the act of smoking. What does it taste like? How does it feel? The idea is to thoroughly experience the process. While smoking, check in with your body and ask yourself how things are going. Is smoking really enjoyable? How does it taste in your mouth and feel in your throat and lungs? Have you had enough for now? Bringing awareness to the act of smoking and listening to your own body will eventually lead to a cessation of smoking.[7]

Excessive alcohol is a major bone killer, as already detailed in Chapter 7. While moderate alcohol intake (a few drinks per week) might not be a problem, excessive alcohol hinders calcium absorption, damages the liver, and can hinder vitamin D metabolism. Take a moment to calculate how much alcohol you drink each week.

Currently I drink _____ alcoholic beverages per week. I can reduce this to _____ drinks this week and _____ drinks next week. My final goal is to reduce my alcohol intake to _____

❖ References

1 Barnard, Neal, *The Power of Your Plate*, (Summertown, TN: Book Publishing Company, 1990).

2 Gebhardt, Susan, and Ruth Matthews, "Nutritive Value of Foods," United States Department of Agriculture, 1981.

3 Leveille, Gilbert A., et al., *Nutrients in Foods*, (Cambridge, MA: The Nutrition Guild, 1983).

4 Zemel, MB, "Calcium utilization: effect of varying level and source of dietary protein," *Am J Clin Nutr* 48 (1988): 880–3.

5 Cummings, Steven, et al., "Risk Factors For Hip Fracture In White Women," *The New England Journal of Medicine* 332.12 (1995): 767–774.

6 Paffenbarger, Ralph S., et al., "The Association Of Changes In Physical-Activity Level And Other Lifestyle Characteristics With Mortality Among Men," *The New England Journal of Medicine* 328.8 (1993): 538–545.

7 Chopra, Deepak, *Perfect Health*, first ed. (New York: Harmony Books, 1990).

Chapter 14

Developing An Alkaline Diet

❖ Your Body's Acid-Alkaline Balance is Very Important

*Y*our body is the greatest chemical manufacturing plant under the sun. For that chemical magic to work perfectly, uncounted factors must be in perfect balance. With only marginal balance we get only marginal results. One of the most important, yet most overlooked internal balances, is that of the acid-base balance.

In Chapter 7, we learned that the chemistry of the human body operates best in an alkaline state and the internal environment of a healthy body is slightly alkaline, maintaining a pH just above 7.0. The countless chemical reactions necessary for life can only occur within a very specific pH range. Because the pH level is so critical, the body has many checks and balances to maintain its pH within a narrow range. One of the major mechanisms for bringing pH back into line when it has become too acid is to draw calcium and other alkalinizing minerals from the bones to buffer this acidity and alkalinize the body. While our bones do not suffer from an occasional withdrawal of calcium for alkalinization, excessive and prolonged acidity can drain bone of calcium reserves and lead to bone thinning.[1] New research now documents the long standing speculation than an acid internal condition leads to a loss of minerals from the body and from the bone in particular.[2]

❖ DIET CAN CONTRIBUTE TO EXCESS ACIDITY

Many organs and systems, especially the kidneys, adrenals and lungs, play important roles in maintaining proper pH. Diet, however, is also important. Everything we ingest is "burned" in the furnace of our digestion. Upon digestion, each food leaves either an acid or alkaline ash, depending on the minerals it contains. On a balanced whole foods diet, the acid and alkaline ash remains in proper proportion and does not adversely affect body pH. An imbalanced diet high in animal protein, sugar, caffeine and processed foods, however, can disrupt pH balance. In our society we consume a very imbalanced diet high in acid-forming foods. This imbalanced diet pushes us towards an acid state, the response to which is a withdrawal of calcium from the bones.

Which Foods Have an Acid-Forming Effect and Which Foods Have an Alkaline-Forming Effect?

The majority of fruits and vegetables leave an alkalinizing effect. Most grains are somewhat acid-forming as are high protein foods. Refined sugar is acid-forming, while nat-

292
. . . .

BETTER BONES, BETTER BODY

ural sea salt is alkaline-forming. The acid and alkaline reactions of various common foods as complied by Dr. Russell Jaffe are illustrated at the end of this chapter. Ideally our diet should be composed of about 35 percent acid-forming foods and 65 percent alkaline-forming foods. Offering a general guideline, Dr. Jaffe suggests that for every 10 foods we eat, six are vegetables (especially leafy greens), two are fruits, one is protein and one is high starch like potatoes.[3] Individuals recovering from illness would do well to raise the alkaline portion of their diet to some 80 percent of all foods.

❖ MONITORING YOUR ACID/ALKALINE BALANCE

The first step in establishing a health-promoting alkaline diet is to assess your current pH. A good measure of average body pH is easily obtained by assessing the pH of your first morning urine. To do this, follow these simple steps:

1. Obtain a packet of pH hydrion test paper. This test tape measures acid-alkaline states and should be marked into one-half point divisions ranging at least from 5.5 to 8.0. Should you not be able to obtain this tape in a local drugstore, see Appendix 4.
2. First thing in the morning, just before your first urination, open the test tape packet and cut off two or three inches of the paper tape. Now wet the test tape with urine.
3. As the tape is moistened with urine it will take on a color. The color relates to the acid or alkaline state of your urine and ranges from yellow to dark

blue. Match the color of your test strip with the color chart on the back of the test tape packet.

4. Jot down the number that corresponds to the color your tape has taken on. Any number below 7 means that your urine is on the acid side. The lower the number, the more acid the condition. For example, a number of 4.5 indicates considerable acidity while 6.0 indicates much less. A number of 7 indicates the neutral state, neither acid or alkaline. The body functions best in an alkaline state. Ideally the first morning urine pH should be neutral or near a pH of 6.5 to 7, (an occasional 7.5 to 8 reading is okay). When the first morning urine is neutral or just slightly acidic, this indicates that the overall cellular pH is appropriately alkaline.

5. If your readings fall below 6.5, you should begin changes aimed at alkalinizing your diet. Below are listed simple dietary modifications that will help alkalinize your diet. In the beginning, because of the acid-forming tendency of the standard American diet, most people will find low pH readings. On the other hand, there will be an occasional person whose pH readings are always highly alkaline (greater than 7.5). A knowledgeable health professional can provide more information for those with this situation. See Appendix 2 for more information.

❖ DEVELOPING AN ALKALINE DIET

Your body is a very complicated chemical processing plant with 60 trillion plus cells involved in some 6 trillion chemical reactions each second. While the chemical processes can occur in an acid environment, this is not ideal. An alkaline internal state is required for ideal chemical functioning and for the achievement of optimal health. If your pH readings are regularly below 6.5, your overall health would improve if you alkalinize your diet by making the following dietary changes:

Take a few minutes and study Illustration 14.1 entitled "Food and Chemical Effects on Acid/Alkaline Body Chemical Balance." This easy-to-use chart clearly details which foods make the body more alkaline and which make it more acid. Note that on the left side of the page are listed the foods and substances that are alkalinizing to the body. To the furthest left are the most alkaline substances like salt, sea vegetables, yams, lentils and limes. Towards the middle of the sheet on the same left side are the lower alkaline substances like ginger tea, oats, Brussels sprouts and oranges. On the right hand side of the page are listed the acid-forming foods. The highest acid-forming foods are to the far right. These include jams, ice cream, walnuts and beef. The lesser acid-forming foods are to the center of the page and include honey, fish, brown rice, kidney beans and figs.

As you are studying this chart, note that most of the favorite American foods and drinks are acid forming. Meats are acid forming as is sugar, coffee, tea, cheese and all dairy products except clarified butter. Wheat is acid forming, as are most grains. No wonder most Americans are in an acid body chemical state. We eat mostly acid-forming foods! On the other hand, most fruits and vegetables are alkaline-forming as are oats, quinoa, wild rice, most spices and most seeds.

If you regularly have a first morning urine lower than 6.5 and are attempting to regain health, a good goal would be to strive for a diet of predominately alkaline-forming foods. For those recovering from disease, ideally the diet should be 80 percent alkaline forming and only 20 percent acid-forming. As one regains health, a 60 percent alkaline to 40 percent acid diet is generally fine. To simplify matters, let your first morning urine pH be your guide. If you are below 6.5 then increase the alkaline foods. If you are 6.5 to 7, you are in a health-promoting acid/alkaline balance.

If you are in an acid state, the first step is to eat more of the alkalinizing vegetables and fruits. For example, strive for two cups of the alkalinizing vegetables at both lunch and dinner. Consider a breakfast of alkaline fruits or oatmeal. Limiting flesh foods will also go a long way towards reducing acidity. In addition, the following simple changes are especially helpful for quickly alkalinizing the body:

✦ Drink the juice of one-half lime, lemon or apple cider vinegar in water a few times during the day. Although these citrus fruits contain organic acids, when metabolized by the body, they leave an alkaline residue. The same holds true for apple cider vinegar made from whole apples which are high in alkalinizing minerals.

✦ Add yams and sweet potatoes to your diet on a regular basis as well as lentils. All these foods help to alkalinize the body quickly.

✦ Make it a point to eat daily at least one cup of alkalinizing greens (kale, mustard and turnip greens, collards or endive). Use lettuce as well, but in addition to these other greens. Also, grated daikon radish is a wonderful alkalinizing condiment.

✦ Learn how to prepare miso and seaweed in soups and other dishes and consume some daily, even if only a small amount. Miso soup with daikon radish, ginger and seaweed is both a great digestant and an alkalinizer.

✦ Favor the alkalinizing grains like oats, quinoa and wild rice.

✦ Enjoy liberal amounts of fruits. In season eat plenty of watermelon and its juice along with the other melons and fruits and berries. If you suffer from gas, bloating or weak digestion, favor cooked fruit and small amounts of fresh juices.

✦ Certain supplements like the buffered vitamin C, magnesium and L-glutamine also alkalinize and should be used in optimum doses as recommended (see Appendix 1).

Be patient and persistent. Remember, an alkaline pH indicates good reserves of the alkaline minerals. It can take time to build up these reserves. Do not be discouraged with a slow movement towards the ideal alkaline state, a pH of 6.5 to 7.

FOOD AND CHEMICAL EFFECTS ON ACID/ALKALINE BODY CHEMISTRY BALANCE

Most Alkaline	More Alkaline	Low Alkaline	Lowest Alkaline
Baking soda	Spices	Herbs (most)	Ginger tea
Sea salt	Cinnamon	Green tea	Sucanat
Mineral water	Molasses	Rice syrup	Úmeboshi vinegar
Umeboshi	Soy sauce	Apple cider	Algae
plums	Kambucha tea	vinegar	Ghee
			Mother's milk
			Oats
			Grain coffee
			Quinoa
			Wild rice
Pumpkin	Poppy seeds	Primrose oil	Avocado oil
seeds	Chestnuts	Sesame seeds	Flaxseed oil
	Pepper	Cod liver oil	Coconut oil
		Almonds	Olive oil
		Sprouts	Other seeds
Lentils	Kohlrabi	Potato	Brussel sprouts
Onion	Parsnip	Bell pepper	Beets
Daikon	Garlic	Mushrooms	Chives/cilantro
taro root	Kale	Cauliflower	Okra
Sea	Parsley	Rutabaga	Turnip greens
vegetables	Endive	Salsify	Squashes
Burdock	Mustard greens	Ginseng	Lettuce
lotus root	Ginger root	Eggplant	Jicama
Sweet	Broccoli	Pumpkin	
potato/yam		Collard greens	
Limes	Grapefruit	Lemons	Oranges
Nectarines	Canteloupe	Pears	Apricots
Persimmons	Honeydew	Avocado	Bananas
Raspberries	Citrus	Pineapple	Blueberries
Watermelon	Olives	Apples	Currants
Tangerines	Loganberries	Blackberries	Raisins
	Mangoes	Cherries	Grapes
		Peaches	Strawberries
		Papaya	

Illustration 14.1 *(Cont.)*

FOOD AND CHEMICAL EFFECTS ON ACID/ALKALINE BODY CHEMISTRY BALANCE

Lowest Acid	Low Acid	More Acid	Most Acid
Curry	Vanilla	Nutmeg	Jam/jelly
Honey	Black tea	Coffee	Table salt
Maple syrup	Alcohol	Saccharin	Yeast
Rice vinegar	Balsamic		hops/malt
	vinegar		Sugar
			Cocoa
			White vinegar
Cream	Cows' milk	Casein, milk	Processed cheese
Yogurt	Aged cheese	protein	Ice cream
Goat/sheep	Soy cheese	30-day cheeses	
cheese	Goat milk	Soymilk	
Eggs	Lamb/mutton	Pork/veal	Beef
Gelatin	Boar/elk	Squid	Pheasant
Organs	Shellfish	Lobster	
Vension	Goose/turkey	Chicken	
Fish			
Wild duck			
Triticale	Buckwheat	Maize	Barley
Millet	Wheat/kamut	Barley groats	
Kasha	Spelt/Teff	Corn	
Amaranth	Farina/	Rye	
Brown rice	Semolina	Oat bran	
	White rice		
Pumpkin	Almond oil	Pistachio seed	Hazelnuts
seed oil	Sesame oil	Chestnut oil	Walnuts
Grape seed	Safflower oil	Pecans	Brazil nuts
oil	Tapioca	Palm kernel oil	Fried foods
Sunflower oil	Seitan		
Pine nuts			
Canola oil			

Illustration 14.1 *(Cont.)*

FOOD AND CHEMICAL EFFECTS ON ACID/ALKALINE BODY CHEMISTRY BALANCE

Lowest Acid	Low Acid	More Acid	Most Acid
Spinach	Tofu	Green peas	Soy beans
Fava beans	Pinto beans	Peanuts	Carob
Kidney beans	White/red	Snow peas	
String beans	beans	Carrots	
Chutney	Azuki beans	Chickpeas	
Rhubarb	Lima beans		
	Chard		
Guava	Plum	Cranberries	
Pineapple	Prune	Pomegranates	
(dry)	Tomatoes		
Figs			
Persimmon			
Cherimoya			
Dates			
	Antihistamines	Psychotropics	Antibiotics

(Ref. Serammune Physicians Lab, Reston, Virginia, 1995). Table prepared by Dr. Russell Jaffe.

❖ References

1 Barzel, U., "Acid Loading and Osteoporosis," *Journal of the American Geriatric Society* 30 (1982): 613.

2 Sebastian, Anthony, et al., "Improved Mineral Balance and Skeletal Metabolism in Postmenopausal Women Treated with Potassium Bicarbonate," *New England Journal of Medicine* 330.25 (1994): 1776–1781.

3 Jaffe, Russell, and Patrick Donovan, "The importance of an alkaline diet," Serammune Physicians Lab, 1993.

Chapter # 15

Exercising Into Bone Health

A great body of research now proves that exercise builds strong bones and the documentation grows daily. It is well known that exercise, especially lifelong exercise, is one of the most important factors in building and maintaining healthy bones. While athletes have stronger bones than sedentary people, even modest exercise benefits bone. A recent Finnish study, for example, suggests that regular physical activity of just four hours a week or more is associated with significantly higher bone mineral density.[1]

While regular lifelong exercise is best for bone, it is never too late to begin building bone density with exercise. A bone building exercise program can be started at any stage of life. Best of all, even a modest exercise program yields impressive results as detailed earlier. When exercise is combined with proper nutritional supplementation, increases in bone density are even greater. Everyone from the athletic youth to the aged confined to wheelchairs have been able to build bone mass with the dynamic duo of exercise and nutrition supplementation.

Remember, bone mass and muscle mass increase and decrease together. As your muscles strengthen, so do your bones. Importantly, both bone and muscle can be substantially rebuilt at any age. The studies on rebuilding lost muscle are just as impressive as those with rebuilding bone. Several studies show that weight training undertaken by sedentary elderly individuals can increase muscle mass by 15 to 20 percent and muscle strength by 200 percent in just 10 weeks.[2] Even more, Dr. William Evans of the Knool Laboratory For Human Performance Research at Penn State University reports that with their exercise program they can make a 95-year-old as strong as a 50-year-old and a 65-year-old as physically fit as a healthy 30-year-old.[2,3,5] The Better Bones, Better Body approach is to use a strong, clinically proven bone-building exercise program along with a comprehensive nutritional supplement program and lifestyle modifications. Our exercise component is modeled after the most successful research studies to date.

❖ SAMPLE EXERCISE PROGRAMS

It is clear that physical activity and the placement of strain on the bones stimulates them to grow dense and strong. From current research, it appears that the exercise programs which yield the greatest bone-building results are those involving strength-training exercises as well as some aerobic component. Let's look at a few of the most successful bone-building exercise programs.

At the University of Toronto, Dr. Chow and colleagues conducted a one year exercise program with postmenopausal women aged 50 to 62. During the study period, women were divided into three groups. One group did no special exercise. The second group undertook aerobic exercise and the third group did a program combining both aerobic and strength-training exercises The aerobic exercise consisted of 5 to 10 minutes warm-up followed by 30 minutes of aerobic activity (walking, jogging, aerobic dance, etc.). Exercise was done at 80 percent maximum heart rate. The combination aerobic and strength-training program consisted of 10 to 15 additional minutes of low intensity strength training. Strength training involved exercises using free weights attached to the wrists and ankles working various muscle groups in the arms, legs and trunk. The women performed 10 repetitions in each muscle group at the maximum weight possible for them. At the end of the year the women doing the aerobic exercise gained 4.1 percent in the calcium bone index and those doing the aerobic exercise plus strength training gained 7.5 percent. The nonexercising control group lost bone calcium during the same period.[7]

Another study from the University of Washington study conducted by Dr. Gail Dalsky further documents the remarkable benefits gained through strenuous exercise. In this study a modest nutrition component was included adding vitamin D and calcium supplements. These research findings again indicate that women can actually build bone mass after menopause. The bone built was spinal trabecular bone and the amount rebuilt was substantial. Over a period of several months, sedentary postmenopausal women participated in an exercise program which consisted of weight bearing and aerobic exercises. They exercised from 50 to 60 minutes, three times a week. Calcium intake was controlled at 1500 mg combined with 50 IU of vitamin D_3. At the end of nine months, exercisers showed a 5.2 percent increase in spine mineral density. After 22 months in the program, the women showed a 6.1 percent increase in bone density. Thus, postmenopausal women actually gained bone density at a time when they otherwise would have rapidly lost bone![8] Every one percent increase in bone mineral yields a six percent decrease in the risk of osteoporotic fracture.[9] The details of Dr. Dalsky's bone building exercise program are as follows:

Illustration 15.1

DR. DALSKY'S CLINICALLY PROVEN-BONE BUILDING PROGRAM

1. Exercise was regular, but just three times per week. Each exercise session lasted one hour. The exercise was strenuous with the aerobic component being done at 70 percent of maximum oxygen uptake.
2. Exercises were of both the weight-bearing, strength-training type (walking, jogging, stair-climbing, weight-lifting) and nonweight-bearing aerobic exercises (cycling, rowing).
3. Bone mineral increases were seen after nine months, but were even greater after 22 months.
4. Calcium intake was controlled at 1500 mg per day, through a combination of diet and calcium supplements. The calcium supplement used was calcium carbonate, not the best form of calcium for building bone. The only other nutrient given was a modest 50 IU vitamin D_3 per day.
5. The gains in bone density were maintained as long as the women did the exercise program. The gains made, however, were largely lost when the women stopped exercising.[8, 10]

A third sample exercise program is a more recent study from the USDA Nutrition Research Center again at Tufts University. These researchers broadened their approach looking not only at how exercise might help bone mass but also how physical training might improve other osteoporosis risk factors such as muscle mass, strength and balance. In this year-long study, postmenopausal women aged 50 to 70 were divided into two groups. The placebo group did only their regular activity while the study group undertook high intensity strength training two days a week. Each exercise session lasted just under an hour with 45 minutes of strength training and 10 minutes warm-up and stretching. The exercises used included hip and knee extensions, lateral pull-downs, back extensions and abdominal flexion using pneumatic resistance machines. Training intensity goal was set at 80 percent of the person's 1RM, "one repetition maximum" (details on how to calculate your 1RM to follow). With this simple, twice-a-week strength-training program, women were able to halt bone loss and even build somewhat over one percent bone mass in both the hip and spine. Sedentary controls lost 2 percent bone mass during this time period. As the author of this study noted, over time this small but steady gain in bone mass will look very good when compared to the ever growing bone losses of non-exercising women. Even more, these active women gained strength, the greatest being a 76 percent increase in upper back and arm strength while the sedentary group did not experience any increase. Exercisers also improved their balance by an average 14 percent while balance in the control group worsened by 8 percent. Each of these factors—bone density, strength and balance—in their own way serves to reduce the risk of osteoporotic fracture.[11]

So, exercise and strength training benefit bone in various ways and even halting bone loss is in itself a significant feat. Remember that the total number of hip fractures would be reduced by one-half if the occurrence of fractures could be delayed by five or six years.[12] Appropriate exercising, even if done for only a few years after menopause, should help delay fractures. Finally, even more bone might be built if all of the bone-building nutrients are used in adequate amounts. Therefore, I suggest your exercise program be accompanied by enough nutritional supplementation to bring your total daily intake of all 18 key bone-building nutrients up to optimum levels. An alkalizing diet and the avoidance of anti-nutrients would yield even more benefits.

Together, proper nutrition, a life-supporting lifestyle and adequate exercise can help build and rebuild one at any life stage. Hopefully, you have already committed yourself to making some bone-building nutritional and lifestyle changes. Now let's go on with developing the exercise component of you personal Better Bones, Better Body Program.

❖ DEVELOPING YOUR OWN PERSONAL EXERCISE PROGRAM

The exercises you choose should be activities you enjoy or that you can learn to enjoy. If you do not currently exercise regularly, begin slowly and build up exercise time and endurance. If your overall health and bone density permit, aim at incorporating both weight-bearing and aerobic exercises into your program. Following Dr. Dalsky's model, include a variety of exercises including walking, jogging, stair climbing, weight lifting and/or cycling. A good combination of strength-building, weight lifting and aerobic exercise enhances cardiovascular fitness while also fortifying bone.[8, 13]

When it comes to weight-bearing exercises, remember that short periods of artificial, unusual loading can produce more new bone than long term routine loading. Unusual and unexpected bursts of demand, like jumping when you otherwise do not jump or lifting weights which are substantially heavier than those things you usually lift, build bone better than routine activities.[14] For example, an unpublished British study found women aged 20 to 50 increased hip bone density by nearly four percent in six months just by doing

50 two-legged jumps each day.[15] It sounds simple enough, so if two-legged jumping is safe for you, do it! Imagine what a daily 10 minute jump rope routine might do for your bones as well as you heart and figure! Actually various researchers in the United States and abroad are looking into jumping as a shortcut to bone strengthening. Equally, if you are in shape for it, a program of short bursts of heavier weight lifting can be designed following the guidelines below. If you are interested in using short bursts of unusual loading to build bone, make sure you pick an activity which is safe and appropriate for you. If needed, a fitness trainer, physical therapist or experienced health professional can help develop your bone-strengthening exercise program.

Judging the adequacy of your personal exercise program is often difficult. One guideline is to exercise at least three times per week for at least one hour. A second guideline is to exercise vigorously enough to gradually increase your aerobic capacity and cardiovascular fitness, as well as muscle strength. Studies document that increased aerobic capacity and increased muscle mass are both associated with an increase in bone density.[16, 17] In addition to the Better Bones, Better Body Guidelines that follow, your local health club or fitness trainer can help you measure gains in both muscle strength and aerobic capacity. Remember to have the strength of your back extensor muscles measured and work to increase their strength. Back extensor muscle strength correlates well with spinal bone density.[18, 19]

All in all, it is fair to assume that if your bone density is less than ideal, you need a more rigorous exercise program. While moderate exercise such as walking might be of some bone-maintaining value, significant bone-building seems to require greater exertion. If your aim is to maintain your bone mass, all sorts of exercise should be of some benefit. If your aim is to build bone, you would do well to develop a rigorous and regular exercise program with a significant weight-lifting component.

Finally remember that exercise is important even if you choose to use hormonal or other drug therapy for osteoporosis. In fact, studies show that taking estrogen alone will only maintain bone mass, while combining exercise with drug therapy can lead to significant bone density increases. In one study conducted by the Center for Climacteric Studies in Gainesville, Florida women who were surgically menopausal gained eight percent in spinal bone density within one year combining a Nautilus muscle-strengthening/endurance program with estrogen therapy.[20]

Illustration 15.2

MY GENERAL EXERCISE COMMITMENT

Currently I spend _____ hours exercising per week, while I spend _____ hours per week in sedentary recreation like watching TV and reading. Steps I can take to increase my physical exercise and activity level are:

1.   4.
2.   5.
3.   6.

Specifically my bone-building exercise program will consist of:

1. The beginning, simple and safe exercises illustrated in 15.6. List the ones you will do and for how many minutes each:

   _____

   _____

2. Weight Bearing Exercise
   walking _____   weightlifting _____
   jogging _____   weight machines _____

hiking _____   stair climbing _____
tennis/racquetball _____   jump rope routine _____
Others of your choice _____

3. Aerobic Type Exercises
   swimming _____   rapid walking _____
   rowing _____   dancing _____
   cycling _____

4. My ultimate goal is to exercise _____ times per week for _____ minutes each session.

   Today I will begin exercising _____ times per week for _____ minutes a session and work my way up to my goal exercise program within _____ weeks.

   I will schedule myself to do my regular exercise program on the following days of the week:

   _____.

❖ BETTER BONES, BETTER BODY GUIDELINES FOR STRENGTH TRAINING

Strength training is a great way to maintain and build bone strength. When beginning a strength-training program one should seek professional guidance with a weight trainer or at a fitness center. Once a program has been designed specifically for you, you can exercise with free weights at home or with the equipment at the fitness center.

An excellent way a trainer can gauge which weights you should use is the 1RM test (one repetition maximum).[11] The 1RM test is defined as the maximum mass of a free weight or other resistance that can be moved by a muscle group through the full range of motion using good form, one time only. This is also referred to as "muscle strength" which is the maximum force that can be exerted one time while maintaining good form.

So the first step is to determine your muscle strength (or the 1RM) weight. Then you begin your weight training program using 50 to 60 percent of that maximum weight. If on a weight machine the maximum weight you can lift in good form in the knee extension movement is 45 pounds, then you begin using 22 to 23 pound weights for that exercise.

Train at least two to three days a week leaving at least one day in between workouts. Prior to each session, be sure you warm up your muscles by doing some stretching and easy resistance exercises such as rowing or using a stationary bike, being sure to warm up the particular muscle groups that will be involved in that training session. When training a specific muscle, controlled repetition should last for six to nine seconds with a three second rest between repetitions. A rest period of 90 to 120 seconds between sets is necessary for the muscle to effectively benefit from the training.[11]

Your goal is eight to ten repetitions per set, accomplishing three sets of each exercise. Over time you can increase your weight to 80 percent of your maximum 1RM strength. Make sure that every few weeks you retest your maximum muscle strength to verify that you are indeed increasing your strength. If you have osteoporosis, be sure your strength-training program is supervised by a health care practitioner.

Illustration 15.3

MY STRENGTH TRAINING EXERCISE PROGRAM

ACTIVITY	1RM	60% 1RM	80% 1RM
Exercises with Machines			
Hip extension			
Leg extension			
Lateral pull-down			
Hamstring curl			
Back extension			

(If you have osteoporosis you can probably do these under supervision, but begin with light weights. Do not try to estimate your 1RM to avoid putting too much strain on your back)

Abdominal flexion

(Do not do if you have significant osteoporosis)

Free Weight Lifting

Biceps curl	Triceps press up	Triceps press back
Military press	Chest press	Lateral lift

Repetitions: Do three sets of 8 to 10 repetitions for each exercise

Number of workouts per week: two or three

❖ BETTER BONES, BETTER BODY GUIDELINES FOR AEROBIC ENHANCEMENT

Aerobics is defined as rhythmic movement using the large muscle groups, over an extended period of time. The purpose is to increase the body's ability to consume and process oxygen. Running, jogging, swimming, stepping, dancing and the like are common activities used in aerobic exercising.

In designing your aerobic program, you need to set a standard of training three to five days per week. Each training session should be from 20 to 60 minutes, working at 55 to 85 percent of your maximum heart rate. You want the exercise to be strenuous enough to gradually increase aerobic capacity, but you do not want it to be too strenuous. The proper exercise level is found by calculating the ideal range for your "work-out heart rate." For the average healthy individual, the formulas to figure out both the lower and higher ends of your ideal "work-out heart beat range" are as follows:

To estimate your *minimum* training heart rate: take 220, minus your age, times .65. When starting an exercise program, this should serve as your upper heart rate level. So if you are 48, your training heart rate would be 112 (220 − 48 × .65 = 112). The formula for calculating your estimated *maximum* training heart rate is 220 minus your age times .85, which would be 146 beats per minute in this example. This would be the upper advisable exercise heart rate level after considerable training.

In both aerobics and strength training, the three keys are frequency, intensity and duration. Remember, we need to work our muscles and bones beyond their normal stress loading to produce a training effect.[21]

Illustration 15.4

MY AEROBIC ENHANCEMENT PROGRAM

65% of my maximum heart rate _____	85% of my maximum heart rate_____

The aerobic activity I chose is:

_____ Walking	_____ Swimming
_____ Jogging/Running	_____ Cycling
_____ Dancing/Step	_____ Other

Number of workouts per week: 3 to 5
Minutes in each session: 20 to 60 minutes at 65 to 85% maximum heart rate

Exercise not only builds bone, but can also be an excellent way to reduce stress and fatigue and to build energy. Those interested in developing energy-enhancing athletic ability at any age would benefit from Dr. John Douillard's audio cassette program called "Invincible Athletics." Using the ancient Vedic knowledge, he has developed a training program that builds aerobic capacity without stressing the heart.[22] See Appendix 5.

❖ SPECIAL EXERCISE NOTE FOR THOSE WITH OSTEOPOROSIS

If you have osteoporosis, exercise is an avenue for rebuilding bone. Exercise combined with good eating and nutritional supplementation is even better. As we begin, however, keep in mind that not all osteoporosis is the same. Many of you may have been told you have osteoporosis because your bone density is just barely two standard deviations lower than that of young women. This does not mean that you will ever suffer a significant osteoporotic fracture. Often, however, just being told you have osteoporosis makes you fear that your bones might break with any unusual activity. In some instances, as when one's bone density is *very* low compared to her age mates or when one is elderly or very unfit, this might be the case. Most women who are told they have osteoporosis, however, still have bones strong enough for them to safely undertake a significant bone-building exercise program. In all cases, you must take care, however, not to put excessive stress on weakened bones and any exercise program should be supervised by your health care practitioner.

You might want to begin with some of the simple and

safe exercises shown in Illustration 15.6 and move into more vigorous exercises as determined by you and your health care practitioner. If you have already experienced a fracture or if you are at high risk for fracture, any exercise program beyond the simple movements illustrated on page 316 should be supervised by your health care practitioner. Also keep in mind that some exercises and types of movement are not safe for those with established osteoporosis and doing them can actually cause more harm than good.

The movements not recommended for those with osteoporosis are illustrated on the next page. Let's begin by reviewing these and then go over some simple exercises that should be safe for most everyone. Also do not forget that practicing good posture, sitting and standing straight and tall, is a form of exercise we all should practice. Doing so strengthens the muscles which support the skeleton. Those who have advanced osteoporosis or who have already suffered an osteoporotic fracture could obtain many helpful exercise hints from a physical therapist and are referred to physical therapist Jeannie Aisenbrey's article on *Exercise in the Prevention and Management of Osteoporosis*[23] as well as to Dr. John Aloia's book, *Osteoporosis: A Guide to Prevention and Treatment.*[24]

Exercises to Avoid if You Have Osteoporosis

Exercises in which you bend over frontwards are called flexion movements. These can put undesired pressure on the spinal vertebra and are not recommended for those with osteoporosis. If you have osteoporosis, take special care to avoid the flexion type exercises illustrated below. Such flexion exercises have actually been shown to increase the incidence of spinal fractures in persons with significant spinal osteoporosis.[25]

Illustration 15.5

EXERCISES NOT RECOMMENDED FOR THOSE WITH OSTEOPOROSIS

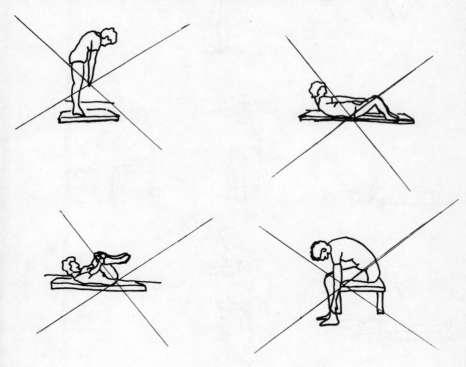

The following exercises are generally considered safe for almost everyone. If you are very weak or find it difficult to stand, do only the exercises which seem appropriate for you and seek assistance with the more difficult ones. For an enjoyable way of building bone mass even among the already

Illustration 15.6

SAFE BEGINNING EXERCISES FOR EVERYONE

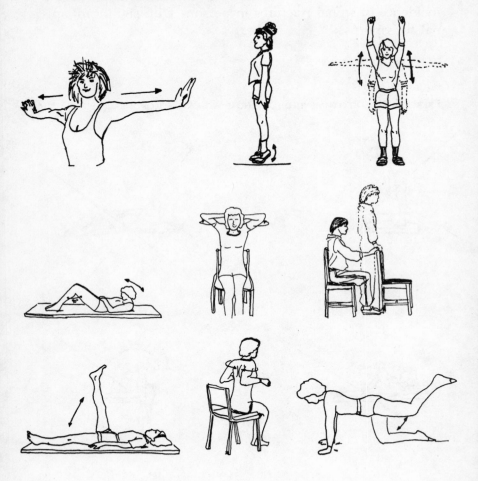

Adapted from Aisenbrey, J., "Exercise in the Prevention and Management of osteoporosis," Physical Therapy *67.7 (1987): 1100-1105.*

fragile you might try the Japanese program of warm water pool exercises. Exercising in a pool of warm water daily not only increases bone mass but can also improve fitness and the quality of everyday life.[26] Remember, even those confined to wheelchairs have been able to build bone mass and reduce fracture incidence with simple exercises like these. If strong enough, begin using light hand weights and doing a little more walking or other aerobic activity each day.

❖ SPECIAL EXERCISE NOTES FOR WOMEN NEAR MENOPAUSE

Many researchers suggest that American women undergo a period of rapid bone loss in the period around menopause (perimenopause). The accelerated bone loss is reported to begin a few years before the last period and continues a few years after the last period. While some women lose little or no bone during this period, many appear to reduce their bone mass at this time of hormonal changes. Osteoporosis authority Dr. Robert Heaney of Creighton University estimates that, averaged over the whole skeleton, American women can lose from 10 to 15 percent of their total bone mass in the first 10 years after menopause.[27] Looking at it another way, other researchers suggest that a women might lose a quarter of all the hip bone density they are going to lose in their lifetime during this perimenopausal period. Even a greater percentage of total spinal bone loss can occur at this time.[28, 29]

Numerous studies document that *postmenopausal* bone loss, that is bone loss which occurs in the period well after a woman's last period, can be halted with nutritional supplements and/or exercise. Little attention, however, has been given to halting bone loss within the first few years before and after menopause. Many researchers, in fact, suggest that this perimenopausal bone loss cannot be halted without the use of hormone drugs. Personally I doubt this is so. While some bone loss may well occur as the female body adjusts to lower estrogen levels, I do not believe that greatly accelerated bone loss needs to be the norm during the perimenopausal period. I have yet to see a comprehensive study attempting to prevent this phase of potentially accelerated bone loss. Hopefully scientists will soon design a multifactorial study aimed at preventing accelerated perimenopausal bone loss. Such a study should include wide ranging nutritional supplementation, exercise, an alkalizing diet and lifestyle interventions.

If you are nearing menopause or a few years past it, you would do well to develop a strong, comprehensive bone-building program. This is a period when you are at high risk of undergoing considerable bone loss. This would not be the time in life to slack off on your nutritional supplements, reduce exercise or get lazy about life-supporting behavioral modifications. Remember, your nutrition program should be comprehensive, including all bone-building nutrients, not just calcium. The exercise component should be regular and rigorous. Studies show that modest exercises like brisk walking are probably not enough even to maintain existing bone. To rebuild bone during the perimenopausal period clearly requires rigorous exercise.[17, 30] On the other hand, even 45 minutes of moderate intensity low impact or high impact strength-building exercise done only two times a week has been found effective in maintaining bone mineral density in early postmenopausal women. Going a step further, postmenopausal women participating in weight training Nautilus-type programs gained more bone density than those who exercised aerobically.[31] Build muscle, build aerobic capacity and build bone!

Finally, if you do suffer from excessively low estrogen or progesterone levels at this time, take measures to correct this situation. Many books, including *The Mend Clinic Guide To Natural Medicine for Menopause and Beyond* which I co-authored, fully detail the many natural life-supporting ways to do this without resorting to dangerous estrogen drugs. See Appendix 5 for a listing of these books.

❖ SPECIAL EXERCISE NOTES FOR YOUTH STILL IN THEIR GROWING YEARS

The seeds of lifelong bone health are sown in youth. It is the very nature of bone to grow to fit perfectly the needs of each individual body. All this is done in youth spontaneously and without any effort on our part. Growth hormones and other factors dictate the irrepressible growth of bone. Young bones will always grow bigger and stronger. The degree of bone size and strength developed, however, varies. Genetics provides each of us with a maximum potential peak bone mass. Our nutrition and physical activity patterns in turn dictate how much of that peak bone mass potential we will actually achieve. Calcium, magnesium, phosphorus, vitamin D—in short all the 18 plus bone-building nutrients—are needed in high amounts during these growing years, a fact that is reflected by the increased in RDAs for adolescents.

Unfortunately, while adolescence is a time of high nutrient need it is often a time of low nutrient intake. This is especially true for girls who early on become aware of our cultural preference for thinness. One recent survey found 81 percent of 10-year-olds said they had already dieted.[32] Low nutrient intake clearly limits the fulfillment of one's peak bone mass potential. Supernutrition during adolescence, on the other hand, nourishes the formation of super strong bones. Several studies show that children who obtain even the RDA of calcium, for example, have greater bone density and fewer fractures than those consuming less calcium.[33-35] Children obtaining significantly more than the RDA for calcium have even stronger bones than those consuming just the RDA or less.[35] These studies show that simple nutritional supplementation with only one mineral, calcium, could go a long way towards reducing the incidence of osteoporosis. Providing all children with adequate levels of *all* the essential nutrients, I believe would go a long way towards eliminating the osteoporosis fracture epidemic. Equally, physical exercise is especially important during the growing years and unfortunately girls begin to turn away from vigorous physical exercise towards more sedentary activities as they enter puberty.

For youth the message is very simple. Seize the opportunity to build super bones! Adequate daily consumption of all essential nutrients, not just calcium, is a great place to start. Appendix 1 outlines the minimal RDA requirements for children. Be sure your child obtains at least the RDA of all nutrients with extra calcium and magnesium for stronger bones. A good bone-building diet would be an alkaline diet that limits the consumption of acid-forming substances like sodas and sugars, fast foods and excess meat. Instead, vegetables, fruits, lentils, almonds, potatoes, sweet potatoes, squashes, all root crops and greens should be consumed in abundance. Daily vigorous exercise is the next ingredient. Hopefully the activities would be fun and done outdoors in the sunshine and open air.

Exercising Into Bone Health

Finally, in our culture children, just as adults, are subject to an unprecedented amount of emotional and psychological stress. Stress drains bone, no matter what size the body it is in. Every effort should be made to reestablish a sense of security, peace and happiness for all children.

About half of our bone mineral is deposited between infancy and puberty and most of the other half settles into place during the great growth spurt between puberty and the end of adolescence. These "growing" years are indeed the time for building lifelong healthy bones. Skeletal consolidation, however, continues through our 20s and into the mid-30s and most of us do not reach our peak bone mass until around the age of 35.[27, 36] So up to age 35 or so you will have nature's help in building bone mass and modest efforts can yield remarkable results. Even women aged 25 to 34 were found to increase spinal bone mass by a whopping 10 to 15 percent with regular exercise and calcium supplementation of 800 to 1,000 mg.

❖ References

1 Cheng, S, et al., "Bone mineral density and physical activity in 50-60 year old women," *Bone & Mineral* 12.2 (1991): 123-32.

2 Evans, William J., "Exercise, Nutrition and Aging," *Journal of Nutrition* 122 (1992): 796-801.

3 Evans, William, "Body Building for the Nineties," *Nutrition Action Health Letter* 5.1 (1992): 5-6.

4 Martin, D., and M. Notelovitz, "Effects of aerobic training on bone mineral density of postmenopausal women," *Journal of Bone & Mineral Research* 8.8 (1993): 931-6.

5 Evans, William, personal communication, Knool Laboratory For Human Performance Research at Penn State University (Dec. 1995).

6 Anon, "Seniors Pump Iron," *Health News & Review* Summer, 1995.

7 Chow, Raphael, et al., "Effect of two randomized exercise programmes on bone mass of healthy postmenopausal women," *BMJ* 295 (1987): 231-234.

8 Dalsky, G., et al., "Weight-Bearing Exercise Training and Lumbar Bone Mineral Content in Postmenopausal Women," *Ann Intern Med* 108.6 (1988): 824-828.

9 Randall, Teri, "Longitudinal Study Pursues Questions of Calcium, Hormones, and Metabolism in Life of Skeleton," *JAMA* 268.17 (1992): 2353-7.

10 Dalsky, G.P., "The role of exercise in the prevention of osteoporosis," *Compr Thor* 15.9 (1989): 30-7.

11 Nelson, Miriam, et al., "Effects of High-intensity Strength Training on Multiple Risk Factors for Osteoporotic Fractures A Randomized Controlled Trial," *JAMA* 272.24 (1994): 1909-1914.

12 Farmer, M., et al., "Race and Sex Differences in Hip Fracture Incidence," *Am J Public Health* 74 (1984): 1374-1380.

13 Block, J.E., et al., "Greater Vertebral Bone Mineral Massing Exercising Young Men," *West Jr Med* 145 (1986): 39.

14 Lanyon, L.E., "Skeletal Responses to Physical Loading," *Physiology and Pharmacology of Bone,* ed. Gregory R. Mundy, and John T. Martin. (Berlin: Springer-Verlag, 1993) 107:485-505.

15 Anon., "Jumping can strengthen bone, reduce fractures," *Medical Tribune* November 25, 1993:

16 Nelson, Miriam, et al., "A 1-y walking program and increased dietary calcium in postmenopausal women: effects on bone," *Am J Clin Nutr* 53 (1991): 1304-11.

17 Sinaki, M., "Exercise and Physical Therapy," *Osteoporosis Etiology, Diagnosis and Management,* ed. B. Riggs, and J. Melton. (New York: Raven Press, 1988).

18 Sinaki, M., et al., "Relationship Between Bone Mineral Density of Spine and Strength of Back Extensors in Healthy Postmenopausal Women," *Mayo Clinic Proceedings* 61.2 (1986): 116-122.

19 Halle, J. S., et al., "Relationship between trunk muscle torque and

bone mineral content of the lumbar spine and hip in healthy postmenopausal women," *Phys Ther* 70.11 (1990): 690-9.

20 Notelovitz, M., et al., "Estrogen therapy and variable-resistance weight training increase bone mineral in surgically menopausal women," *Journal of Bone & Mineral Research* 6.6 (1991): 583-90.

21 Binder, Joy, personal communication, Certified Fitness Trainer, Syracuse NY, (1995).

22 Douillard, John, *Invincible Athletics,* audiotapes ed. (Lancaster, MA: Sports Organization Of Maharishi Ayur-Veda, 1991).

23 Aisenbrey, J., "Exercise in the Prevention and Management of Osteoporosis," *Physical Therapy* 67.7 (1987): 1100-1105.

24 Aloia, John, *Osteoporosis: A Guide to Prevention and Treatment,* (Champagne, IL: Human Kinetics, 1989).

25 Sinaki, M., and B. Mikkelsen, "Postmenopausal Spinal Osteoporosis: Flexion Versus Extension Exercises," *Archives of Physical Medicine and Rehabilitation* 65 (1984): 593-596.

26 Tsukahara, N., et al., "Cross-sectional and longitudinal studies on the effect of water exercise in controlling bone loss in Japanese postmenopausal women," *Journal of Nutritional Science & Vitaminology* 40.1 (1994): 37-47.

27 Heaney, R., and J. Barger-Lux, *Calcium and Common Sense,* (New York: Doubleday, 1988).

28 Nordin, et al., "Relative contributions of years since menopause, age, and weight to vertebral density in postmenopausal women.," *J Clin Endocrinol Metab* 74.1 (1992): 20-23.

29 Hedlund, L.R., and J.C. Gallagher, "Increased Incidence of Hip Fracture in Osteoporotic Women Treated with Sodium Fluoride," *J Bone Miner Res* 4 (1989): 223-5.

30 Cavanaugh, D.J., and C.E. Cann, "Brisk walking does not stop bone loss in postmenopausal women," *Bone* 9.4 (1988): 201-204.

31 Notelovitz, M., "How Exercise Affects Bone Density," *Contemporary Ob/Gyn* 27 (1986): 108-116.

32 Manfred, Erica, "No More Food Fights," *New Age Journal.* November/December (1995): 55-62.

33 Verd, S., et al., "Dietary calcium and bone health," *Am J Dis Ch* 146 (1992): 660-1.

34 Chan, G., et al., "The effect of dietary calcium supplementation in pubertal girls' growth and bone mineral status," *Clin Res* (1992).

35 Johnston, C., et al., "Calcium Supplementation and Increases in Bone Mineral Density in Children," *The New England Journal of Medicine* 327 (1992): 82-88.

36 Fulton, Rachel, "Boning Up!" *Working Mother* 1995: 47-50.

Chapter 16

Promoting Endocrine Health

❖ CARING FOR YOUR
- THYROID • PARATHYROID • ADRENALS • OVARIES
- KIDNEYS • PANCREAS • LIVER

*W*orking together, the endocrine glands form the automatic pilot in control of many body functions, including bone-building and maintenance. Recognizing this, a wise person protects and nourishes these important glands. Listed below are a series of things you can do to maximize endocrine health.

For the Health of My Thyroid I Can:

✦ Increase intake of iodine-rich foods such as fish, seafood, sea vegetables (like kelp and nori) and green leafy vegetables.

✦ Get the RDA for all nutrients, especially zinc and copper.

◆ Consume high quality essential fatty acids (as in cold pressed safflower, sesame, sunflower or flaxseed oils and fresh nuts and seeds).

◆ Use thyroid medications only if truly necessary and in the lowest effective doses.

◆ Begin the practice of yoga postures and exercises, such as shoulder stands and inverted postures which increase blood flow to thyroid gland.

◆ Identify sources of chronic emotional stress and seek solutions to such problems.

For the Health of My Parathyroid Gland I Can:

◆ Eliminate or reduce: soft drinks, sugar, excess meat, processed foods like luncheon meats, baked goods and boxed mixes with phosphate additives.

◆ Increase consumption of: fresh or frozen vegetables, fresh fruits, dried beans (lentils, kidney beans, chickpeas, split peas, etc.), almonds and fresh nuts.

For the Health of My Adrenal Glands I Can:

◆ Eliminate or severely restrict my consumption of: sugar, sodas, chocolate, caffeine, alcohol and white flour products.

◆ Increase intake of: whole grains (brown rice, oatmeal, barley, millet, buckwheat, etc.), fresh fruits, fresh vegetables and dried beans.

◆ Be regular in eating and avoid skipping meals.

✦ Do relaxing exercise 20 minutes daily, even if simply walking.

✦ Learn and practice breathing exercises and/or meditation.

✦ Seek solutions to chronic worry and stress.

✦ Obtain adequate rest and avoid "pushing myself."

✦ Enjoy regular sleep, getting to bed by 10:30 PM.

✦ Correct any tendency towards hypoglycemia.

✦ Use extra vitamin C (one to three grams per day) along with pantothenic acid (100-500 mg).

✦ Use nettles and/or dandelion root tea, 3-4 cups per week.

For the Health of My Ovaries I Can:

✦ Consume a whole-foods diet very low in animal fat and limited in total fats (both animal and vegetable sources).

✦ Severely restrict my intake of fried foods.

✦ Strive for healthy, normal menstrual periods and seek assistance for correcting menstrual irregularities.

✦ Rest during my periods if fatigued.

✦ Avoid exposure to sexually transmitted diseases.

✦ Avoid ovary removal if at all possible.

For the Health of My Kidneys I Can:

✦ Keep the kidneys well-nourished with fresh, whole foods.

♦ Maintain proper intakes of magnesium and vitamin B_6 in particular.

♦ Drink at least eight glasses of pure water per day.

♦ Reduce or eliminate sugar, coffee, excessive protein and excessive salt.

For the Health of My Liver I Can:

♦ Use plenty of fresh vegetables and their juices. The dark green and leafy greens such as dandelion and turnip greens, collards and kale are especially good for the liver, as are artichokes.

♦ Choose vegetables, grains and beans over meats whenever possible and limit intake of fat.

♦ Drink plenty of pure water. Hot water, plain or with ginger or lemon, is preferable. Dandelion root tea is also helpful.

♦ Consume enough fiber and water so that you have at least one bowel movement a day. With adequate fiber and water the stool will float.

♦ Exercise regularly in the fresh air.

♦ Avoid alcohol.

♦ Avoid smoking or exposure to smoke.

♦ Avoid exposure to pesticides, herbicides, chemical solvents or toxic vapors.

♦ Avoid unnecessary medication and all "recreational" drugs.

♦ Use saunas and or steam baths and skin brushing to detoxify through the skin.

For the Health of My Pancreas I Can:

+ Eat a whole foods diet free from sugar, alcohol, coffee, white flour and excessive fats.
+ Consume foods high in chromium and zinc (or use supplements of these in RDA quantities).
+ Eat regular meals and snacks as necessary.
+ Exercise daily in the fresh air and sunshine when possible.
+ Avoid excessive mental work and excessive worry.

Chapter 17

Rethinking the Role of Estrogen Replacement for Osteoporosis

❖ Estrogen Replacement and Osteoporosis

*I*t is hard to imagine a book on osteoporosis written in 1996 which did not discuss hormone replacement therapy. Indeed at this time, estrogen replacement therapy represents the first line medical treatment for preventing and halting excessive bone loss. From the Better Bones, Better Body perspective, however, the risks of estrogen supplementation far outweigh its rather limited beneficial effects on bone. Furthermore, as this book details, there exist many ways to achieve greater bone benefits which are fully life-supporting and good for the entire body.

Interestingly, today it appears the pharmaceutical industry is also looking for alternatives to estrogen drugs as the preferred treatment for osteoporosis. The main reason for this marketing shift is new, rather definitive research linking estrogen use with increased incidence of breast cancer. As reported recently in the *Wall Street Journal,* a new trend toward non-hormonal drugs for osteoporosis is well underway. Currently at least 22 non-hormonal osteoporosis drug treatments are in development. One such drug is Fosamax produced by the Merck pharmaceutical company. Fosamax recently gained FDA approval for the treatment of osteoporosis. One would expect that Merck's new non-hormonal treatment for osteoporosis would be pitted against the estrogens currently used such as the best-selling Premarin produced by American Home Products, another pharmaceutical giant. This, however, does not appear to be the case. On the contrary, the two pharmaceutical mega-corporations have reportedly struck a deal whereby they will divide the market, both working together to promote Premarin for treating menopausal symptoms and the new Fosamax for osteoporosis treatment and prevention.[1] In regards to osteoporosis, the move is away from estrogen drugs. The new non-hormonal osteoporosis drugs are a topic well worth discussing. More about this new medical approach to osteoporosis in the next chapter.

Even though new non-hormonal osteoporosis drugs are on the horizon, estrogen drugs today still represent the primary medical approach for both prevention and treatment of osteoporosis. Each year within the United States alone, millions of women are told to use estrogens for bone health promotion. In addition, doctors, the pharmaceutical companies and the media are suggesting that the use of estrogen drugs benefits heart health. Thus, now more than ever we need an updated critique of the pros and cons of estrogen therapy. Before beginning this critique, however, let's briefly review the history of estrogen drugs, the ideology surrounding their use and the Better Bones, Better Body perspective on hormone replacement therapy.

The History of Estrogen Drug Use

Since its development in 1938, synthetic estrogen has been experimented with for a wide variety of female health concerns. Most of these estrogen experiments ended in disaster. In the 1940s the now infamous estrogen known as DES (diethylstilbestrol) was developed and given to prevent miscarriage and promote fetal well-being. In 1949 it was claimed "to make a normal pregnancy more normal."[2] This premature claim proved not to be true. DES was of no help in pregnancy. Furthermore, by the early 1970s DES was found to cause cancer in the offspring of women who used it. Later it was also implicated in promoting cancer in the women themselves.[3] Today, women who used DES even more than 30 years ago have a 35 percent greater risk of breast cancer than women who never used DES.[4] Thus DES, the first estrogen "miracle drug," was also the first hormone product to be named a human carcinogen. Unfortunately, between 1947 and 1971, two million pregnant women in the United States were given DES.

Soon after it was found useless in pregnancy maintenance, DES was declared useful for exactly the opposite purpose, that of a morning-after contraceptive pill. Once again without adequate testing it was applied for this purpose with deleterious results and its use for this purpose was discontinued, this time by the manufacturers themselves.

In the 1950s the combination estrogen/progestin birth control pill (BCP) was developed and first experimented with on Puerto Rican women and then the United States population at large. By 1962 there were early reports of life-threatening strokes and blood clots among women using the first generation of birth control pills and by 1967 the FDA required that drug manufacturers note on the label the suspected risks of using this drug. In 1968 British studies confirmed the suspected link between BCP use and risk of blood clots in the brain, lungs and veins. In 1970 the Senate examined studies suggesting that the birth control pill increased a woman's risk of breast cancer, stroke and high blood pressure as well as blood clots. Also at this time certain types of birth control pills were taken off the U.S. market as they were found to cause cancer in dogs. By 1989 studies linked even the newer, lower-dose BCP to increased incidence of breast cancer.[5-7]

During the 1960s the use of estrogen drugs postmenopausally became fashionable following drug company sponsored publications by Dr. Robert Wilson promising "forever young with forever estrogen."[8] By the mid-1970s an estimated 30 percent of all postmenopausal women in the United States were using estrogen replacement drugs.[9] Without adequate testing, estrogen became one of the top five prescription drugs in the United States.[10] By 1975, however, estrogen replacement was shown to cause endometrial cancer in a significant number of women using it. Sales plummeted and through consumer group litigation the FDA was forced to prepare package inserts clarifying known risks and declaring that estrogens would not keep users feeling or looking young.[11-13] Thus the first wave of postmenopausal estrogen therapy came to an abrupt halt and today it is unacceptable practice to give estrogen alone to women with an intact uterus.

The development of synthetic progestin and the finding that estrogen-induced endometrial cancer could be largely prevented by the addition of this ovarian hormone provided the foundation for a second wave of postmenopausal estrogen use. Additionally, FDA approval of estrogen for osteoporosis prevention and treatment added great impetus to this second wave. In the mid-1990s we are experiencing what I believe will be known as the crest of this second wave. While no one knows exactly how many women in the U.S. currently use estrogen replacement therapy, an educated guess might be as high as 30 percent of postmenopausal women. [13-16] For example, osteoporosis researchers Drs. Riggs and Melton of the Mayo Clinic conducted a random survey of women living in Rochester, Minnesota. In this survey they found that the proportion of women receiving replacement estrogen within 20 years after menopause increased from 4 percent in 1980 to 33 percent in 1992.[15]

Looking back it seems fair to say that the history of estrogen replacement therapy is one large scale experimentation with female health, conducted without the informed consent of the women involved. In 1977, researchers Barbara and Gideon Seaman concluded that, in most cases, synthetic hormones have taken from life much more than they have given and that to use hormones is to tamper with the unknown at the most profound level of biochemistry.[17] In the upcoming section we explore whether the situation is any different today.

The Ideology Surrounding Estrogen Supplementation

At first, synthetic estrogen was employed as a replacement hormone only for those women who had undergone ovary removal. Thus estrogen was replaced in women who had been made estrogen deficient by removal of their estrogen-producing gland, the ovaries. Soon, however, an interesting concept developed which greatly expanded the estrogen market. This concept was that menopause induced a state of estrogen deficiency and that this deficiency should be corrected with estrogen drugs. This idea was made popular by Wilson and others during the first estrogen replacement boom, then faded under the impact of the estrogen-uterine cancer link. Now this belief is once again in vogue. Nature, it is argued, made a mistake in lowering a woman's production of sex hormones at menopause. Luckily science is here to correct that mistake. I do not see a mistake on nature's part. Rather I believe that nature in all her wisdom has struck a delicate balance between the need for, and exposure to, these powerful sex hormones.

❖ THE BETTER BONES, BETTER BODY PERSPECTIVE ON HORMONE REPLACEMENT THERAPY

Fully recognizing the unparalleled intelligence, organizing power and healing potential of our magical bodies, the Better Bones, Better Body Program seeks to optimize health through the maintenance and regeneration of full, normal functioning. Ideally, replacement of function must occur only when regeneration proves impossible. Further, from this perspective everything done to benefit bone should also benefit the entire body. Long term health of the breast, uterus, ovaries or liver should not be jeopardized for the sake of bone. From this perspective, the use of hormone drugs as a first line approach to osteoporosis would be limited to cases such as:

✦ Women who have undergone ovary removal.
✦ Women who have experienced premature reduc-

tion in, or loss of, ovarian hormone functioning due to uterus removal or other causes.

✦ Postmenopausal women who are experiencing severe life-disrupting symptoms of estrogen deficiency and who cannot or choose not to undertake a life-supporting program to regenerate endocrine well-being.

It is likely that this Better Bones, Better Body perspective on hormone therapy is at variance with other things you have been told or heard. Let's review the pros and cons of hormone therapy so that you may draw your own conclusions.

The Pros of Estrogen Replacement Therapy

Pro #1. **Estrogen replacement has been shown to halt bone loss and reduce the risk of fracture.**

What the research shows:

✦ Estrogen significantly reduces the rate of bone loss in most, but not all, women. In some 10 to 20 percent of all cases bone loss continues unabated even on estrogen therapy.[18]

✦ While estrogen significantly reduces bone loss in most women, dramatic bone loss begins once again immediately upon cessation of estrogen use.[19]

✦ In 1992 a monumental meta-analysis of all English language studies on the effect of estrogen therapy estimated that estrogen use reduced the risk of hip fracture by 25 percent.[20] As calculated by the American College of Physicians this means that only 2 to 3 percent of all postmenopausal women will avoid hip fracture by taking estrogen therapy.[21, 22]

✦ A recent large study of nearly 10,000 women, however, further refined our idea of exactly how much estrogen therapy reduces hip fractures, the most serious type of osteoporotic fracture. In 1995, Dr. Cummings from the University of California in San Francisco and colleagues reported that:[23, 24]

1. For the 9,516 women studied *as a whole* neither previous nor current use of estrogen therapy resulted in a significant reduction in risk for hip fracture.
2. For estrogen therapy to reduce the risk of hip fracture, the following conditions must be met:
   ✦ Estrogen therapy must be begun within five years after menopause
   ✦ Estrogen therapy must be continued lifelong
   ✦ Estrogen users must not have a history of osteoporosis or fractures upon beginning therapy.
3. If all the above conditions are met, they report a 30 to 40 percent reduction in hip fracture risk.
   ✦ As for other osteoporotic fractures, estrogen therapy is reported to reduce the incidence of all osteoporotic fractures together by 30 to 50 percent.[20]
   ✦ The latest research indicates that all in all, seven years of continuous ERT are needed to have a significant impact on bone mineral density. With seven years of hormone use the average bone density at all sites is only *slightly* higher in women on estrogen that in women not using the drug.[25]
   ✦ Finally, If a woman takes ERT for seven years after menopause and then stops using the drug, there will be no significant positive effect on bone density by the time she reaches the age of

75 when hip fractures begin to occur with greater frequency. Thus, it now appears that life long replacement use is necessary to produce any significant preservation of bone mass.[19, 23-25]

Interpreting the Research

Estrogen therapy may reduce somewhat the fracture rate, but often only under very specific conditions and always only at the expense of very serious risks. The Better Bones, Better Body approach represents a safer and more life-supporting means of building and maintaining bone mass.

Hip fractures are the most serious, costly and life-threatening of all the consequences of osteoporosis. Lifelong estrogen therapy begun within five years of menopause, and continued lifelong, in women with no history of osteoporosis or fracture has been recently reported by Dr. Cummings and colleagues to reduce the risk of hip fracture by 30 percent.[23] On the other hand as previously described in Chapter 9, the same study reports a 30 percent reduction in risk of hip fracture from walking for exercise or having an increase in weight since the age of 25. Similarly older women who tended to stand on their feet for four or more hours a day had a 70 percent lower risk than those who stood for less time. Other indices of general fitness also were linked with lower risk of a hip fracture and women who self-rated themselves as having a higher level of health experienced 70 percent less risk than those who rated themselves as having poor health.

Lifelong estrogen use is but one way of reducing hip fracture by about 30 percent and it is the only way which carries with it so many risks including an increased incidence of breast cancer.

Pro #2. Estrogen drugs reduce or eliminate various symptoms of menopausal imbalance including hot flashes, vaginal dryness, urethrial atrophy and irritation.

Most, but not all women, find that estrogen therapy corrects these common symptoms generally associated with estrogen deficiency. However, while estrogen therapy can correct many common symptoms of menopausal imbalance, many other fully safe and life-supporting approaches bring as great a benefit without the risks that estrogen drugs carry. References for those seeking to develop a program of natural alternatives to estrogen drugs are given in Appendix 5.

Pro #3. Estrogen supplementation reduces selected heart disease risk factors and thus some researchers suggest that estrogen supplementation can reduce the incidence of coronary heart disease.

Some, but not all researchers, suggest that current estrogen use is associated with between a 35 and 45 percent reduction in risk of heart disease and a 28 percent reduction in the rate of death from coronary disease.[20, 26-29]

Here it is important to remember that to date the evidence for estrogen heart-sparing effect is largely circumstantial. Most of it comes from observational studies which suggest that women on estrogen replacement had fewer heart attacks than women free of this drug therapy. These studies do not prove that estrogen was the reason for the lower incidence of heart attacks. It could be, for example, that women who used hormones also had better health habits or closer medical supervision. In fact, it will take decades of very carefully planned controlled studies to determine if postmenopausal estrogen use actually lowers the incidence of heart disease. Moreover, to me it is very unlikely that estrogen replacement will prove to improve overall longevity.

The one controlled study completed to date on estrogen and heart disease risk factors, known as the Postmenopausal Estrogen/Progestin Interventions Trial (PEPI), reports only modest gains in two risk factors and only under very specific treatment conditions. These gains in beneficial HDL cholesterol and fibrinogen, I would add, can be easily matched and superseded with simple, hazard-free nutrition and lifestyle modifications. While space does not permit further elaboration here, analysis of the PEPI Trial and estrogen's proposed heart-sparing benefits is available from the Nutrition Education and Consulting Service (See Appendix 2). Suffice it here to say that the same fully life-supporting means taken to build strong bones will also reduce the risk factors for and incidence of heart disease.

Now, let us move our attention to the other side of the argument and look at the downside of estrogen drug use as taken from the *Physicians Desk Reference* and other sources.

The Cons of Estrogen Replacement Therapy

Con #1. **Unopposed ERT directly and significantly increases a woman's risk of endometrial (uterine) cancer.**

A woman's risk of endometrial cancer is increased up to 15 times by using postmenopausal estrogen alone.[30] This estrogen-endometrial cancer link was reported as early as 1946 and became fully acknowledged by the medical community in 1976 bringing an end to the first wave of postmenopausal estrogen replacement therapy. In women with a uterus, the standard dose of estrogen used alone causes endometrial hyperplasia in 5 to 25 percent of women per year and irregular bleeding in 35 to 40 percent per year. In the recent much publicized PEPI Trial one in three women on estrogen alone developed potentially precancerous uterine lesions.[31]

Con #2. **ERT use substantially increases a woman's risk for breast cancer.**

Over the years numerous researchers have reported this finding while others denied it. I believe that the link now appears undeniable. For example:

✦ In 1987 Henderson summarized that overall studies using population-based controls (as opposed to hospital population controls) consistently demonstrated a 50 to 70 percent increased risk of breast cancer after long-term use of estrogen.[32, 33]

✦ In 1986 large scale Italian studies found that women who have ever used non-contraceptive estrogens have a nearly doubled risk of breast cancer, with the risk increasing with duration of use.[34]

✦ Reporting more moderate findings, a large scale British study in 1987 calculated it took some 20 years of estrogen use to increase the risk of breast cancer by 50 percent. In this study elevations in breast cancer associated with long-term estrogen use were apparent across all menopausal subgroups. That is, long-term use had the same negative effect on women who had undergone natural menopause as it did on women who underwent hysterectomy with ovary removal. Hormones exerted particularly adverse effects in those initiating use subsequent to a diagnosis of benign breast disease.[35]

✦ In 1989 a study of 23,000 Swedish women found

that nine or more years of estrogen at least doubled the risk of breast cancer. Shorter term use of
estrogen for menopausal symptoms was also
found to increase breast cancer risk by 10 percent.[36]
This groundbreaking study also found that the addition of a progestin offered no protection against
the development of breast cancer. In fact, the risk
of breast cancer was four times higher among
women who took estrogen combined with a progestin for more than four years. This finding was
in strong contrast to the claim made by some
American scientists that synthetic progestin might
offer protection against breast cancer.[37]

✦ Again a Danish study of nearly 1,500 women
found a 36 percent increased risk of breast cancer
in women who have ever used combination estrogen and progestin hormone therapy, with a
trend toward increased risk with increased duration of use. This study also looked at combined
estrogen and testosterone use and found women
on this combination to have well over twice the
incidence of breast cancer as women not on any
hormones.[38]

Over the years, all of the above studies and many more
supporting the estrogen-breast cancer link have been refuted
or minimized by segments of the medical and pharmaceutical community. The results of a recent large U.S. study, however, are undeniable. Findings of the 1995 Harvard Nurses'
Health Study were published in the *New England Journal of
Medicine*. This study of 121,700 women watched since 1976
reported a significant increase of breast cancer risk among
women who have ever used estrogen and nearly a 50 percent higher risk of breast cancer for women on long-term

hormone replacement therapy as compared with never users.[39] The details of this study are summarized below.

Illustration 17.1

ESTROGEN USE AND BREAST CANCER RISK
DETAILS OF THE HARVARD NURSES HEALTH STUDY, 1995[39, 40]

- ✦ Current ERT use was associated with a 32 percent increased risk of breast cancer.
- ✦ Current users of estrogen hormone therapy for five to nine years had a 46 percent increased risk.
- ✦ The older the postmenopausal women, the greater the risk. With five plus years use, women aged 60 to 64 had a 71 percent higher risk.
- ✦ The risk of death from breast cancer was increased 45 percent among women who had taken estrogen for five or more years.
- ✦ The addition of a progestin did not reduce the risk of breast cancer, but increased it. For current users, the risk of breast cancer with ERT plus progestin was increased by 41 percent as compared to women not on the combined hormone therapy.
- ✦ It is not known how long the increased risk for breast cancer will persist after hormone supplementation is discontinued.

In addition, other studies have shown that the estrogen-induced risk increases for women with a family history of breast cancer. A meta-analysis of 16 studies found women with a family history of breast cancer who used ERT had a two to six times higher risk of breast cancer (average 3.4) than those never to use the drug.[41]

In closing this section we are reminded of the words of

Dr. Graham Colditz, director of the Harvard Nurses' Health Study and principal investigator of this research. In 1994 he commented; "Should breast cancer be the price we pay for reduced risk of heart disease and fractures? I believe the answer is no. Alternative approaches to preventing heart disease are available, this is not so for breast cancer."[42]

Con #3. ERT use is associated with an increased incidence of ovarian cancer.

For several years selected researchers have questioned the link between estrogen replacement and ovarian cancer. Now, as with the estrogen-breast cancer link, the data appears conclusive. In a seven year follow-up study of 240,073 women, "any" estrogen use gave rise to a 15 percent increased risk of fatal ovarian cancer. For six to ten years of estrogen use, there was a 40 percent increased risk and with over 11 years of drug use there was a 70 percent increase. Little work has been done on the estrogen replacement-ovarian cancer link, yet this is important as more women in the United States die each year of ovarian cancer than of endometrial cancer.[43]

Con #4. ERT use increases the risk of gallbladder disease by some 250 percent.

Estrogen, through its action on the liver, affects bile production and composition, resulting in a greatly increased incidence of gallstones and gallbladder disease. Current users of estrogen replacement experience nearly three times greater risk of gallbladder disease than non-users. Furthermore, it appears that this increased risk of gallbladder disease continues even after discontinuation of estrogen therapy.[44]

Con #5. ERT users have been found to have twice the rate of fibrocystic breast disease as non-estrogen users.

Studies now show that the degree of risk for fibrocystic breast disease is related to the length of time estrogen drugs are used.[45] One study reported a five-fold increased risk of fibrocystic breast disease for women using postmenopausal estrogens for 10 to more.[46] while another found the greatest increase in benign breast disease among women using the drugs for 15 years or more.[47] These increases are important as fibrocystic disease can place a women at higher risk for breast cancer. Also when the breasts are thickened by cysts it is more difficult to detect breast cancer from mammograms.[48]

Con #6. ERT increases incidence of systemic lupus erythematosus.

Again it was the Harvard Nurses' Health Study that found ever-users of estrogen replacement to have twice the risk of lupus as non-users. Current users have two and one-half times the risk and past users, some 80 percent extra risk.[49]

Con #7. Women on unopposed estrogen have a significantly higher incidence of abnormal uterine bleeding than do non-users.

In a recent study at a large medical center, the prevalence of abnormal bleeding was found to reach 61.3 percent in postmenopausal estrogen users, while the rate was only 17.7 percent in patients not using estrogen.

Con #8. Use of ERT greatly increases likelihood that a women will have to undergo a hysterectomy.

There is a significantly higher prevalence of hysterectomy amongst postmenopausal women as confirmed by the recent PEPI Intervention Trial.

Con #9. Oral ERT may reduce circulating testosterone.

Because of increased liver production of sex-binding globulin which binds free testosterone, estrogen drugs have been found to reduce circulating testosterone by some 30 percent.[50]

Con #10. **ERT may well have adverse effects on nutrients**.

As with estrogen containing oral contraceptives, replacement estrogen is likely to deplete folic acid and lower vitamins B_6, B_{12} and C while increasing absorption of iron, copper and vitamin K. Estrogen is also reported to exert an antagonistic effect on vitamin E.[51, 52]

Con #11. **The cumulative effect of decades of oral contraceptive use combined with postmenopausal estrogen and progestins is unknown.**

There has been no attempt made to calculate the cumulative effects upon women's health of decades of unnatural exposure to estrogen and progestin supplementation from both oral contraceptive use and postmenopausal replacement therapy. It is not unreasonable to suggest that the ever-raising rate of breast cancer may well be related to this unprecedented hormone exposure.

Other adverse effects of ERT include bloating, headaches, depression, breast tenderness, yeast infections and blood sugar fluctuations. ERT also causes fibroid tumors to grow, increases blood pressure in some women and can aggravate asthma in postmenopausal women with the condition.

The Pros of Progestin Therapy

As if the estrogen story were not in itself complicated enough, the situation is even further exacerbated by the addition of a progestin agent necessary to limit the carcinogenic effects of estrogen on endometrial tissue. During a woman's reproductive years, the ovarian hormones estrogen and progesterone work together to maintain the menstrual cycle and provide for reproduction. At menopause a woman's ovarian production of estrogen all but ceases and ovarian progesterone production totally ceases. When given to women in menopause, estrogen affects the body in many ways including stimulating overgrowth of the endometrial cells which line the uterus. It is now clear that this "unopposed estrogen" stimulation of the endometrium frequently induces endometrial cancer. A progestin given along with the estrogen drugs provides for a sloughing off of the endometrial build-up and thus in most cases prevents the development of endometrial cancer in women using estrogen drugs. Thus, good medicine now demands that any woman with an intact uterus receive a progestin drug along with estrogen therapy.

The natural hormone produced by the human body is known as "progesterone." Synthetic progesterone drugs, on the other hand, are known as "progestins" or "progestogens". Synthetic progestins, of which Provera is the most popular, are the hormones used in connection with synthetic hormone replacement therapy. In the past few years natural progesterone drugs have also become available. These drugs are pharmaceutical grade hormones made from plant derivatives, extracted from wild yam or soy, that are identical in chemical structure to the human progesterone hormone. Natural progesterone is now available as over-the-counter topical cream and oils and in prescription pills made of up "micronized progesterone". One of the progestin agents tested in the PEPI Trial, this natural form of progesterone was found to be more effective than synthetic progestins at preserving estrogen's benefits on HDL cholesterol and fibrinogen. While both natural progesterone and the synthetic progestins protect the endometrium from overstimulation by estrogen, they differ in many other of their actions. More about the benefits of this new natural progesterone later.

While generally protecting a woman from estrogen-induced endometrial cancer, these powerful progestin drugs also bring with them an array of undesired side effects. Since the use of a progestin drug is obligatory whenever estrogen drugs are given to a woman with a uterus, we need to review the pros and cons of progestin therapy.

Pro #1. The giving of a progestin along with estrogen replacement greatly reduces endometrial overgrowth and associated endometrial cancer commonly induced by estrogen given alone.

The recent PEPI study confirms this observation that most, but not all endometrial overstimulation is eliminated by the addition of a progestin. Specifically in this study 46 women developed precancerous endometrial overgrowths. Forty-one of these women were on estrogen alone while three were taking the combination estrogen with progestin.[31]

Pro #2. The addition of a progestin does not limit estrogen's positive effect on bone.

Because a progestin must be added to the estrogen program for all women with a uterus, the question arises as to whether the progestin will alter estrogen's bone-sparing effects. The answer appears to be no. In fact, several studies now suggest that the synthetic progestins, and even more so natural progesterone, stimulate an increase in bone density.[53, 54]

Pro #3. The addition of a progestin appears not to negate totally estrogen's beneficial effects on beneficial HDL cholesterol and fibrinogen.

Over the years various studies have suggested that progestin drugs might have adverse effects on blood fats, raising the bad cholesterol (LDL) while lowering the good cholesterol (HDL).[55-58] If this were true, the addition of a progestin could negate estrogen's beneficial effect on HDL, the good cholesterol.

The 1995 NIH sponsored PEPI Trial found that the addition of progestins did not totally negate estrogen's beneficial effects on these two risk factors for heart disease. While estrogen alone provided the most improvement in these risk factors, some slight benefit did remain after the addition of the synthetic progestins. Natural micronized progesterone spared more of estrogen's beneficial effects. What all this means for hormone consumers is that if you are banking on the much touted heart protective benefits of estrogen and you have an intact uterus, be sure your physician prescribes natural micronized progesterone or another form of natural progesterone along with the estrogen drug. As a rule today, the synthetic progestin Provera rather than natural progesterone is given along with estrogen.

The Cons of Progestin Therapy

Progestins are newer drugs and we know less about their full effects than we do about estrogens. What we do know, however, gives great cause for concern. The following is a summary of the warnings regarding the use of the commonly prescribed synthetic progesterone Provera given in *The Physicians Desk Reference*, 1995.

Illustration 17.2

POTENTIAL SIDES EFFECTS OF PROVERA (MEDROXYPROGESTERONE)

Precautions:

- ✦ May cause fluid retention, epilepsy, migraine, asthma, cardiac or renal dysfunction.
- ✦ May cause breakthrough bleeding or menstrual irregularities.
- ✦ May cause or contribute to depression.
- ✦ The effect of prolonged use of this drug on pituitary, ovarian, adrenal, hepatic or uterine function is unknown.
- ✦ May interfere with body's ability to process sugar; diabetic patients must be carefully monitored.
- ✦ May increase the thrombotic disorders associated with estrogens.

Adverse Reactions:

- ✦ May cause breast tenderness and discharge.
- ✦ May cause sensitivity reactions such as hives, itching, swelling or rash.
- ✦ May cause acne and abnormal hair growth.
- ✦ Swelling, weight changes (increase or decrease).
- ✦ Cervical erosions and changes in cervical secretions.
- ✦ Jaundice.
- ✦ Mental depression, fever, nausea, insomnia or sleepiness.
- ✦ Severe acute allergic reactions.
- ✦ Thrombophlebitis and pulmonary embolism.
- ✦ Breakthrough bleeding, spotting, amenorrhea or changes in menses.

When taken with estrogens, the following have been observed:

- ✦ Rise in blood pressure, headache, dizziness, nervousness, fatigue.
- ✦ Changes in libido, abnormal hair growth, thyroid chemical changes.
- ✦ Premenstrual-like syndrome, changes in appetite.
- ✦ Symptoms of urinary tract infection without actual infection.
- ✦ Severe skin conditions.

Will Postmenopausal Progestin/Progesterone Therapy Increase the Risk of Breast Cancer?

For some time selected serious and authoritative researchers have suggested the possibility that progesterone also induces breast cell division and that estrogen and progesterone together might stimulate breast cancer development more than estrogen alone.[59] Few studies, however, have addressed the question of breast cancer risk and estrogen/progestin hormone therapy. The studies that do exist report conflicting results. Some show an increased risk of breast cancer, others do not. For example, two large scale case-controlled studies showed an increased risk among women who had used estrogen plus a progestin while a third study did not.[20, 60, 61] Beyond this, a large scale Swedish study reported a fourfold increase in the risk of breast cancer in women who had used estrogen plus progestins for six years or more.[36] Similarly, a large population-based controlled Danish study found sequential therapy with estrogen and progestin to be associated with an increased risk of breast cancer.[38] The large scale 1995 Harvard Nurses' Health Study also found an increased risk of breast cancer among women using combined hormone therapy.[39] Grady and her colleagues conclude that, "Evidence concerning the effect of estrogen plus progestins on breast cancer risk is limited, but there is some reason to worry about increased risk with long-term use."[20]

❖ IS POSTMENOPAUSAL HORMONE REPLACEMENT WORTH IT? WHAT THE EXPERTS NOW SAY

If you are wondering what the research community thinks about hormone replacement therapy, consider a review published in the *Annals Of Internal Medicine*, December, 1992. The article, "Hormone Therapy to Prevent Disease and Prolong Life in Postmenopausal Women," was co-authored by Dr. Grady of the University of California and seven other foremost estrogen researchers. In this study they reviewed all English language literature since 1970 on the effects of estrogen therapy and estrogen plus progestin therapy on endometrial cancer, breast cancer, coronary heart disease, osteoporosis and stroke. They then extrapolated this vast data to calculate lifetime probabilities of selected diseases and estimate overall longevity with and without hormone therapy. In essence they ask "Is hormone replacement therapy worth it or not?"

Despite all the hoopla about the benefits of hormone replacement therapy for osteoporosis prevention and treatment, the conclusion of this exhaustive study came to quite a different conclusion: "Hormone therapy should probably be recommended for women who have had a hysterectomy and for those with coronary heart disease or at high risk for coronary heart disease. For other women, the best course of action is unclear."[20] When all risks and benefits were considered, no basis at all was found for recommending estrogen or combined hormone therapy for osteoporosis prevention. Note also that these scientists' endorsement of hormone therapy for heart health promotion was rather limited, suggesting that only those with coronary heart disease, or those at high risk for coronary heart disease, would experience an overall benefit from use of these drugs.

This very tempered and limited endorsement of estrogen is especially significant as it was authored by some of the best known advocates of estrogen therapy. It is also perhaps worthy of note, however, that this study was funded in part by the Merck Company, producer of the new Fosamax drug for osteoporosis. Here again our attention is called to the need for public interest research and product development. For decades the conventional medical community insisted that the scientific data on estrogen's risks and benefits clearly demonstrated these drugs to be the therapy of choice for osteoporosis prevention and treatment. Now as a new non-hormonal osteoporosis drug becomes available a new interpretation of the same scientific data yields a polar opposite conclusion.

I agree with the conclusion by Dr. Grady and colleagues that for the average women concerned with osteoporosis, the risks of hormone therapy outweigh its benefits. For those concerned with osteoporosis, this book is dedicated to the development of effective, safe ways to build and rebuild bone mass. In addition, the Better Bones Better Body perspective suggests that there are also better ways than estrogen therapy to deal with heart disease. In fact this program espouses dietary and lifestyle modifications which are good for every cell of your body that will reduce your risk of heart disease as well as osteoporosis much more than estrogen drugs. While space does not permit for details here, the full Better Bones, Better Body approach to promoting heart health is available from the Nutrition Education and Consulting Service (See Appendix 2).

❖ THE NEW NATURAL PROGESTERONE TREATMENT FOR OSTEOPOROSIS

When it comes to hormone therapy for osteoporosis the new kid on the block is definitely a substance known as "natural progesterone." Unlike the synthetic progestins, natural progesterone has a molecular configuration identical to the hormone produced by the ovaries. Introduced directly to the public in over-the-counter topical creams, natural progesterone has become an "underground" self-help treatment for two major categories of ailments: (1) Alleviation of various female disorders related to relative estrogen dominance and progesterone deficiency such as PMS, fibrocystic breast disease, vaginitis, ovarian cysts, endometriosis and uterine fibroid tumors and; (2) Prevention, halting and reversal of bone loss.[54]

It is now known that the bone-building cells (osteoblasts) have receptors for progesterone and that progesterone stimulates bone growth.[62] While no long-term scientific studies exist on the use of natural progesterone for osteoporosis, many physicians have found it of significant benefit. The clinician most experienced in using natural progesterone to build bone is Dr. John Lee of Sebastopol, California. For more than 15 years Dr. Lee has been using natural transdermal progesterone creams for osteoporosis with exceptional success.[54] He has found natural progesterone capable of reversing excessive bone loss and preventing new fractures among women with established osteoporosis. The greatest bone-building benefits reportedly are seen in the women with most bone loss.

Dr. Lee reports that with or without estrogen therapy, natural progesterone builds bone. In cases of severe osteoporosis he reports bone density increases of 10 to 15 percent in six months and an average 15 percent in three years with little occurrence of new fractures.[54, 63, 64] Although many of the women in his study continued on their estrogen therapy while adding the natural progesterone, others dropped the estrogen totally. Both groups seemed to gain bone while on progesterone. I have seen no evidence that women with good bone density experience additional bone-building benefits from progesterone therapy, but studies on natural progesterone have barely begun.

While I have yet to see other published studies reporting the exceptionally high degree of progesterone-induced bone mass increases reported by Dr. Lee, many other clinicians informally report significant bone-building benefits from natural progesterone.[65-68] Hopefully the conventional medical community will soon conduct clinical trials with this promising natural substance. For now, given that natural progesterone appears much more effective and safer than estrogen or synthetic progestins, women with osteoporosis seeking hormonal treatment would do well to read and refer their health care practitioner to Dr. Lee's book, *Natural Progesterone, The Multiple Roles Of A Remarkable Hormone.*[54]

In closing this section it is wise to recall the basic Better Bones, Better Body tenet that "health lies in balance and perfect health lies in perfect balance." Hormones, even "natural" ones, are powerful substances and should be given in the appropriate doses according to individual need. As Dr. Serafina Corsello, director of the Corsello Centers for Nutritional and Complementary Medicine in New York City emphasizes, any individual hormone therapy should address the needs of the entire endocrine system. She likens endocrine functioning to a symphony orchestra in which all instruments must be individually tuned as the basis for a perfect performance. When administrating hormone therapy she emphasizes the importance of "balancing the triad." By this she means balancing the adrenals, thyroid and ovaries, each individually and then one with each other. She regularly tests and adjusts the adrenal hormones when needed using natural extracts and DHEA. This is done concomitantly with the ovarian hormones estradiol, estrone, progesterone and testosterone; and those of the thyroid. Self-administration of hormones or the prescription of hormone therapy without proper testing can create an even greater imbalance.[68]

What About Natural Estrogen?

As "natural" progesterone is more bio-compatible, more effective and safer than synthetic progestins one might wonder, Is there a "natural" estrogen? The answer is yes and this too is an under-explored area which promises to yield great health benefits. Estrogen is an interesting substance and actually some 20 different estrogens are produced by the ovaries. Those produced in greatest quantity are estradiol (the predominant estrogen in premenopausal women), estrone (a metabolite of estradiol which predominates postmenopausally) and estriol (also a metabolite of estradiol which is produced in large amounts during pregnancy).

In this country, the most common conventional estrogen therapy used today is conjugated equine estrogen processed from the urine of pregnant horses. These horse estrogens are really a cocktail of estrogens containing some estradiol and estrone as is made in humans and an enormous amount of equilin, a horse estrogen that doesn't occur at all in humans.[69] The pharmaceutical industry considers this horse estrogen formula "natural" because it contains some estradiol and estrone as produced by the human body. Holistically minded physicians, however, take exception to this use of the term "natural" because of the high content of non-human horse estrogen in these drugs.[65, 69] There are also many chemically compounded estrogen hormone drugs the pharmaceutical industry calls "synthetic" such as ethinyl estridial as in Estinyl or Feminone and esterfied estrogens as in Evex and Menest.

Currently, attention is being drawn towards several forms of "natural estrogen" therapy. The first concerns plant substances known as phytoestrogens, which are plant compounds having an estrogen-like effect. For example, compounds like isoflavones and phytosterols found in soy and other foods have a mild estrogenic effect. Many attribute the near absence of hot flashes in Japan to their lifelong high soy intake. The herbs dong quai, licorice root, alfalfa, red clover, fennel seed and black cohosh are all known to exhibit phytoestrogen activity. For centuries these herbs have been used to alleviate menopausal symptoms. Several supplement companies produce herbal formulas containing these phytoestrogens for use during the menopausal transition.

The second new form of "natural estrogen" concerns chemical substances with the same molecular structure as those hormones produced by the ovaries. Sapogenins from soy and wild yam are extracted and these are then synthesized into a compound with the same chemical structure as one of the three major human estrogens. Selected conventional estrogens such as Estrace and the estradiol patch use the natural micronized estradiol estrogen and various pharmacies compound a variety of natural estrogens for physicians. See Appendix 4 for suppliers.

The third and newest "natural estrogen" is a hormone

replacement formula which includes all three of the common human estrogens: estradiol, estrone and estriol. The formula, called "Tri-Est," contains 80 percent estriol, 10 percent estradiol and 10 percent estrone. This combination of estrogens was developed by Dr. Jonathan Wright of Kent, Washington. He prefers the higher levels of estriol for several reasons. First it is a weak estrogen adequate for relieving the symptoms of estrogen deficiency, yet not as over-stimulating as estradiol. Secondly some early research suggests that estriol might be cancer protective.[70-72] While little follow-up work has been done on this latter possibility, there is a European study on osteoporosis which suggests that postmenopausal estriol use might be associated with a decreased risk of breast cancer.[38] To my knowledge, estriol's effect on bone loss has not been studied.

Estriol-centered formulas are reportedly used more commonly in Europe than in the United States and are suggested by some to be safer and more bio-compatible than the estradiol-centered estrogens commonly used in the United States.[65, 66, 73] Further research on estriol-centered formulas appears warranted. A wide variety of natural estrogen formulas can be ordered by your physician through special suppliers. See Appendix 4 for a list of suppliers. Those interested in learning more about the new natural estrogen formula can refer to Dr. Alan Gaby's book, *Preventing and Reversing Osteoporosis*[66] and my co-authored publication, *The Mend Clinic Guide to Natural Medicine for Menopause and Beyond*.[74]

The Better Bones, Better Body Perspective On Natural Hormone Therapy

First, it appears obvious that when hormone therapy is required the most natural, bio-compatible forms of that hormone should be used when at all possible. For this reason, studies on the efficacy, safety and clinical benefits of natural progesterone, natural estrogen-like plant compounds and estriol-centered estrogen formulas are long overdue.

It is essential, however, for those using either natural or conventional hormones to undergo regular medical examinations and, if osteoporosis is a concern, regular bone density measurements. Also women on any form of hormone therapy should consider having their hormone levels measured to ensure that they are receiving a dose that is appropriate for them as a distinct biochemical individual. Interestingly, your physician carefully monitors your blood when you take thyroid hormone or insulin, yet estrogen and progestins are given to millions without the slightest consideration about measuring to see if the dose given is the correct amount for that particular woman. Therefore, it should not come as a total surprise that overdosing with estrogen drugs might be common. Diagnos-Techs, Inc. is a laboratory in Kent, Washington specializing in measurement of hormone levels directed by Dr. Elias IIyia. Having analyzed the estrogen levels in hundreds of women, Dr. IIyia reports it to be the rule that women on conventional estrogen replacement therapy exhibit excessively high estrogen levels.[75] For the same reason, one's progesterone level should be measured if natural progesterone or synthetic progestins are taken. Hormones are potent substances with considerable individual variation in absorption.[76] Their use should be carefully monitored, rather than just relying on symptom relief to indicate dosage. Recognizing the value of accurate hormone dosing, selected laboratories now offer estrogen and progesterone measurements easily obtained from saliva samples which can be used to individualize postmenopausal hormone supplementation should you chose to use these drugs. See Appendix 4 for a listing of these laboratories.

❖ References

1 Tanouye, Elyse, "Merck's Osteoporosis Warnings Pave the Way for Its New Drug," *Wall St. Journal* (June 28 1995): B1;B4.

2 Seaman, Barbara, and Gideon Seaman, M.D. *Women and the Crisis in Sex Hormones,* fifth edition (New York: Bantam Books, 1981) 621.

3 Greenberg, E., "Breast Cancer in Women Given Diethylstilbestrol in Pregnancy," *New England Journal of Medicine* 311.22 (1984): 1393-1398.

4 Anon., "DES and Cancer," *USA Today* (April 28, 1993).

5 Stadel, B., et al., "Oral Contraceptives and Premenopausal Breast Cancer in Nulliparous Women," *Contraception* 38.3 (1988): 287-299.

6 Kay, Clifford R., "Breast Cancer and the Pill-A Further Report from the Royal College of General Practitioners OC Study," *British Journal of Cancer* 58 (1988): 675-80.

7 Miller, D., et al., "Breast Cancer Before Age 45 and Oral Contraceptive Use: New Findings," *American Journal of Epidemiology* 129.2 (1989): 269-280.

8 Wilson, R., *Forever Young,* (New York: Evans, 1966).

9 Stadel, B., and N. Weiss, "Characteristics of Menopausal Women: A Survey of King and Pierce Counties in Washington, 1973-74," *Am J Epidemiology* 102 (1975): 209-216.

10 National Women's Health Network, *Taking Hormones and Women's Health: Choices, Risks, Benefits,* (Washington, D.C.: National Women's Health Network, 1989).

11 Ford, A., "Hormones: Getting out of Hand," *Adverse Effects: Women and the Pharmaceutical Industry,* ed., K. McDonnell. (Toronto: Women's Educational Press, 1986) 27-40.

12 Anon., "Hormone Replacement Therapy Overview," *The Network News-National Women's Health Network,* May/June (1989).

13 Coney, Sandra, *The Menopause Industry,* (Emeryville, CA: Publishers Group West, 1994) 369.

14 Henkel G., *Making the Estrogen Decision.* (New York: Fawcett Columbine, 1992).

15 Riggs, Lawrence B., "Letter to the Editor," *The New England Journal of Medicine* (1993): 66.

16 Riggs, B.L., and L.J. Melton, "The Prevention and Treatment of Osteoporosis," *New England Journal of Medicine* 327 (1992): 620-627.

17 Seaman, B., and G. Seaman, *Women and the Crisis in Sex Hormones,* (New York: Bantam Books, 1977).

18 Lindsay, R., personal communication, Continuing Education Course on Osteoporosis: Harvard University, (1987).

19 Ettinger, Bruce M.D., and Deborah Grady, M.D., "The Waning Effect of Postmenopausal Estrogen Therapy on Osteoporosis," *The New England Journal of Medicine* 329.16 (1993): 1192-1193.

20 Grady, Deborah, et al., "Hormone Therapy to Prevent Disease and Prolong Life in Postmenopausal Women," *Annals of Internal Medicine* 117.12 (1992): 1016.

21 Anon., "Menopause," *Harvard Women's Health Watch* May (1995).

22 Robb-Nicholson, Celeste, "By the Way, Doctor," *Harvard Women's Health Watch* (July 1995).

23 Cummings, Steven, et al., "Risk Factors For Hip Fracture In White Women," *The New England Journal of Medicine* 332.12 (1995): 767-774.

24 Cauley, Jane, et al., "Estrogen Replacement Therapy and Fractures in Older Women," *Annals of Internal Medicine* 122.1 (1995): 9-17.

25 Felson, David T., et al., "The Effect of Postmenopausal Estrogen Therapy on Bone Density In Elderly Women," *New England Journal of Medicine* 329.16 (1993): 1141-1146.

26 Silverberg, E., and J. Lubora, "Cancer Statistics, 1989," *CA - A Cancer Journal for Clinicians* 39.1 (1989): 3-20.

27 Wilson, P. R. Garrison, and W. Castelli, "Postmenopausal Estrogen

Use, Cigarette Smoking, and Cardiovascular Morbidity in Women Over 50—The Framingham Study," *The New England Journal of Medicine* 313.17 (1985): 1038-1043.

28 Wilson, P., "Prospective Studies: The Framingham Study," *Long-Term Effects of Estrogen Deprivation, ed.* Postgraduate Medicine. (New York: McGraw-Hill, Inc., 1989) 51-52.

29 Stampfer, Mei, et al., "Postmenopausal Estrogen Therapy and Cardiovascular Disease: Ten-Year Follow-Up from the Nurses' Health Study," *New England Journal of Medicine* 325.11 (1991): 756-761.

30 Peterson, H., N. Lee, and G. Rubin, "Genital Neoplasia," *Menopause: Physiology and Pharmacology, ed.* D. Mishell. (Chicago: Year Book Medical Publishers, 1987) 275-298.

31 PEPI, "Effects of Estrogen or Estrogen/Progestin Regimens on Heart Disease Risk Factors in Postmenopausal Women," *JAMA* 273.3 (1995): 199-208.

32 Henderson, B., R. Ross, and M. Pike, "Breast Neoplasia," *Menopause: Physiology and Pharmacology, ed.* D. Mishell. Yearbook Medicine Publishers, 1987) 261.

33 Ross, R., et al., "A Case-Control Study of Menopausal Estrogen Therapy and Breast Cancer," *JAMA* 243.16 (1980): 1635-1639.

34 LaVecchia, C., et al;., "Non-Contraceptive Oestrogens and the Risk of Breast Cancer in Women," *Int J Cancer* 38 (1986): 853-858.

35 Brinton, L., R. Hoover, and J. Fraumeni, "Menopausal Oestrogens and Breast Cancer Risk: An Expanded Case-Control Study," *Br J Cancer* 54.5(Nov) (1986): 825-832.

36 Bergkvist, L., et al., "The Risk of Breast Cancer After Estrogen and Estrogen-Progestin Replacement," *The New England Journal of Medicine* 321.5 (1989): 293-297.

37 Gambrell, R., "Sex Steroid Hormones and Cancer," (Chicago: Year Book Medical Publishers, 1984) 1-63.

38 Ewertz, Marianne, "Influence Of Non-Contraceptive Exogenous And Endogenous Sex Hormones On Breast Cancer Risk In Denmark," *Int. J. Cancer* 42 (1988): 832-838.

39 Colditz, Graham, et al., "The Use of Estrogens and Progestins and the Risk of Breast Cancer in Postmenopausal Women," *The New England Journal of Medicine* 332.24 (1995): 1589-1593.

40 McPherson, Klim, "Breast cancer and hormonal supplements in postmenopausal women," *BMJ* (September 16, 1995).

41 Steinberg, Karen K., et al., "A Meta-analysis of the Effect of Estrogen Replacement Therapy on the Risk of Breast Cancer," *JAMA* 265.15 (1991): 1985.

42 Colditz, Graham, "Heart Disease And Hormone Supplementation," May/June ed. (Network News: 1994) 4-5.

43 Rodriguez, C., "Estrogen replacement therapy and fatal ovarian cancer," *Am J Epidemiol* 141 (1995): 828-35.

44 Petitti, D., et al., "Increased Risk of Cholecystectomy in Users of Supplemental Estrogen," *Gastroenterology* 94.Jan (1988): 91-95.

45 Canny, P., et al., "Fibroadenoma and the Use of Exogenous Hormones. A Case-control Study," *Am J Epidemiol* 127.3 (1988): 454-461.

46 Berkowitz, Gertrud S, et al., "Estrogen Replacement Therapy and Fibrocystic Breast Disease In Postmenopausal Women," *American Journal of Epidemiology* 121.2 (1985): 238-245.

47 Trapido, E., et al., "Estrogen Replacement Therapy and Benign Breast Disease," *J Natl Cancer Inst* 73.5 (1984): 1101-1105.

48 Stomper, P.C., et al., "Mammographic changes associated with postmenopausal hormone replacement therapy: a longitudinal study.," *Radiology* 174.2 (1990): 487-90.

49 Sanchez-Guerrero, Jorge M. D., et al., "Systemic Lupus Erythematosus And Estrogen Therapy," *Annals of Internal Medicine* 122.6 (1995): 430-432.

50 Cutler, W., *Hysterectomy: Before & After*, (New York: Harper & Row, 1988).

51 Roe, D., *Drug-induced Nutritional Deficiencies*, (Westport, Conn: The Avi Publishing Co., Inc., 1976).

52 Killeen, R., S. Ayres, and R. Mihan, "Polymyositis: Response to Vitamin E," *Southern Medical Journal* 69.10 (1976): 1372-1373.

53 Prior, Jerilynn C., "Progesterone and the prevention of osteoporosis," *The Canadian Journal of Ob/Gyn & Women's Health Care* 3.4 (1991): 178-184.

54 Lee, John R., *Natural Progesterone. The Multiple Roles of a Remarkable Hormone*, (Sebastopol, CA: BLL Publishing, 1995) 105.

55 Fraser, D., et al., "The Effects of the Addition of Nomegestrol Acetate to Post-Menopausal Oestrogen Therapy," *Maturitas* 11 (1989): 21-34.

56 Barrett-Connor, E., "Postmenopausal Estrogen, Cancer and Other Considerations," *Women Health* 11. 3/4 (1986): 179-195.

57 Riggs, B., "Practical Management of the Patient with Osteoporosis," *Osteoporosis Etiology, Diagnosis and Management,* (New York: Raven Press, 1988) 481-490.

58 Ottoson, U.B., et al., "Subfractions of high-density lipoprotein-cholesterol during estrogen replacement therapy: a comparison between progestogens and natural progesterone," *Am J Obstet Gynecol* 151 (1985): 756-50.

59 Key, T., and M. Pike, "The Role of Oestrogens and Progestagens in the Epidemiology and Prevention of Breast Cancer," *Eur J Cancer Clin Oncol* 24.1 (1988): 29-43.

60 Palmer, JR., et al., "Breast cancer risk: results from the case-control surveillance study.," *Am J Epidemiol* 134 (1991): 1375-85.

61 Kaufman, D.W., et al., "Estrogen replacement therapy and the risk of breast cancer: results from the case-control surveillance study," *Am J Epidemiol* 134 (1991): 1375-85.

62 Prior, J.C., "Progesterone as a bone-trophic hormone," *Endocrine Reviews* 11 (1990): 386-398.

63 Lee, J.R., "Osteoporosis reversal. The role of progesterone," *Int Clin Nutr Rev* 10.3 (1990): 384-91.

64 Lee, J.R., "Is natural progesterone the missing link in osteoporosis prevention and treatment?" *Medical Hypotheses* 35 (1991): 316-18.

65 Wright, Jonathan V. M.D., "On Call for Hormone Replacement Therapy, You Can't Beat the Real Thing," *Let's Live* (1995).

66 Gaby, Alan R. Ph.D., *Preventing and Reversing Osteoporosis,* (Rocklin: Prima Publishing, 1994) 304.

67 Milner, Martin, personal communication, Center for Natural Medicine Portland, Oregon (1995).

68 Corsello, Serafina, personal communication, The Corsello Centers for Nutritional-Complementary Medicine (1996).

69 Barnard, Neal D., "Hormone Replacement Increases Cancer Risk," *Good Medicine.* Autumn (1995): 14-15.

70 Follingstad, A., "Estriol, the Forgotten Estrogen?" *Journal of American Medical Association* 239 (1978): 29-30.

71 Lemon, Henry M., et al., "Reduced Estriol Excretion in Patients With Breast Cancer Prior to Endocrine Therapy," *JAMA* 196.13 (1966): 112-120.

72 Lemon, H.M., "Pathophysiologic considerations in the treatment of menopausal patients with oestrogens; the role of oestriol in the prevention of mammary carcinoma," *Acta Endocrinol Suppl* 233 (1980): 17-27.

73 Pelton, Ross, et al., *How to Prevent Breast Cancer*, (New York: Simon & Schuster, 1995).

74 Maas, Paula, et al., *The Mend Clinic Guide to Natural Medicine for Menopause and Beyond*, (New York: Dell, 1997 (forthcoming)).

75 Ilyia, Elias, personal communication (1995).

76 Barnes, R., and R. Lobo, "Pharmacology of Estrogens," *Menopause: Physiology and Pharmacology*, ed. D. Mishell. Yearbook Medicine Publishers, 1987) 301.

Chapter **18**

. . . .

Fosamax and Final Thoughts

*I*f you are a middle-aged or older woman whose doctor is a member of the conventional medical community, it is very likely you have been told to use drug therapy to reduce your risk of osteoporosis. To date estrogen therapy has been the primary drug used to reduce bone loss. With the recent FDA approval of the bisphosphonate, alendronate, another player has entered into the field. This new drug is manufactured by Merck and goes under the trade name of Fosamax. Bisphosphonates as a group are considered by many to represent the next generation of osteoporosis treatment.[1] Like estrogen, the bisphosphonate drugs act to limit bone breakdown but do not stimulate bone formation.[2] Although the drug has been just recently approved, we are already witnessing a carefully orchestrated campaign to promote its use by making osteoporosis and the need for bone density testing a household concern.[3-6]

I am not sure that such a strong publicity campaign is in the public interest. From the onset, the manufacturers of this new drug have suggested to physicians that all women with a bone density two standard deviations or more below that of normal young women could benefit from lifelong use of this drug.[7] According to osteoporosis authority Dr. Robert Melton of the Mayo Clinic, some 45 percent of all Caucasian women aged 50 years and over in this country have a bone mass at least at one site which is two standard deviations below that of normal young women.[8] So, from the pharmaceutical point of view, 45 percent of all Caucasian women and an unknown percentage of minority women are candidates for lifelong bone stabilizing drug therapy. This by itself is a rather frightening proposition. In fact, the drug has been found to decrease the incidence of vertebral fractures, but it is not known if it will reduce the incidence of hip and other non-vertebral fractures. Nor is it known if the drug is safe or effective over the long haul, yet it must be used indefinitely in order to maintain its benefits. As Dr. Sambrook states in a recent *New England Journal of Medicine* editorial of November, 1995 ". . . because bisphosphonates accumulate in the skeleton for prolonged periods, long-term safety remains a question. Other questions, such as the long-term effect of the new bisphosphonates on bone turnover and mechanical strength, also remain to be answered."[2] Earlier bisphosphonate drugs like Editronate have been shown to be inadequate. Should this drug prove effective with minimal adverse effects it would be a boon for many older individuals at high risk for fracture. In this case it would best be used in conjunction with a life-supporting bone regeneration program as described in this book. Should it prove ineffective, we would have yet another case of mass experimentation with women's health.

No matter what the fate of this or any other new drug therapy however, the Better Bones, Better Body Program represents another direction. Our direction concerns working with nature for the regeneration of our full health potential, including the potential of lifelong healthy bones.

Over ten years ago I began what I intended to be a brief research project looking into a common disorder known as osteoporosis. As an anthropologist I was struck by the rather alarming frequency of this disease within our culture and I wondered what the incidence was in other cultures. Certainly the indigenous and traditional peoples I had worked with exhibited no signs of weak bones at any age. What began as a "brief" project turned into a decade-long endeavor now known as The Osteoporosis Education Project. What began as "thinking about" osteoporosis turned into a massive "rethinking" the entire nature and causes of excessive bone loss. This rethinking in turn clarified in my mind the need for a new, comprehensive, fully life-supporting approach to building bone health in our culture.

In this book I have woven together my vision of such a life-supporting program from the best research findings of the medical, nutritional and anthropological sciences. It is my hope that the scientific community will direct its research dollars to a comprehensive study of the efficacy of a Better Bones, Better Body approach which incorporates at a minimum:

+ Optimum intake of all essential bone-building nutrients
+ Reduction in anti-nutrients and bone-damaging lifestyle factors
+ Adequate weight-bearing exercise
+ A bone-sparing alkaline diet
+ Holistic endocrine health optimization

It is clear to me that the compelling public interest dictates broad testing of such a common sense approach.

Evaluating The Success of Your Bone Building Program

It is important that your bone-building program be successful and that you actually achieve your goals of halting and reversing bone loss. This is especially true if you are at high risk of suffering an osteoporotic fracture or if you have already fractured a bone. Every program to enhance bone health, be it our Better Bones, Better Body Program or any other program, should be carefully monitored. Each individual is different. It could be that a program excellent for others is not appropriate in your case. Poor results also might mean you need to improve your compliance, that is to adhere to the program more strictly. On the other hand, a lack of success could be due to an overlooked bone-depleting disease or other factor which should be addressed medically.

The best way to measure the success of your personal program is to obtain a bone density scan of the spine and hip. Ideally a baseline scan should be taken before beginning your program and follow-up measurements done to gauge the success of your efforts. In the beginning, follow-up exams are usually scheduled at one year. Later they can be spread out more if your results are right on target. For accuracy, it is important that the baseline and follow-up exams are done on the same type of equipment. Today, in 1996, the state-of-the-art bone scan device is known as the DEXA scanner. It is accurate, uses low levels of radiation, and measures both spongy trabecular and dense cortical bone. Just as you need to take the time to develop your personalized bone-building program, so you should also make it a priority to measure its success and review the results with your health care professional. Any bone-building program that is not producing the desired results should be modified.

Keep in mind also that osteoporosis is not only a big public health problem, but it is also big business. Currently sales for estrogen and other osteoporosis drugs total one billion dollars and this figure is expected to soar to 3.3 billion dollars within the next five years. Premarin, the most popular of all estrogen drugs, is currently the number one best-selling drug in the country. Sales of this drug alone totaled $853 million in 1994. Worldwide sales of the new bisphosphonate drug Fosamax recently approved for osteoporosis treatment are expected to exceed one billion dollars a year.[3-6] It is not unlikely that a commonsense, life-supporting approach that yields no great profits to any one party might get lost when such huge profits are at stake.

Finally remember that within each of us operates a vast intelligence beyond our comprehension; an intelligence capable of orchestrating six trillion distinct yet coordinated reactions each second; an intelligence which provides for balanced functioning and instantaneous communication between our 60-odd trillion cells; an intelligence undaunted by the task of producing a living, thinking human being from whatever food, air, water and sunlight we give it. The development and maintenance of a multi-purpose skeletal system just right for the demands we place on it, at any point in our life, is but one comparatively simple expression of this vast intelligence. For lifelong healthy bones we need only pause amid our hectic daily lives and seek ways to reestablish internal balance and nourish the flow of intelligence already within us.

❖ References

1 Christiansen, Claus, "Treatment of Osteoporosis," *Treatment of the Postmenopausal Woman: Basic and Clinical Aspects,* ed. Rogerio A. Lobo. (New York: Raven Press, 1994) 183–195.

2 Sambrook, Philip N., "The Treatment of Postmenopausal Osteoporosis," *The New England Journal of Medicine* 333.22 (1995): 1495–6.

3 Tanouye, Elyse, "Osteoporosis Drug, Made by Merck Gets Boost from Panel," *Wall Street Journal* July 14 (1995).

4 Tanouye, Elyse, "Merck's Osteoporosis Warnings Pave, the Way for It's New Drug," *Wall St. Journal* June 28 (1995): B1;B4.

5 Tanouye, Elyse, "Delicate Balance Estrogen Study Shifts Ground For Women—And for Drug Firms," *Wall Street Journal* (1995): 1;A8.

6 Zones, Jane, "Osteoporosis Campaign to Generate Big Bucks," *The Network News* 20.5 (1995): 1;4.

7 Merck & Co., Inc., FOSAMAX package insert and research data, Merck & Co., Inc., (1995)

8 Melton, L., et al., "How many women have osteoporosis?" *J Bone Miner Res.* 7 (1992): 1005-1010.

❖ Appendices

Appendix 1

Recommended Dietary and Nutrient Guidelines

❖ BACKGROUND INFORMATION ON THE RDAs

Since 1943 the National Academy of Sciences has published Recommended Dietary Allowances, known as the RDAs. The RDAs are defined as specified intake levels of essential nutrients considered to be adequate to meet the known nutritional needs of practically all healthy people.[1] The emphasis is on providing "adequate" levels for "practically all healthy" people and from this arises great controversy. Many scientists are concerned as to whether the recommended guidelines should be aimed at providing just adequate levels to prevent deficiency diseases, or if nutrient intake levels should be set higher, closer to levels known to promote optimum health. Also, there is growing concern with the fact that many segments of our society are not "healthy" and have special needs beyond the RDAs.

Every six to 10 years the Academy revises the RDAs to reflect updated scientific data. Amid much controversy the 1989 RDA revisions lowered recommended intakes for six nutrients including vitamins B_6, B_{12}, folic acid, iron, magnesium and zinc. Also the Academy failed to raise the calcium RDA for postmenopausal and elderly women, as was strongly recommended by many nutritional professionals. Many progressive nutritionists have called the present RDAs "obsolete and out of touch."[2] Studies on bone health confirm that optimum health-promoting nutrient intake levels are often well above the current RDAs.

ADULT GUIDELINES FOR TOTAL NUTRIENT INTAKE FROM COMBINED FOOD AND SUPPLEMENT SOURCES

NUTRIENT	RDA 1989*	MORE OPTIMUM INTAKE**
Calcium	800-1200 mg	1000-1500 mg
Chromium	50-200 mcg	200 mcg
Copper	2-3 mg	2-3 mg
Folic Acid	180-200 mcg	400 mcg
Iodine	150 mcg	——
Iron	10-15 mg	10-18 mg
Magnesium	280-350 mg	500-600 mg
Manganese	2.5-5 mg	15 mg
Niacin	15-19 mg	——
Pantothenic Acid	4-7 mg	100-200 mg
Phosphorus	800-1200 mg	800-1200 mg
Potassium	1875-5625 mg	4000-5625 mg

1 Brown, Judith, The Science of Human Nutrition, (New York: Harcourt Brace Jovanovich, Inc., 1990).

2 Somer, Elizabeth, "In Search of the Balanced Diet," The Nutrition Report. August (1986):58.

Pyridoxine, B$_6$	1.6-2 mg	25 mg
Riboflavin	1.3-1.7 mg	25 mg
Selenium	50-200 mcg	100-200 mcg
Thiamin	1-1.5 mg	25 mgg
Vitamin A	800-1000 IU	10,000 IU
Vitamin B$_{12}$	2 mcg	——
Vitamin C	60 mg	1,000-3,000 mg
Vitamin D	5-10 IU	400 IU
Vitamin E	8-10 IU	400 IU
Vitamin K	70-140 mcg	——
Zinc	12-15 mg	22 mg

* RDA values are for nonpregnant, nonlactating adults. For nutrients without RDAs the designated "Safe and Adequate" levels were used.

** Partially adapted from Werbach, *Nutritional Influence on Illness*, Third Line Press, 1989 and Lieberman and Bruning, *The Real Vitamin and Mineral Book: Going Beyond the RDAs*, Avery, 1990.

RECOMMENDED DIETARY ALLOWANCES FOR CHILDREN (1989)

	INFANTS 0.0-0.5 YEARS	INFANTS 0.5-1.0 YEARS	CHILDREN 1-3 YEARS	CHILDREN 4-6 YEARS	CHILDREN 7-10 YEARS	YOUNG TEEN 11-14 YEARS
Protein, g	13	14	16	24	28	46
Vitamin A, mcg	375	375	400	500	700	1000
Vitamin C, mg	35	35	45	45	45	50
Vitamin D, IU	300	400	400	400	400	400
Vitamin E, mg	3	4	6	7	7	10
Thiamin, B$_1$, mg	0.3	0.4	0.7	0.9	1.0	1.3
Riboflavin, B$_2$, mg	0.4	0.5	0.8	1.1	1.2	1.5
Niacin, B$_3$, mg	5	6	9	12	13	17
Pyridoxine, B$_6$ mg	0.3	0.6	1.0	1.1	1.4	1.7

....
Appendix 1

Folate mcg	25	35	50	75	100	150
Vitamin B$_{12}$, mcg	0.33	0.5	0.7	1.0	1.4	2
Calcium, mg	400	600	800	800	800	1200
Phosphorus, mg	300	500	800	800	800	1200
Magnesium, mg	40	60	80	120	1270	270
Iron, mg	6	10	10	10	10	12
Zinc, mg	5	5	10	10	10	15
Iodine, mcg	40	50	70	90	120	150
Selenium, mcg	10	15	20	20	30	40

ESTIMATED SAFE AND ADEQUATE DIETARY INTAKE OF OTHER VITAMINS AND MINERALS

Copper, mg	0.5-0.7	0.7-1.0	1.0-1.5	1.5-2.0	2.0-2.5	2.0-3.0
Manganese, mg	0.5-0.7	0.7-1.0	1.0-1.5	1.5-2.0	2.0-3.0	2.5-5
Chromium, mg	0.01-0.04	0.02-0.06	0.02-0.08	0.03-0.12	0.05-.2	0.05-0.2
Potassium, mg	350-925	425-1275	550-1650	775-2325	1000-3000	1525-4575

Appendix **2**

·················

Services and Products of the Nutrition Education and Consulting Service

❖ PUBLICATIONS

Nutrition News and Notes

A bi-monthly newsletter highlighting hot-breaking nutrition news with a self-help program on the back side. Send a self-addressed stamped envelope for a sample.

The Nutrition Detective Workbook: A Self-Help Program for Assessing and Maximizing Your Nutrient Status

This highly illustrated workbook guides you to identification and correction of nutritional deficiencies. Includes wholesome food sources of major nutrients.

Is The Right Food Wrong For You? A Self-Help Program to Detect and Overcome Food Allergies

A simplified self-help program for uncovering and managing food and chemical sensitivities.

Estrogen Therapy For Osteoporosis and Heart Health: Is It Worth It?

A critique questioning the value of estrogen drugs for the prevention and treatment of osteoporosis and the promotion of heart health. This booklet contains a thorough review of the findings of the NIH 1995 Postmenopausal Estrogen/Progestin Interventions Trial (PEPI).

Meditation Audiocassette

A 20-minute meditation and visualization tape for optimizing mind/body functioning.

❖ LECTURE AND CONSULTING SERVICES:

✦ Individual nutrition consulting appointments via telephone or in person.
✦ Contract lectures and workshops.
✦ Computerized 3-day diet analysis.

❖ PRODUCTS

Nutritional Supplements

Contact NECS for Dr. Susan Brown's choice of selected nutrient supplements.

Body Chemistry Balancing pH Test Kit

Self-Help Kit For Development of the Health Promoting Alkaline Diet which includes:

✦ Hydrion pH paper.
✦ Audiocassette by Dr. Brown on why and how to develop an alkaline diet.
✦ Written instructions on developing and maintaining an alkaline diet.

Vitamin C Adequacy Test Kit

Includes instructions for vitamin C flush test and Vitamin C adequacy urine testing strips.

For information on these services and products contact:
The Nutrition Education and Consulting Service, East Genesee Medical Building, 1200 E. Genesee Street, Suite 310, Syracuse, NY 13210 (315) 471-0264.

❖ KEEPING UP WITH THE NEW RESEARCH ON OSTEOPOROSIS:

Information on osteoporosis changes daily. In this book you have the most up-to-date information I know of. I am sure, however, that research now in progress will yield information of additional benefit to you. The following groups can help you keep up with the latest information.

National Women's Health Network
1325 G St., NW
Washington, DC 20005
Write for information on their *Network News* Newsletter.

Osteoporosis Education Project
East Genesee Street Medical Building
1200 E. Genesee Street, Suite 310
Syracuse, New York 13210
(315) 471-0264
Send a self-addressed stamped envelope requesting information on updates.

Appendix **3**
. . . .

Wholesome Food Sources of Selected Nutrients

CALCIUM: YOUR BEST WHOLESOME FOOD SOURCES

RDA 800-1,200 mg	AMOUNT	CONTENT IN MG
VEGETABLES (fresh, cooked)		
Bok choy	1 cup	74
Broccoli	1 cup	136
Carrots	1 cup	51
Collards	1 cup	210
Kale and dandelion greens	1 cup	148
Mustard greens	1 cup	193
Okra	1 cup	148

Parsley, dried	¼ cup	72
Parsley, raw	1 cup	31
Turnip greens	1 cup	266
GRAINS		
Amaranth grain, boiled	1 cup	276
Amaranth flour	1 cup	407
Barley, pearled	1 cup	57
Millet flour	1 cup	92
Rice, white or brown, cooked	1 cup	20-22
Soy bean flour, low fat	1 cup	165
Teff, grain or flour	1 cup	407
LEGUMES, cooked		
Chick peas	½ cup	75
Cowpeas, black eyed peas	½ cup	106
Green beans & lima beans	½ cup	31
Hummus	½ cup	62
Kidney beans and black beans	½ cup	35
Navy beans	½ cup	48
Peanuts	½ cup	68
Pinto beans	½ cup	41
Soybeans	½ cup	66
Soy milk	½ cup	25
Tofu	½ cup	155
Dairy		
American cheese	1 oz.	175
Buttermilk	1 cup	288
Cheddar cheese	1 oz.	204
Cottage cheese	1 cup	130
Milk	1 cup	300
Monterey jack cheese	1 oz.	212

Swiss cheese	1 oz.	270
Yogurt, low-fat, plain	1 cup	415
Yogurt, whole milk, plain	1 cup	275
FRUITS (not a good source of calcium)		
NUTS & SEEDS		
Almond butter	¼ cup	172
Almonds	¼ cup	150
Brazil nuts	¼ cup	100
Sesame seeds, whole	¼ cup	352
Soybean nuts, roasted	¼ cup	116
ANIMAL PROTEIN		
Oysters	4 oz.	107
Canned salmon with bones	4 oz.	90
Canned sardines with bones	3 oz.	372
Scallops	10 pieces	280
OTHER GOOD CALCIUM SOURCES		
Blackstrap molasses	1 Tbs.	137
Bone marrow of chicken thigh bone (bones must be well cooked to extract calcium)	1 bone	250-300
SEAWEED (dried)		
Arame	1 oz.	375
Hijiki	1 oz.	450
Wakame	1 oz.	425

Sources: Gebhardt, Susan, and Ruth Matthews, "Nutritive Value of Foods," United States Department of Agriculture, 1981. Leveille, Gilbert A., et al., *Nutrients in Foods*, (Cambridge, MA: The Nutrition Guild, 1983) Rockwell, Sally, *Calcium Without The Cow*, (Seattle: Diet Design, 1996).

MAGNESIUM: YOUR BEST WHOLESOME FOOD SOURCES

RDA 280-350 MG	AMOUNT	CONTENT IN MG
VEGETABLES		
Bean sprouts	½ cup	98
Collards, cooked	1 cup	44
Corn, fresh/canned	1 cup	52/8
Kale, cooked	1 cup	40
Peas, cooked	1 cup	34
Potato, baked with skin	1 med.	34
Spainch, cooked	1 cup	106
Winter squash, cooked	1 cup	64
GRAINS, cooked		
Flour, white enriched	1 cup	34
Flour, whole wheat	1 cup	136
Oatmeal	1 cup	117
Rice, white enriched	1 cup	16
Rice, wild	1 cup	238
Soy flour	1 cup	144
Wheatena	1 cup	50
LEGUMES, COOKED		
Great northern beans	½ cup	33
Kidney & lima beans	½ cup	44
Lentils	½ cup	134
Peanuts	¼ cup	63
Soybeans	½ cup	74
Soy milk	1 cup	46
Soy protein, texturized	¾ cup	74
Split peas	½ cup	134
Tofu	3½ oz.	76

Appendix 3

DAIRY (not generally a good source of magnesium)		
FRUITS (not generally a good source of magnesium)		
NUTS & SEEDS		
Almonds & cashews	¼ cup	95
Brazil nuts	¼ cup	88
Hazel nuts	¼ cup	59
Pecans	¼ cup	32
Sesame seeds	1 Tbs.	18
Walnuts	¼ cup	36
ANIMAL PROTEIN (not generally a good source except seafood)		
Seafood		
Cod, haddock, mackerel, pike, salmon, snapper	3 oz.	30-34
Oysters	3 oz.	36
Shrimp	3 oz.	48
OTHER		
Kelp	1 Tbs.	104

Sources: Gebhardt, Susan, and Ruth Matthews, "Nutritive Value of Foods," United States Department of Agriculture, 1981. Leveille, Gilbert A., et al, *Nutrients in Foods*, (Cambridge, MA: The Nutrition Guild, 1983).

MANGANESE: YOUR BEST WHOLESOME SOURCES

RDA 2-5 MG	AMOUNT	CONTENT IN MG
VEGETABLES		
Artichoke	3.5 oz.	0.36
Asparagus	4.7 oz.	0.26
Beet greens	3.5 oz.	1.30
Beets	4.7 oz.	1.27
Chard, Swiss	4.8 oz.	0.45
Green beans (fresh or frozen)	3.5 oz.	0.31
Lettuce, Boston	2.6 oz.	0.40
Parsley	1 oz.	0.28
Peas (frozen/canned)	3.5 oz.	0.22/0.28
Spinach (frozen/canned)	3.5 oz.	0.53/0.65
Turnip greens	5.1 oz.	2.1
Data on other vegetables is not available, but manganese content is likely to vary. For example, broccoli, cabbage, carrots, cauliflower, celery, cucumber, lettuce, and onions range from 0.07-0.19 mg of manganese per serving.		
GRAINS (cooked)		
Bread, rye	1 slice-1 oz	0.33
Bread, whole wheat	1 slice-1 oz.	0.59
Flour, buckwheat	½ cup	1.20
Flour, dark rye	½ cup	4.30
Flour, soy defatted	½ cup	2.90
Pasta (macaroni, egg noodles)	3.5 oz.	0.24-0.26
Rice, brown	½ cup	1.60
Rice, white enriched	½ cup	1.05
Tapioca	5.3 oz. = 1 cup	1.04

Wheat germ, toasted	1 oz. = 2 Tbs.	2.81
CEREALS		
Barley, pearled	1 oz.	0.48
Oatmeal	3.5 oz.	0.93
Oats, puffed; Cheerios	3.5 oz.	4.07
Raisin bran	3.5 oz.	3.36
Wheat flakes, Total	1.1 oz.	0.49
Wheat shredded	3.5 oz.	2.99
Data on other grains and cereals is not available, but likely to be similar.		
Legumes (cooked)		
Beans (pinto, black-eyed peas, lima, red, kidney, navy)	3.5 oz.	0.51-0.67
Peanuts, (dry roasted or peanut butter)	3.5 oz.	1.82-2.08
Data on other beans is not available, but manganese content is likely to be similar.		
DAIRY (generally not a good source of manganese)		
FRUIT		
Apple juice	1 cup	0.28
Avocado	1 = 9.5 oz.	0.45
Blackberries	1 cup	1.86
Blueberries	1 cup	0.41
Currants	1 cup	0.29
Figs, dried	10	0.73
Grape juice	1 cup	0.91
Grapes	1 cup	0.66
Loganberries	1 cup	1.83
Peaches, dried	10 halves	0.39
Pineapple canned	3.5 oz.	1.04

Pineapple, fresh	1 slice = 3 oz.	1.79
Pineapple juice	1 cup	0.80
Raisins, prunes	3.5 oz.	0.29-0.35
Raspberries	1 cup	1.24
Strawberries	3.5 oz.	0.39
Manganese content in other fruits is not available. Content varies, for example, apples, cherries, grapes, melons, oranges, peaches, pears and plums only average 0.26-0.89 mg per serving.		
NUTS		
Almonds/almond butter	1 oz.	0.54
Brazil nuts	1 oz.	0.79
Hazelnuts	1 oz.	1.20
Pecans	1 oz.	1.34
Walnuts	1 oz.	0.51
Animal Protein (not generally a good source)		
Other		
Tea (brewed from a bag)	7.0 oz.	0.42

Sources: Leveille, Gilbert A., et al, *Nutrients in Foods,* (Cambridge, MA: The Nutrition Guild, 1983). Kirschmann, John D., and Lavon J. Dunne, *Nutrition Almanac,* (New York: McGraw-Hill, 1984). Kies, C., *Nutritional Bioavailability of Manganese,* ed. Kies (Washington: American Chemical Society, 1987). Bucci, L.R., "Manganese: Its Role in Nutritional Balance," *Today's Chiropractic* 17.2 (1988): 23.

ZINC: YOUR BEST WHOLESOME FOOD SOURCES

RDA 10-15 MG	AMOUNT	ZINC IN MG
VEGETABLES (not a good source of zinc)		
Alfalfa sprouts, raw	1 cup	1.0
Brussel sprouts, cooked	1 cup	0.54
Sauerkraut	1 cup	1.88
Sweet potato, baked	1 med.	1.0
WHOLE GRAINS		
Bran, wheat	⅓ cup	3.8
Cornmeal, ground flour	½ cup	1.3
Oatmeal	1 cup	1
Wheat germ	¼ cup	4.40
Cerals, fortified with zinc		
Bran flakes	1 cup	5.10
Oatmeal	1 cup	2.50
Raisin bran	1 cup	3.50
Raisin Rice and Rye	1 cup	4.70
LEGUMES (cooked)		
Beans, black	½ cup	.96
Beans, pinto	½ cup	1.3
Beans, kidney-limas-white	½ cup	.9
Chick peas	½ cup	1.3
Navy beans	1 cup	2.02
DAIRY		
American, cheddar, Swiss	1 oz.	0.8
Cottage cheese, lowfat	½ cup	0.5
Edam cheese	1 oz.	1.1
Milk	1 cup	1.0
Ricotta cheese	½ cup	1.6

FRUITS (generally not a good source of zinc)		
NUTS & SEEDS		
Cashews	¼ cup	1.5
Peanut butter	2 Tbs.	.9
Peanuts & pecans	¼ cup	1.1
Pumpkin seeds, dried	1 oz.	2.12
Sesame seeds, toasted	1 oz.	3.2
Sunflower seeds	¼ cup	1.7
ANIMAL PROTEIN		
Beef, cooked	3 oz.	4.1
Beef, liver	3 oz.	4.25
Chicken giblets	½ cup	3.4
Chicken, dark/light	3 oz.	2.0/1.0
Chili, with beans	1 cup	4.10
Crab, Alaskan king	3 oz.	4.9
Egg	1 whole	0.72
Lamb	3 oz.	3.5
Lobster	3 oz.	2.05
Oysters, Eastern	1 average	11.2
Pork	3 oz.	3.4
Turkey, dark	3 oz.	3.3
Turkey, roasted light meat	3 oz	1.5

Sources: Gebhardt, Susan, and Ruth Matthews, "Nutritive Value of Foods," U.S. Department of Agriculture, 1981. Leveille, Gilbert A., et al, *Nutrients in Foods*, (Cambridge, MA: The Nutrition Guild, 1983).

Boron: Your Best Wholesome Food Sources

RDA (none given). Researchers suggest 3 mg as possibly an appropriate minimum. Amount given is a standard serving size.	Amount	Boron in mg
VEGETABLES		
Avocado	3.5	1.12
Broccoli	3.6	.257
Carrots	3.0	.219
Celery	3.1	.197
Parsley (dried)	1.0	.26
Squash (summer)	3.6	.218
Squash (winter)	3.6	.271
Spinach, canned	3.6	.257
GRAINS (not generally a good source of boron)		
LEGUMES, cooked		
Blackeyed peas	3.0	.409
Lima beans	3.3	.323
Pinto beans	3.0	.285
Kidney beans	3.2	.289
DAIRY (Not a good source of boron)		
FRUITS		
Apple (red, with peel, raw)	4.8	.377
Apple juice, canned	4.4	.295
Apple sauce, canned	4.3	.294
Cherries	3.7	.712
Grape juice, canned	4.4	.465
Grapes	5.6	.736
Orange	4.6	.284

Peach	3.0	.390
Pears, raw	5.8	.607
Plum, raw	4.6	.557
Prune juice	4.5	.664
Prunes	.9	.537
Raisins, dried	2.5	1.390
Strawberries	5.2	.200
NUTS & SEEDS		
Almonds	1.0	.644
Peanut butter/Peanuts	1.0	.386
ANIMAL PROTEIN (not a good source of boron)		
Other		
Wine	4.1	.415

Sources: Hunt, CD, et al, "Concentration of boron and other elements in human foods and personal-care products," *J Am Diet Assoc* 91.5 (1991): 558-68.
Anderson, David L, et al, "Concentrations and Intakes of H, B, S, , Na, C1, and NaC1 in Foods," *Journal of Food Composition and Analysis* 7 (1994): 59-82.
Nielsen, F., C. Hunt, and L. Mullen, "Effect of Dietary Boron on Mineral, Estrogen, and Testosterone Metabolism in Postmenopausal Women," *FASEB J* 1 (1987): 394-397. Yeung, Jeff E., "Boron—Becoming Recognized as an Esential Mineral," *Vitamin Research Products* 3.5 (1988)

VITAMIN K₁: YOUR BEST WHOLESOME FOOD SOURCES

RDA 70-140 mcg	Mcg Vit. K$_1$ per 1 standard serving (3½ oz)
Kale	729
Green tea	712
Turnip greens	650
Spinach	415
Broccoli	200
Lettuce	129
Cabbage	125
Watercress	57
Asparagus	57
Oats	20
Green peas	19
Whole wheat	17
Green beans	14

Source: *Vital Communications*, Vol. 1, #1, Spring 1993.

Appendix **4**
....

Product Suppliers

❖ SUPPLIERS OF LABORATORY TESTS AND INFORMATION CONSULTANTS

Tests For Hidden Hypersensitivities and Delayed Immune Responses

Serammune Physicians Laboratory
1890 Preston White Drive
Reston, VA 22091
800-553-5472

Suppliers of the Elisa/Act test, a comprehensive and unique white blood cell test that can identify a wide range of delayed hypersensitivities. Some 350 items are tested including foods, chemicals, additives, preservatives, colors and toxic metals. Along with test results comes a comprehensive program for recovering immune competence.

Urinary Tests For Bone Resorption

Great Smokies Diagnostic Laboratory
18A Regent Park Blvd.
Ashville, NC 28806
1-800-522-4762/704-253-0621

Meridian Valley Clinical Lab
515 Harrison St.,
Kent, WA 98042
800-234-6825/206-859-8700

MetaMetrix Medical Laboratory
5000 Peachtree Blvd.
Norcross, GA 30071
404-446-5483/800-221-4640

Ostex International
2203 Airport Way South
Seattle, WA 98134
206-292-8082/1-800-99-OSTEX

Laboratories Offering the New Saliva Tests for Hormone Levels

Diagnos-Techs, Inc.
6620 South 192nd Place
Kent, WA 98032
1-800-87-TESTS/206-251-0596
        This laboratory works only with physicians, but the
        interested public can receive information on these

tests from Dr. Rebecca Wynsome (see Information
Consultants). Send a SASE for information.

National BioTech Laboratory
3212 NE 125th Street
Seattle, WA 998125
800-846-6285/206-363-6606

Aeron Life Cycles Laboratory
1933 Davis St., Suite 310
San Leandro, CA 94577
800-631-7900

❖ NUTRIENT SUPPLEMENT SUPPLIERS

Nutrition Education and Consulting Service (NECS)
1200 E. Genesee Street
Syracuse, NY 13210
315-471-0264

>   Send a SASE for information on the products com-
>   monly recommended by Dr. Brown. These include
>   several hydroxyapatite formulas, adrenal glandulars
>   and various products from the Seraphim company
>   (unique magnesium blend, liquid choline citrate to
>   enhance magnesium absorption and a fully buffered
>   Vitamin C powder).

NEEDS
527 Charles Ave. 12A
Syracuse, NY 13209
800-634-1380/315-488-6300

>   A mail order supplement company offering a wide
>   range of nutrition products.

Allergy Resources
P.O. Box 444
Guffey, CO 80820
800-USE-FLAX/719-689-2969
> A mail order company that offers a wide range of nutrition and health products.

❖ Suppliers of Plant-Derived Progesterone and Estrogen Products

Biotanica
PO. Box 1285
Sherwood, OR 97140
1-800-572-4712/503-625-4824
> This company sells Dr. Tori Hudson's herbal formulas for menopause and PMS.

Phyto-Pharmica
825 Challenger Drive
Green Bay, WI 54311
1-800-553-2370
> Manufactures and distributes the formulas of Dr. Michael Murray including Fem-Tone, Remifemin and other formulas for menopause.

Maharishi Ayur-Ved Products International, Inc.
P.O. Box 541, 417 Bolton Road
Lancaster, MA 01523
1-800-255-8332
> Produces two Ayurvedic herbal formulas for menopause called Golden Transition.

Pioneer Nutritional Formulas, Inc.
PO. Box 259
Shelburne Falls, MA 01370
413-625-8212/1-800-458-8483

> Produces a high-potency herbal support product for menopause.

Professional & Technical Services Inc.
5200 SW Macadam Ave.
Portland, OR 97201-6103
503-226-1010/800-648-8211

> Distributes natural progesterone cream and other natural hormone products.

Women's International Pharmacy
5708 Monona Drive
Madison, WI 53716-3152
608-221-7800/800-279-5708

> A compounding pharmacy providing physicians with a wide range of natural hormone products.

❖ Information Consultants

As the need for specialized information arises selected health professionals offer long distance education/information services to other health professionals and individual patients. Among those offering education services relevant too the topics of this book are:

Susan E. Brown, Ph.D.
Nutrition Education and Consulting Services
1200 East Genesee Street
Syracuse, NY 13210
315-471-0264

> Offers education services to health professionals

and the interested public in natural approaches to osteoporosis prevention and reversal and natural menopausal well-being. Telephone consultations and lecture services are available.

Dr. Mary Jo Cravata
PO. Box 3629
San Rafael, CA 94901
415-459-1529

A chiropractor specializing in Ayurvedic medicine. She offers an audio tape introduction to Ayurvedic medicine.

Dr. Martin Milner
1313 SE. 39th Ave.
Portland OR 97214
503-232-7751

Offers education services on the development of natural hormone menopausal and osteoporosis programs.

Sally Rockwell Ph.D.
Diet Design
PO. Box 31065
Seattle, WA. 98103
206-547-1814

Specializes in high calcium nutrition programs for those with dairy and other food sensitivities and offers a publication, *Calcium Without The Cow*, detailing non-dairy sources of calcium.

Dr. Rebecca Wynsome
150 Nickerson St.
Seattle WA 98109
206-283-1383

Specializes in the use and interpretation of salivary tests for hormone levels and natural hormone treatment.

Appendix **5**
·····················

Additional References

Books on Recovering Natural Menopausal Well-being

Barbach, Lonnie, *The Pause: Positive Approaches to Menopause,* (New York: Dutton/Penguin, 1993).

Coney, Sandra, *The Menopause Industry: A Guide to Medicine's "Discovery" of the Mid-Life Woman,* (New York: Penguin Books, 1991).

Gittleman, Ann Louise, *Super Nutrition for Menopause,* (New York: Pocket Books, 1993).

Kamen, Betty Ph.D., *Hormone Replacement Therapy Yes or No?* (Novato: Nutrition Encounter, Inc., 1993).

Lee, John R, *Natural Progesterone. The Multiple Roles Of A Remarkable Hormone*, (Sebastopol, CA: BLL Publishing, 1995).

Murray, Michael T., *Menopause: How You Can Benefit from Diet, Vitamins, Minerals, Herbs, Exercise and Other Natural Methods*, (Rocklin, CA: Prima Publishing, 1994).

Northrup, Christiane, *Women's Bodies, Women's Wisdom*, (New York: Bantam Books, 1994).

Ojeda, Linda Ph.D., *Menopause Without Medicine*, second ed. (Alameda: Hunter House, 1992).

Ryneveld, Edna Copeland, *Secrets of a Natural Menopause*, (St. Paul: Llewellyn Publications, 1995).

Seaman, B., and G. Seaman, *Women and the Crisis in Sex Hormones*, (New York: Bantam Books, 1977).

Smith, Trevor, *Homeopathy For The Menopause*, (Worthing, Sussex, England: Insight, 1994).

Weed, Susan W., *Menopausal Years*, (Woodstock: Ash Tree Publishing, 1992).

Books on Ayurvedic Medicine

Douillard, John, audiotape set. *Invincible Athletics: Awakening the Athlete in Everyone.* The Maharishi Ayur-Veda fitness course and handbook with an introduction by Deepak Chopra, M.D. This tape can be purchased from:

Dr. John Douillard
3065 Center Green Dr.
Boulder, CO 80301
303-442-1164.

Heyn, Brigit, *Ayurveda The Indian Art of Natural Medicine & Life Extension*, (Rochester, VT: Healing Arts Press, 1990).

Lad, Vasant, *Ayurveda The Science of Self-Healing A Practical Guide*, (Santa Fe NM: Lotus Press, 1985).

Chopra, Deepak, *Perfect Health*, *(New York:* Harmony Books 1990).

Books on Chinese Medicine

Connelly, Dianne M., *Traditional Acupuncture: The Law Of The Five Elements*, (Columbia, MD: The American City Building, 1979).

Kaptchuk, Ted J., *The Web That Has No Weaver: Understanding Chinese Medicine*, (NewYork: Congdon & Weed Inc., 1983).

Wolfe, Honora Lee, *Second Spring: A Guide to Healthy Menopause Through Traditional Chinese Medicine*, first ed. (Boulder: Blue Poppy Press, 1990) 181.

Index

active bone loss *see* bone loss
adrenal glands, 104, 182–185, 326–327
adrenal glandular products, 255
adrenal hormones, 183
  see also corticosteroids;
    glucocorticoids
aerobics, 307, 311–312
aging
  and bone loss, 40–41
  see also elderly
alcohol, 259
  and bone health, 155–156
  consumption, 288–289
  and nutrient absorption, 155
alkaline diet, 259, 290–299
  and fractures, 261
alkaline phosphate, and magnesium,
  85
alkaline/acid balance *see* pH balance
alkalinization, 295–296
allergies *see* food allergies
alpha-linolenic acid, 111
aluminum, and bone health, 162, 166
amenorrhea, 149
amylase, 249
ancestral diet, 80
androgens, 31, 184, 187
androstenedione, 179
anemia, 168
animal protein, and bone health,
  122–125
anorexia, 48, 158–159
antacids, aluminum-containing, 162
anticonvulsants, 164
antinutrients *see* alcohol; caffeine; salt;
  sugar
antibiotics, 163
  and vitamin K, 108
arthritis, 87
  and calcium, 246
asthma, 87
atherosclerosis, 109
athletes, and diet, 48, 149, 159
Ayurveda, 72, 73–74

Ayurveda *(continued)*
  books about, 404–405
  and digestion, 271–272

bacteria *see* intestinal flora
balance
  of body systems, 21–22
  and exercise, 305
balanced diet, 238
beta-carotene, 103
betaine hydrocholoric acid, 249
Better Bones, Better Body Program,
  10–11, 197, 219–232, 368
  design guidelines, 248–259
  dietary principles, 237–239
  intervention areas, 231, 276–289
bilary cirrhosis, 252
bioflavanoids, 260
birth control pills, 332–333, 346
bisphosphonate alendronate *see*
  Fosamax
bitters, and digestion, 271–272
blood calcium, 26
  and calcitonin, 179
  deficiency, and biomedical reactions,
    18–19
  and parathyroid hormone, 179
blood clots, and oral contraceptives, 333
blood minerals, 49
body systems, balance, 21–22
body weight, and bone health,
  157–158, 243–244
bone
  and calcium metabolism, 26
  degeneration *see* bone loss
  density *see* bone mass
  functions of, 25–27
  generation *see* bone building
  life cycle, 24–25
  mineral reserves, 68, 133
  remodeling *see* bone remodeling
  resorption *see* bone loss
  structure, 27–29, 38
  see also cortical bone; trabecular bone

bone building, 5, 19–20, 68, 219–232
  and diet, 235–241
  and essential nutrients, 239–240,
    246–247
  and exercise, 143–145, 301–321
  and progesterone, 354
  and silica, 89–90
  and vitamin C, 253–254
  and vitamin D, 253
  and youth, 220
  see also bone remodeling
bone building programs, 225–232
  evaluating, 369–370
  guidelines, 229–231
bone cartilage, and manganese, 92–93
bone collagen, 27, 89, 122, 213
  and manganese, 92–93
  and vitamin C, 101
bone loss, 24–25, 213–215
  and aging, 40–41
  and dietary excesses, 121–134
  and endocrine imbalance, 178–191
  factors in, 63–64, 230
  and fractures, 259–260
  and lack of exercise, 140–149
  and lifestyle factors, 153–172
  measurement of, 213–215, 397
  and nutrient inadequacies, 77–79,
    80–113
  perimenopausal, 260–261, 317,
    318–319
  postmenopausal, 247, 317–318
  signs of, 200–215
  see also osteoporosis
bone marrow, 25
  disorders, and osteoporosis, 52
bone mass, 24, 38
  and body weight, 157–158, 243–244
  and estrogen, 67
  and fractures, 208, 226
  and genetics, 319
  measurement of, 206–212, 369
  and muscle mass, 145–146, 302, 307
  and progesterone, 348
  standards, 208–209, 214
  see also osteoporosis
bone protein *see* bone collagen
bone remodeling, 23–24, 29–31, 39
boron, 95–98, 260
  consumption, 240
  food sources, 393–394
  and vegetarians, 254
breast cancer
  and estrogen therapy, 331, 341–344
  and progestin/progesterone, 351

cadmium, 166
caffeine, 258–259
  and bone health, 128, 130–132
  and calcium, 131
  consumption, 278–280
  in foods, 279
  and magnesium, 131
calcitonin, 31, 179, 182
  and magnesium, 85
calcitriol, 100
calcium, 81–84
  absorption, 168–169
  and bone health, 77, 81
  and boron, 96
  and cadmium, 166
  and caffeine, 131
  consumption, 83, 239
    anthropological data, 62–63
    and youth, 320
  deficiency, 205
    and osteoporosis, 61–64
  and fat, 110, 129
  food sources, 383–385
  and glucocorticoid hormones, 183
  imbalance, 245–246
  and iron, 249, 255
  and magnesium, 86
  and phosphorus, 125
  and protein, 123
  recommended dosage, 63, 82
  and smoking, 154
  and sodium, 127
  storage of, 26
  and sugar, 128
  supplementation, 87, 161, 246, 250,
    252, 303
    timing of, 255
  and vitamin A, 103
  and vitamin D, 98, 100, 102
  and youth, 262
  and zinc, 91
  see also blood calcium
calcium carbonate, 249
calcium citrate, 249, 250
calories, consumption, 237
Camde Nutri-Calc Plus Program, 237
cancer, 140
  see also breast cancer; endometrial
    cancer; ovarian cancer
Candida, 163
carbon dioxide, 133
cardiovascular disease, 140
  and calcium, 246
  and estrogen therapy, 339–340
  and exercise, 142

cardiovascular fitness, 147, 307
cells, 17–18
  see also osteocyte
chemotherapy, 39, 163–164
children *see* youth
Chinese medicine, 72–73, 190, 405
chromium, 282
collagen *see* bone collagen
compression fractures, 36
connective tissue disorders, 53
copper, 94–95
  consumption, 239
  and youth, 262
cortical bone, 24, 28–29
corticosteroids, 102, 160–161
cortisol, 167, 183
cortisone, 160
coumadin, and vitamin K, 107
crystalline minerals, 27
crystallization process, 20

degenerative diseases, 5, 140
  and fat, 120
  and sugar, 128
depo medroxyprogesterone, 164
DES *see* diethylstilbestrol, 332
DEXA scan, 369
diabetes, 140–141
diet, 79–80
  adequacy of, 235–236
  ancestral, 80
  and athletes, 159
  balanced, 238
  and bone health, 121–134, 236–237
  elimination, 274
  nutrient content, 46–47
  and osteoporosis, 256–259
  standard American, 157–158, 237
  varied, 238–239
  see also alkaline diet
diethylstilbestrol, 332
dieting, 157
digestion, 266–275
  aids, 249, 256, 270
    in vitamin supplements, 251
  and bone health, 168–170
  and hydrochloric acid, 271
  improvement program, 269–270
diuretics, 162
dowager's hump, 36, 204
drugs
  and bone health, 53, 159–164
  psychotrophic, 164
dual photon absorptiometry,
  207

dual x-ray absorptiometry, 207
dynamic strain, and bone health, 147

eating, 267–268
elderly
  and protein malnutrition, 257
  and vitamin D, 257–258
electromagnetic fields, 39–40
elimination diet, and food allergies,
  274
Eliza/Act Test, 274, 395
endocrine glands, 325–329
  and bone health, 63–64, 178–191
  and osteoporosis, 52
endometrial cancer, and estrogen therapy, 340–33
endurance exercise, 147
energy production, and phosphorus,
  26
essential fatty acids, 110–112
  and youth, 262
estradiol, 179, 356
estriol, 356
estrogen, 31, 185
  and bone health, 6, 64–67, 186
  esterfied, 357
  function, 65
  levels of, 259–260
  and menopause, 64–65, 335
  "natural" formulations, 356–358
  and progestin, 342
  and smoking, 154
  supplementation *see* estrogen
    therapy
  suppliers, 399–400
  and testosterone, 342
  and tubal ligation, 48
  and vegetarian women, 64–65
estrogen therapy, 224, 247, 260, 380
  benefits, 336–340
  and breast cancer, 331
  history, 332–334
  and osteoporosis, 330–360
  risks, 340–346
  usage, 334
estrone, 179, 356
ethinyl estridial, 357
exercise
  and bone health, 39, 140–149,
    222–223, 301–321
  and cardiovascular disease, 142
  endurance, 147
  evaluation studies, 302–306
  and girls, 320
  and HDL, 142

exercise *(continued)*
  and osteoporosis, 313–317
  and perimenopausal women, 260,
    317–319
  training effect, 307, 312
  weight-bearing, 147, 306–307
  and women, 47, 260, 317–319
  and youth, 148, 263, 319–321

fast foods, and magnesium deficiency,
    87–88
fatigue
  and adrenal glandular products,
    255
  and exercise, 313
fats
  and bone health, 129–130
  and calcium absorption, 110, 129
  consumption, 130, 240, 283–285
  and degenerative diseases, 120
  and magnesium absorption, 129
fatty acids *see* essential fatty acids;
    trans fatty acids
ferrous fumerate, 249
ferrous gluconate, 249
ferrous sulfate, 249
fibrinogen, and progestin, 348
fibrocystic breast disease, and estrogen
    therapy, 344–345
fitness, and bone health, 203
flexion movements, 314–315
fluoride, 88–89
fluorine, 239
folic acid, 109–110, 240
food allergies, 170, 255, 272–275
foods
  acidity, 291–292, 298–299
  alkalinity, 291–292, 297
  boron content, 393–394
  caffeine content, 279
  calcium content, 383–385
  consumption guidelines, 241
  fat content, 283–284
  magnesium content, 386–387
  manganese content, 388–390
  nutrient content, 383–395
  preparation, 267
  protein content, 278
  salt content, 286–287
  sugar content, 281
  vitamin K content, 395
  whole, 237–238
  zinc content, 391–392
Fosamax, 331, 353, 366–370
fractures, 141
  and alkaline diet, 261

fractures, *(continued)*
  consequences, 4
  and corticosteroids, 160
  and estrogen therapy, 338
  and Fosamax, 367
  and osteoporosis, 36–39
  risk assessment, 197–215, 210–212
    checklist, 198–199
  statistics, 3–4
  and vitamin K, 106
  see also compression fractures; hip
    fractures; spinal fractures; wedge
    fractures

gallbladder disease, and estrogen ther-
    apy, 344
gastrointesinal disorders, and osteopo-
    rosis, 53
genetics, and bone mass, 319
girls, and exercise, 320
glucocorticoids, and calcium absorp-
    tion, 183
glucose tolerance factor, 282
growth hormone, 31
gums, 202

Harvard Nurses Health Study, 343
HDL cholesterol
  and exercise, 142
  and progestin, 348–349
heart disease *see* cardiovascular disease
heavy metals, and bone health, 39,
    165–166
height, loss of, 203–204
high blood pressure, 141
hip fractures, 4
  and bone density, 226
  and estrogen therapy, 338–339
  Japanese women, 38
  and osteoporosis, 258
  rate, 42, 45
  risks, 51, 208, 210
  and smoking, 153
homocysteine, 104, 109
hormone therapy
  and balance, 355–356
  monitoring, 359–360
  value, 352–353
  see also estrogen therapy; progestin
    therapy
hormones
  and bone health, 178–191
  measurement tests, 398
  see also adrenal hormones; systemic
    hormones
hot flashes, 261

hydrochloric acid, 104, 128–129
  and calcium absorption, 169
  and digestion, 271
hydrogenation, 120
hyperadrenalism, 183
hyperparathyroidism, 98, 180–181
hypoglycemia
  and adrenal glandular products, 255
  and pantothenic acid, 254
hysterectomy
  and estrogen therapy, 345
  and osteoporosis, 48

immobilization renal disease, and
    osteoporosis, 53
information consultants, 400–402
insulin, 31
intestinal flora, 108, 163
Invincible Athletics, 313
iron, and calcium, 246, 249, 255
isoflavones, 357

Japanese Dietary Guidelines, 239
jaw bone loss, 201–202
jumping, 307

Kapha element, 73
kidney disease, and magnesium
    supplementation, 252
kidney stones, 87
  and calcium, 246
kidneys, 189–191, 327–328
  mineral utilization function, 72
  and parathyroid hormone, 18
  and vitamin D metabolism, 18, 85,
    190

L-histidine, and digestion, 272
laboratory tests, 396–398
lactic acid, 133
lactose, 170
  and copper metabolism, 94
lead, 165–166
lifestyles, 5, 153–172
  see also diet; exercise
linoleic acid, 111
liver, 328
  and smoking, 154

magnesium, 85–88
  absorption, and fat, 129
  and bone health, 205
  and caffeine, 131
  and calcium, 86, 246, 252
  consumption, 239
  food sources, 386–387

magnesium *(continued)*
  functions, 26–27
  and kidney disease, 252
  storage of, 26
  supplementation, 86, 87, 252, 255
  and youth, 262
manganese, 92–93
  and calcium, 246
  consumption, 239
  food sources, 388–390
  and youth, 262
medications *see* drugs
meditation, 167–168, 380
medroxyprogesterone *see* Provera
menopausal disorders
  and estrogen therapy, 339
  and herbs, 357
  and progesterone, 354
menopause
  and bone health, 24–25
  books about, 403–404
  and the drug industry, 261–262
  and estrogen levels, 64–65, 335
  and osteoporosis, 6
menstrual cycle, 185
menstrual irregularities, and
    osteoporosis, 48–49
metabolism, and boron, 95
metals *see* heavy metals
methionine, 109
microcrystalline hydroxyapatite, 161,
    252
microglobulins, 31
milk alkali syndrome, 246
milk protein, 170
minerals
  bone reserves, 26–27, 68, 133
  consumption, 46–47
  and kidney function, 72
  and pH balance, 133
  supplementation, 244–245, 251
  see also blood minerals
multi-vitamins
  guidelines, 248–250
  nutrient content, 251
  and osteoporosis, 257–258
muscle mass, and bone density,
    145–146, 302, 307
muscle strength, 202–203, 307,
    309–311

nutrients
  balance of, 244–245
  and bone health, 39, 77–79, 205–206
  bone-building, 246–247
  consumption, 239–240

nutrients *(continued)*
  women, 79
    youth, 262–263
  education, 379
  essential, 80–113
  and estrogen therapy, 346
  food sources, 383–395
  maximizing, 235–263
  and osteoporosis, 46, 53, 256–259
  RDAs, 239–240, 376–377
  supplementation, 161, 221–222
Nutrition Education and Consulting
    Service, 379–382

obesity, and youth, 148
oral contraceptives, 332–333, 346
osteoblasts, 20, 27, 103, 186
osteocalcin, 106
osteoclasts, 27, 29
osteocyte, 19
osteomalacia, 98
osteoporosis, 3, 38–39, 50, 219
  anthropological data, 41–44
  and athletes, 48
  costs, 4
  definition, 35
  and diet, 256–259
  and drug therapy, 370
  and estrogen levels, 6, 64–67
  and estrogen therapy, 330–360
  and exercise, 313–317
  factors in, 7–8, 46–50, 61–74
  and food allergies, 273
  and fractures, 36–39, 258
  and magnesium deficiency, 86
  and men, 45–46
  and menopause, 6
  and multi-vitamin supplementation,
    257–258
  and nutrient intake, 256–259
  primary, 52
  research studies, 227–229, 382
  reversal of, 221
  secondary, 52–53
  and youth, 48
ovarian cancer, and estrogen therapy,
    344
ovaries, 185–189, 327
  malfunction, and bone health, 188
  removal
    and bone health, 47–48, 188
    and estrogen therapy, 335

PABA, 260
pancreas, 329
pancreatic enzymes, 271

pantothenic acid, 254
  and perimenopausal women, 260
para-amino salicylic acid, 163
parathyroid gland, 179–181, 326
parathyroid hormone, 31, 179–180
  and magnesium, 85
  and vitamin D, 18, 85
PEPI Trial, 340
pepsin, 249
perimenopause, 259–262
  and exercise, 317–319
periodontal disease, and vitamin C,
    253–254
pernicious anemia, 168
pH balance, 132–134, 290, 291
  test kit, 381
  testing, 292–293
phosphates, and processed foods, 126
phosphorus, 84–85
  and bone health, 125–126
  and calcium, 125, 246
  consumption, 239
  and energy production, 26
  and hyperparathyroidism, 180
  and vitamin D, 98
photon absorptiometry, 206–207
physical activity *see* exercise
phytoestrogens, 260, 357
phytohormones, 261
phytoprogesterones, 260
phytosterols, 357
Pitta element, 73
pool exercises, 317
Postmenopausal Estrogen/Progestin
    Interventions Trial, 340
posture, 314
potassium, and sodium, 127
potassium bicarbonate, 134
prednisone, 160
Premarin, 331, 370
primary osteoporosis, 52
processed foods, 237, 258
  and magnesium deficiency, 87–88
  and phosphates, 126
  and sodium, 126
progesterone, 185, 347
  and bone health, 186–187, 348
  and breast cancer, 351
  deficiency, 165
  and osteoporosis, 354–356
  suppliers, 399–400
progestin, 347
  and breast cancer, 351
  and estrogen, 342
  and fibrinogen, 348
  and HDL cholesterol, 348–349

progestin *(continued)*
  synthetic, 333–334
progestin therapy
  benefits, 346–349
  risks, 349–350
progestogen, 347
protein, 112–113
  and calcium, 123
  consumption, 240, 276–277
  in foods, 278
  malnutrition in the elderly, 257
  see also animal protein; bone
    collagen; milk protein
Provera, 347, 349
psychotrophic drugs, 164

quantitative computed tomography,
  207

radiation, and bone health, 39
RDA *see* recommended dietary
  allowances
receding gums, 50
recommended dietary allowances, 78,
  375–378
red blood cells, 25
regeneration response, 8–9
remodeling *see* bone remodeling
resorption *see* bone loss
rickets, 98

salt *see* sodium
sapogenins, 357
secondary osteoporosis, 52–53
sedatives, 259
serum manganese, 93
sex hormones *see* estrogen; testosterone
silica, 89–90
  and bone health, 254–255
  consumption, 239
single photon absorptiometry, 206
skin, transparency of, 204–205
sleep
  and calcium, 255
  and magnesium, 255
smoking, 287–288
  and bone health, 153–154
  and calcium absorption, 154
  and hip fractures, 153
  and liver function, 154
  and vitamin C, 154
sodium, 258
  and bone health, 126–127
  and calcium, 127
  consumption, 285–287
  and potassium, 127

sodium *(continued)*
  and processed foods, 126
  storage of, 26
spices, 267
spinal fractures, 4, 42, 203–204
  risks, 208
spinal trabecular bone, 307
  and exercise, 303
standard American diet, 157–158, 237
steroid therapy, and osteoporosis, 49
stooping, 36
strength training *see* muscle strength
stress
  and bone health, 167–168
  and exercise, 313
  and youth, 321
strokes, and oral contraceptives, 333
sugar, 258
  and bone health, 128–129
  and calcium absorption, 128
  consumption, 280–282
  and degenerative diseases, 128
  and magnesium deficiency, 87–88
sunlight exposure, 171
supplements, 244–245
  and bone health, 161, 221–222, 247
  and osteoporosis, 257–258
  and perimenopausal women, 260
  program design, 248–259
  suppliers, 381, 398–399
surgery
  and osteoporosis, 47
  see also hysterectomy; ovaries,
    removal
Sweet Tooth Blues, 282
synthetic progestin, 333–334
systemic bone loss, 50
systemic hormones, 31–32
systemic lupus erythematosus, and
  estrogen therapy, 345

teeth, 202
testosterone
  and bone health, 189
  and estrogen, 342
  and estrogen therapy, 345–346
  and smoking, 154
thyroid gland, 181–182, 325–326
thyroid hormones, and bone health,
  161–162
thyroxin, 31, 181
tobacco *see* smoking
Total Body Burden concept, 70–71
trabecular bone, 24, 28–29
  and anorexia, 158
  magnesium content, 86

trabecular bone *(continued)*
  and mineral loss, 50
traditional Chinese medicine, 72–73,
      190, 405
trans fatty acids, 120
transferrin, 31
Tri-Est, 358
tubal ligation, and estrogen, 48
type 1 collagen *see* bone collagen

urine tests, 213–215
uterine bleeding, and estrogen therapy,
      345
uterine cancer *see* endometrial cancer

vasectomy, and bone health, 189
Vata element, 73
vegetarians
  and bone health, 123–124
  and boron, 254
  and estrogen levels, 64–65
vitamin A, 103–104
  consumption, 240
vitamin B2, 31
vitamin B6, 104–105, 245
  consumption, 240
vitamin B12, 108–109
  consumption, 240
  and digestion, 272
vitamin C, 101–102
  and bone health, 206, 253–254
  consumption, 240
  and perimenopausal women, 260
  and periodontal disease, 253–254
  and smoking, 154
vitamin D, 31, 98–101
  and bone health, 164, 171, 253
  and boron, 96
  consumption, 240
  and the elderly, 257–258
  and magnesium, 85

vitamin D *(continued)*
  metabolism, 18, 190
  recommended dosage, 99–100
  supplementation, 161, 303
  toxicity, 101, 103, 253
vitamin D resistance syndrome, 85
vitamin E, 245
vitamin K1, and bone health, 255
vitamin K, 106–108
  and calcium, 246
  consumption, 240
  food sources, 395
vitamins
  supplementation, 244–245
  and youth, 262–263
  see also multi-vitamins; supplements

warfarin, and vitamin K, 107
wedge fractures, 36
weight, and bone health, 157–158,
      243–244
weight-bearing exercise, 147, 306–307
whole foods, 237–238
women
  and exercise, 47, 317–319
  nutrient consumption, 79
  perimenopausal, 259–262

youth
  and calcium consumption, 320
  and exercise, 148, 319–321
  and nutrient consumption, 262–263
  and obesity, 148
  and osteoporosis, 48
  RDAs, 377–378
  and stress, 321

zinc, 91–92
  and bone health, 205–206
  consumption, 239
  deficiency, 257
  food sources, 391–392

About the Author

Susan E. Brown, Ph.D., CCN is a medical anthropologist and certified nutritionist who has consulted widely on socio-economic, cultural, educational and health issues. She has taught in North and South American universities and authored numerous academic and popular articles.

Currently Dr. Brown directs the Osteoporosis Education Project and the Nutrition Education and Consulting Service in Syracuse, New York. She lectures widely on osteoporosis prevention and reversal and teaches the use of a holistic, natural program for the regeneration of bone health.

In addition to a busy private practice, Dr. Brown serves as a consultant to various medical groups including Serammune Physicians Laboratory, Reston, Virginia and North Medical Family Physicians, Syracuse, New York.

Dr. Brown is co-author of a forthcoming text entitled *The Mend Clinic Book of Natural Remedies for Menopause and Beyond* (Winter, 1997) and has written numerous articles in English and Spanish.

She received her Ph.D. from the University of Michigan in 1972 and is the recipient of two Fulbright-Hays Scholar Awards and an Organization of American States Research Fellowship. Dr. Brown is also a member of Sigma Xi, the honorary scientific research organization of North America.